Mometrix
TEST PREPARATION

CTRN®

Exam Secrets Study Guide

DEAR FUTURE EXAM SUCCESS STORY

First of all, **THANK YOU** for purchasing Mometrix study materials!

Second, congratulations! You are one of the few determined test-takers who are committed to doing whatever it takes to excel on your exam. **You have come to the right place.** We developed these study materials with one goal in mind: to deliver you the information you need in a format that's concise and easy to use.

In addition to optimizing your guide for the content of the test, we've outlined our recommended steps for breaking down the preparation process into small, attainable goals so you can make sure you stay on track.

We've also analyzed the entire test-taking process, identifying the most common pitfalls and showing how you can overcome them and be ready for any curveball the test throws you.

Standardized testing is one of the biggest obstacles on your road to success, which only increases the importance of doing well in the high-pressure, high-stakes environment of test day. Your results on this test could have a significant impact on your future, and this guide provides the information and practical advice to help you achieve your full potential on test day.

Your success is our success

We would love to hear from you! If you would like to share the story of your exam success or if you have any questions or comments in regard to our products, please contact us at **800-673-8175** or **support@mometrix.com**.

Thanks again for your business and we wish you continued success!

Sincerely,
The Mometrix Test Preparation Team

Need more help? Check out our flashcards at:
http://MometrixFlashcards.com/CTRN

Written and edited by the Mometrix Exam Secrets Test Prep Team
Printed in the United States of America

Table of Contents

Introduction

Thank you for purchasing this resource! You have made the choice to prepare yourself for a test that could have a huge impact on your future, and this guide is designed to help you be fully ready for test day. Obviously, it's important to have a solid understanding of the test material, but you also need to be prepared for the unique environment and stressors of the test, so that you can perform to the best of your abilities.

For this purpose, the first section that appears in this guide is the **Secret Keys**. We've devoted countless hours to meticulously researching what works and what doesn't, and we've boiled down our findings to the five most impactful steps you can take to improve your performance on the test. We start at the beginning with study planning and move through the preparation process, all the way to the testing strategies that will help you get the most out of what you know when you're finally sitting in front of the test.

We recommend that you start preparing for your test as far in advance as possible. However, if you've bought this guide as a last-minute study resource and only have a few days before your test, we recommend that you skip over the first two Secret Keys since they address a long-term study plan.

If you struggle with **test anxiety**, we strongly encourage you to check out our recommendations for how you can overcome it. Test anxiety is a formidable foe, but it can be beaten, and we want to make sure you have the tools you need to defeat it.

Secret Key 1: Plan Big, Study Small

There's a lot riding on your performance. If you want to ace this test, you're going to need to keep your skills sharp and the material fresh in your mind. You need a plan that lets you review everything you need to know while still fitting in your schedule. We'll break this strategy down into three categories.

Information Organization

Start with the information you already have: the official test outline. From this, you can make a complete list of all the concepts you need to cover before the test. Organize these concepts into groups that can be studied together, and create a list of any related vocabulary you need to learn so you can brush up on any difficult terms. You'll want to keep this vocabulary list handy once you actually start studying since you may need to add to it along the way.

Time Management

Once you have your set of study concepts, decide how to spread them out over the time you have left before the test. Break your study plan into small, clear goals so you have a manageable task for each day and know exactly what you're doing. Then just focus on one small step at a time. When you manage your time this way, you don't need to spend hours at a time studying. Studying a small block of content for a short period each day helps you retain information better and avoid stressing over how much you have left to do. You can relax knowing that you have a plan to cover everything in time. In order for this strategy to be effective though, you have to start studying early and stick to your schedule. Avoid the exhaustion and futility that comes from last-minute cramming!

Study Environment

The environment you study in has a big impact on your learning. Studying in a coffee shop, while probably more enjoyable, is not likely to be as fruitful as studying in a quiet room. It's important to keep distractions to a minimum. You're only planning to study for a short block of time, so make the most of it. Don't pause to check your phone or get up to find a snack. It's also important to **avoid multitasking**. Research has consistently shown that multitasking will make your studying dramatically less effective. Your study area should also be comfortable and well-lit so you don't have the distraction of straining your eyes or sitting on an uncomfortable chair.

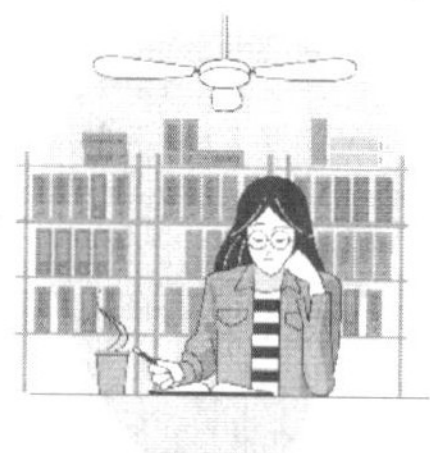

The time of day you study is also important. You want to be rested and alert. Don't wait until just before bedtime. Study when you'll be most likely to comprehend and remember. Even better, if you know what time of day your test will be, set that time aside for study. That way your brain will be used to working on that subject at that specific time and you'll have a better chance of recalling information.

Finally, it can be helpful to team up with others who are studying for the same test. Your actual studying should be done in as isolated an environment as possible, but the work of organizing the information and setting up the study plan can be divided up. In between study sessions, you can discuss with your teammates the concepts that you're all studying and quiz each other on the details. Just be sure that your teammates are as serious about the test as you are. If you find that your study time is being replaced with social time, you might need to find a new team.

Secret Key 2: Make Your Studying Count

You're devoting a lot of time and effort to preparing for this test, so you want to be absolutely certain it will pay off. This means doing more than just reading the content and hoping you can remember it on test day. It's important to make every minute of study count. There are two main areas you can focus on to make your studying count.

Retention

It doesn't matter how much time you study if you can't remember the material. You need to make sure you are retaining the concepts. To check your retention of the information you're learning, try recalling it at later times with minimal prompting. Try carrying around flashcards and glance at one or two from time to time or ask a friend who's also studying for the test to quiz you.

To enhance your retention, look for ways to put the information into practice so that you can apply it rather than simply recalling it. If you're using the information in practical ways, it will be much easier to remember. Similarly, it helps to solidify a concept in your mind if you're not only reading it to yourself but also explaining it to someone else. Ask a friend to let you teach them about a concept you're a little shaky on (or speak aloud to an imaginary audience if necessary). As you try to summarize, define, give examples, and answer your friend's questions, you'll understand the concepts better and they will stay with you longer. Finally, step back for a big picture view and ask yourself how each piece of information fits with the whole subject. When you link the different concepts together and see them working together as a whole, it's easier to remember the individual components.

Finally, practice showing your work on any multi-step problems, even if you're just studying. Writing out each step you take to solve a problem will help solidify the process in your mind, and you'll be more likely to remember it during the test.

Modality

Modality simply refers to the means or method by which you study. Choosing a study modality that fits your own individual learning style is crucial. No two people learn best in exactly the same way, so it's important to know your strengths and use them to your advantage.

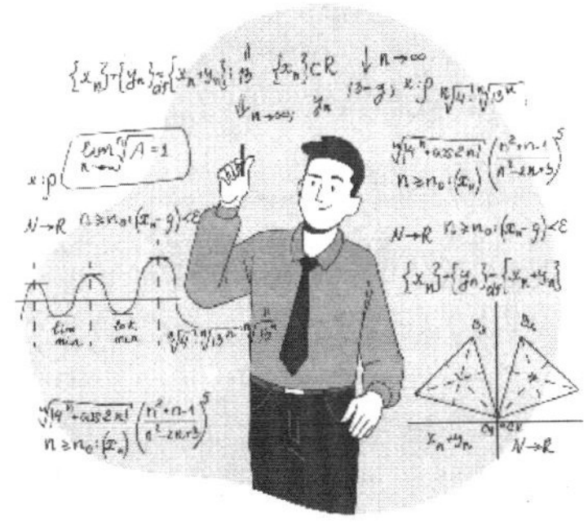

For example, if you learn best by visualization, focus on visualizing a concept in your mind and draw an image or a diagram. Try color-coding your notes, illustrating them, or creating symbols that will trigger your mind to recall a learned concept. If you learn best by hearing or discussing information, find a study partner who learns the same way or read aloud to yourself. Think about how to put the information in your own words. Imagine that you are giving a lecture on the topic and record yourself so you can listen to it later.

For any learning style, flashcards can be helpful. Organize the information so you can take advantage of spare moments to review. Underline key words or phrases. Use different colors for different categories. Mnemonic devices (such as creating a short list in which every item starts with the same letter) can also help with retention. Find what works best for you and use it to store the information in your mind most effectively and easily.

Secret Key 3: Practice the Right Way

Your success on test day depends not only on how many hours you put into preparing, but also on whether you prepared the right way. It's good to check along the way to see if your studying is paying off. One of the most effective ways to do this is by taking practice tests to evaluate your progress. Practice tests are useful because they show exactly where you need to improve. Every time you take a practice test, pay special attention to these three groups of questions:

- The questions you got wrong
- The questions you had to guess on, even if you guessed right
- The questions you found difficult or slow to work through

This will show you exactly what your weak areas are, and where you need to devote more study time. Ask yourself why each of these questions gave you trouble. Was it because you didn't understand the material? Was it because you didn't remember the vocabulary? Do you need more repetitions on this type of question to build speed and confidence? Dig into those questions and figure out how you can strengthen your weak areas as you go back to review the material.

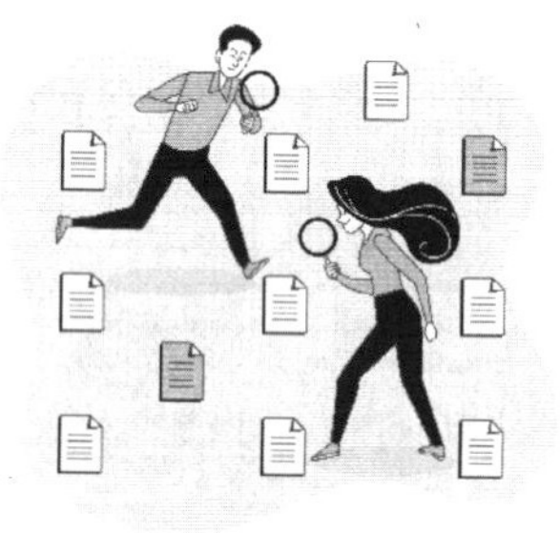

Additionally, many practice tests have a section explaining the answer choices. It can be tempting to read the explanation and think that you now have a good understanding of the concept. However, an explanation likely only covers part of the question's broader context. Even if the explanation makes perfect sense, **go back and investigate** every concept related to the question until you're positive you have a thorough understanding.

As you go along, keep in mind that the practice test is just that: practice. Memorizing these questions and answers will not be very helpful on the actual test because it is unlikely to have any of the same exact questions. If you only know the right answers to the sample questions, you won't be prepared for the real thing. **Study the concepts** until you understand them fully, and then you'll be able to answer any question that shows up on the test.

It's important to wait on the practice tests until you're ready. If you take a test on your first day of study, you may be overwhelmed by the amount of material covered and how much you need to learn. Work up to it gradually.

On test day, you'll need to be prepared for answering questions, managing your time, and using the test-taking strategies you've learned. It's a lot to balance, like a mental marathon that will have a big impact on your future. Like training for a marathon, you'll need to start slowly and work your way up. When test day arrives, you'll be ready.

Start with the strategies you've read in the first two Secret Keys—plan your course and study in the way that works best for you. If you have time, consider using multiple study resources to get different approaches to the same concepts. It can be helpful to see difficult concepts from more than one angle. Then find a good source for practice tests. Many times, the test website will suggest potential study resources or provide sample tests.

Practice Test Strategy

If you're able to find at least three practice tests, we recommend this strategy:

Untimed and Open-Book Practice

Take the first test with no time constraints and with your notes and study guide handy. Take your time and focus on applying the strategies you've learned.

Timed and Open-Book Practice

Take the second practice test open-book as well, but set a timer and practice pacing yourself to finish in time.

Timed and Closed-Book Practice

Take any other practice tests as if it were test day. Set a timer and put away your study materials. Sit at a table or desk in a quiet room, imagine yourself at the testing center, and answer questions as quickly and accurately as possible.

Keep repeating timed and closed-book tests on a regular basis until you run out of practice tests or it's time for the actual test. Your mind will be ready for the schedule and stress of test day, and you'll be able to focus on recalling the material you've learned.

Secret Key 4: Pace Yourself

Once you're fully prepared for the material on the test, your biggest challenge on test day will be managing your time. Just knowing that the clock is ticking can make you panic even if you have plenty of time left. Work on pacing yourself so you can build confidence against the time constraints of the exam. Pacing is a difficult skill to master, especially in a high-pressure environment, so **practice is vital**.

Set time expectations for your pace based on how much time is available. For example, if a section has 60 questions and the time limit is 30 minutes, you know you have to average 30 seconds or less per question in order to answer them all. Although 30 seconds is the hard limit, set 25 seconds per question as your goal, so you reserve extra time to spend on harder questions. When you budget extra time for the harder questions, you no longer have any reason to stress when those questions take longer to answer.

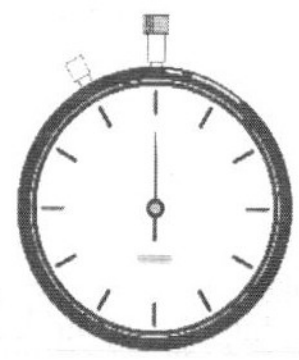

Don't let this time expectation distract you from working through the test at a calm, steady pace, but keep it in mind so you don't spend too much time on any one question. Recognize that taking extra time on one question you don't understand may keep you from answering two that you do understand later in the test. If your time limit for a question is up and you're still not sure of the answer, mark it and move on, and come back to it later if the time and the test format allow. If the testing format doesn't allow you to return to earlier questions, just make an educated guess; then put it out of your mind and move on.

On the easier questions, be careful not to rush. It may seem wise to hurry through them so you have more time for the challenging ones, but it's not worth missing one if you know the concept and just didn't take the time to read the question fully. Work efficiently but make sure you understand the question and have looked at all of the answer choices, since more than one may seem right at first.

Even if you're paying attention to the time, you may find yourself a little behind at some point. You should speed up to get back on track, but do so wisely. Don't panic; just take a few seconds less on each question until you're caught up. Don't guess without thinking, but do look through the answer choices and eliminate any you know are wrong. If you can get down to two choices, it is often worthwhile to guess from those. Once you've chosen an answer, move on and don't dwell on any that you skipped or had to hurry through. If a question was taking too long, chances are it was one of the harder ones, so you weren't as likely to get it right anyway.

On the other hand, if you find yourself getting ahead of schedule, it may be beneficial to slow down a little. The more quickly you work, the more likely you are to make a careless mistake that will affect your score. You've budgeted time for each question, so don't be afraid to spend that time. Practice an efficient but careful pace to get the most out of the time you have.

Secret Key 5: Have a Plan for Guessing

When you're taking the test, you may find yourself stuck on a question. Some of the answer choices seem better than others, but you don't see the one answer choice that is obviously correct. What do you do?

The scenario described above is very common, yet most test takers have not effectively prepared for it. Developing and practicing a plan for guessing may be one of the single most effective uses of your time as you get ready for the exam.

In developing your plan for guessing, there are three questions to address:

- When should you start the guessing process?
- How should you narrow down the choices?
- Which answer should you choose?

When to Start the Guessing Process

Unless your plan for guessing is to select C every time (which, despite its merits, is not what we recommend), you need to leave yourself enough time to apply your answer elimination strategies. Since you have a limited amount of time for each question, that means that if you're going to give yourself the best shot at guessing correctly, you have to decide quickly whether or not you will guess.

Of course, the best-case scenario is that you don't have to guess at all, so first, see if you can answer the question based on your knowledge of the subject and basic reasoning skills. Focus on the key words in the question and try to jog your memory of related topics. Give yourself a chance to bring the knowledge to mind, but once you realize that you don't have (or you can't access) the knowledge you need to answer the question, it's time to start the guessing process.

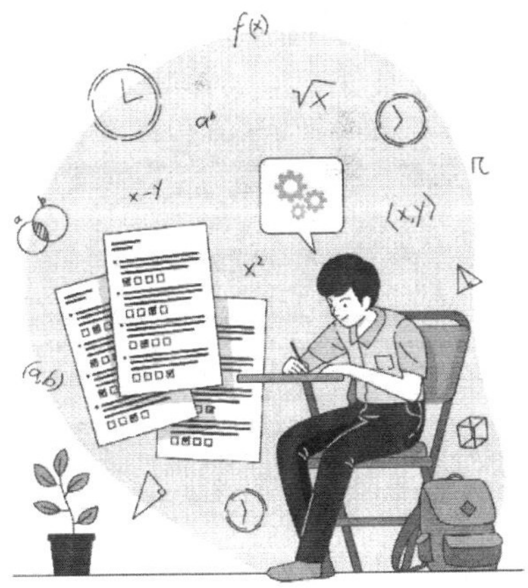

It's almost always better to start the guessing process too early than too late. It only takes a few seconds to remember something and answer the question from knowledge. Carefully eliminating wrong answer choices takes longer. Plus, going through the process of eliminating answer choices can actually help jog your memory.

Summary: Start the guessing process as soon as you decide that you can't answer the question based on your knowledge.

How to Narrow Down the Choices

The next chapter in this book (**Test-Taking Strategies**) includes a wide range of strategies for how to approach questions and how to look for answer choices to eliminate. You will definitely want to read those carefully, practice them, and figure out which ones work best for you. Here though, we're going to address a mindset rather than a particular strategy.

Your odds of guessing an answer correctly depend on how many options you are choosing from.

Number of options left	5	4	3	2	1
Odds of guessing correctly	20%	25%	33%	50%	100%

You can see from this chart just how valuable it is to be able to eliminate incorrect answers and make an educated guess, but there are two things that many test takers do that cause them to miss out on the benefits of guessing:

- Accidentally eliminating the correct answer
- Selecting an answer based on an impression

We'll look at the first one here, and the second one in the next section.

To avoid accidentally eliminating the correct answer, we recommend a thought exercise called **the $5 challenge**. In this challenge, you only eliminate an answer choice from contention if you are willing to bet $5 on it being wrong. Why $5? Five dollars is a small but not insignificant amount of money. It's an amount you could afford to lose but wouldn't want to throw away. And while losing $5 once might not hurt too much, doing it twenty times will set you back $100. In the same way, each small decision you make—eliminating a choice here, guessing on a question there—won't by itself impact your score very much, but when you put them all together, they can make a big difference. By holding each answer choice elimination decision to a higher standard, you can reduce the risk of accidentally eliminating the correct answer.

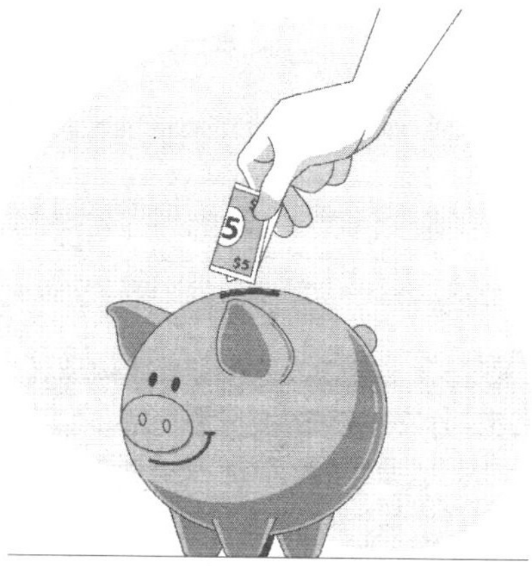

The $5 challenge can also be applied in a positive sense: If you are willing to bet $5 that an answer choice *is* correct, go ahead and mark it as correct.

Summary: Only eliminate an answer choice if you are willing to bet $5 that it is wrong.

Which Answer to Choose

You're taking the test. You've run into a hard question and decided you'll have to guess. You've eliminated all the answer choices you're willing to bet $5 on. Now you have to pick an answer. Why do we even need to talk about this? Why can't you just pick whichever one you feel like when the time comes?

The answer to these questions is that if you don't come into the test with a plan, you'll rely on your impression to select an answer choice, and if you do that, you risk falling into a trap. The test writers know that everyone who takes their test will be guessing on some of the questions, so they intentionally write wrong answer choices to seem plausible. You still have to pick an answer though, and if the wrong answer choices are designed to look right, how can you ever be sure that you're not falling for their trap? The best solution we've found to this dilemma is to take the decision out of your hands entirely. Here is the process we recommend:

Once you've eliminated any choices that you are confident (willing to bet $5) are wrong, select the first remaining choice as your answer.

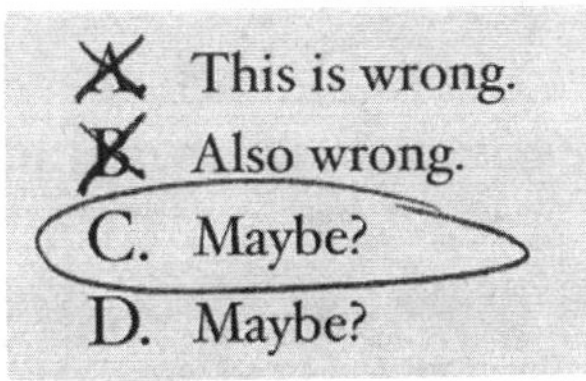

Whether you choose to select the first remaining choice, the second, or the last, the important thing is that you use some preselected standard. Using this approach guarantees that you will not be enticed into selecting an answer choice that looks right, because you are not basing your decision on how the answer choices look.

This is not meant to make you question your knowledge. Instead, it is to help you recognize the difference between your knowledge and your impressions. There's a huge difference between thinking an answer is right because of what you know, and thinking an answer is right because it looks or sounds like it should be right.

Summary: To ensure that your selection is appropriately random, make a predetermined selection from among all answer choices you have not eliminated.

Test-Taking Strategies

This section contains a list of test-taking strategies that you may find helpful as you work through the test. By taking what you know and applying logical thought, you can maximize your chances of answering any question correctly!

It is very important to realize that every question is different and every person is different: no single strategy will work on every question, and no single strategy will work for every person. That's why we've included all of them here, so you can try them out and determine which ones work best for different types of questions and which ones work best for you.

Question Strategies

✓ Read Carefully

Read the question and the answer choices carefully. Don't miss the question because you misread the terms. You have plenty of time to read each question thoroughly and make sure you understand what is being asked. Yet a happy medium must be attained, so don't waste too much time. You must read carefully and efficiently.

✓ Contextual Clues

Look for contextual clues. If the question includes a word you are not familiar with, look at the immediate context for some indication of what the word might mean. Contextual clues can often give you all the information you need to decipher the meaning of an unfamiliar word. Even if you can't determine the meaning, you may be able to narrow down the possibilities enough to make a solid guess at the answer to the question.

✓ Prefixes

If you're having trouble with a word in the question or answer choices, try dissecting it. Take advantage of every clue that the word might include. Prefixes can be a huge help. Usually, they allow you to determine a basic meaning. *Pre-* means before, *post-* means after, *pro-* is positive, *de-* is negative. From prefixes, you can get an idea of the general meaning of the word and try to put it into context.

✓ Hedge Words

Watch out for critical hedge words, such as *likely, may, can, often, almost, mostly, usually, generally, rarely,* and *sometimes.* Question writers insert these hedge phrases to cover every possibility. Often an answer choice will be wrong simply because it leaves no room for exception. Be on guard for answer choices that have definitive words such as *exactly* and *always.*

✓ Switchback Words

Stay alert for *switchbacks.* These are the words and phrases frequently used to alert you to shifts in thought. The most common switchback words are *but, although,* and *however.* Others include *nevertheless, on the other hand, even though, while, in spite of, despite,* and *regardless of.* Switchback words are important to catch because they can change the direction of the question or an answer choice.

✓ Face Value

When in doubt, use common sense. Accept the situation in the problem at face value. Don't read too much into it. These problems will not require you to make wild assumptions. If you have to go beyond creativity and warp time or space in order to have an answer choice fit the question, then you should move on and consider the other answer choices. These are normal problems rooted in reality. The applicable relationship or explanation may not be readily apparent, but it is there for you to figure out. Use your common sense to interpret anything that isn't clear.

Answer Choice Strategies

ANSWER SELECTION

The most thorough way to pick an answer choice is to identify and eliminate wrong answers until only one is left, then confirm it is the correct answer. Sometimes an answer choice may immediately seem right, but be careful. The test writers will usually put more than one reasonable answer choice on each question, so take a second to read all of them and make sure that the other choices are not equally obvious. As long as you have time left, it is better to read every answer choice than to pick the first one that looks right without checking the others.

ANSWER CHOICE FAMILIES

An answer choice family consists of two (in rare cases, three) answer choices that are very similar in construction and cannot all be true at the same time. If you see two answer choices that are direct opposites or parallels, one of them is usually the correct answer. For instance, if one answer choice says that quantity x increases and another either says that quantity x decreases (opposite) or says that quantity y increases (parallel), then those answer choices would fall into the same family. An answer choice that doesn't match the construction of the answer choice family is more likely to be incorrect. Most questions will not have answer choice families, but when they do appear, you should be prepared to recognize them.

ELIMINATE ANSWERS

Eliminate answer choices as soon as you realize they are wrong, but make sure you consider all possibilities. If you are eliminating answer choices and realize that the last one you are left with is also wrong, don't panic. Start over and consider each choice again. There may be something you missed the first time that you will realize on the second pass.

AVOID FACT TRAPS

Don't be distracted by an answer choice that is factually true but doesn't answer the question. You are looking for the choice that answers the question. Stay focused on what the question is asking for so you don't accidentally pick an answer that is true but incorrect. Always go back to the question and make sure the answer choice you've selected actually answers the question and is not merely a true statement.

EXTREME STATEMENTS

In general, you should avoid answers that put forth extreme actions as standard practice or proclaim controversial ideas as established fact. An answer choice that states the "process should be used in certain situations, if..." is much more likely to be correct than one that states the "process should be discontinued completely." The first is a calm rational statement and doesn't even make a definitive, uncompromising stance, using a hedge word *if* to provide wiggle room, whereas the second choice is far more extreme.

BENCHMARK

As you read through the answer choices and you come across one that seems to answer the question well, mentally select that answer choice. This is not your final answer, but it's the one that will help you evaluate the other answer choices. The one that you selected is your benchmark or standard for judging each of the other answer choices. Every other answer choice must be compared to your benchmark. That choice is correct until proven otherwise by another answer choice beating it. If you find a better answer, then that one becomes your new benchmark. Once you've decided that no other choice answers the question as well as your benchmark, you have your final answer.

⊘ Predict the Answer

Before you even start looking at the answer choices, it is often best to try to predict the answer. When you come up with the answer on your own, it is easier to avoid distractions and traps because you will know exactly what to look for. The right answer choice is unlikely to be word-for-word what you came up with, but it should be a close match. Even if you are confident that you have the right answer, you should still take the time to read each option before moving on.

General Strategies

⊘ Tough Questions

If you are stumped on a problem or it appears too hard or too difficult, don't waste time. Move on! Remember though, if you can quickly check for obviously incorrect answer choices, your chances of guessing correctly are greatly improved. Before you completely give up, at least try to knock out a couple of possible answers. Eliminate what you can and then guess at the remaining answer choices before moving on.

⊘ Check Your Work

Since you will probably not know every term listed and the answer to every question, it is important that you get credit for the ones that you do know. Don't miss any questions through careless mistakes. If at all possible, try to take a second to look back over your answer selection and make sure you've selected the correct answer choice and haven't made a costly careless mistake (such as marking an answer choice that you didn't mean to mark). This quick double check should more than pay for itself in caught mistakes for the time it costs.

⊘ Pace Yourself

It's easy to be overwhelmed when you're looking at a page full of questions; your mind is confused and full of random thoughts, and the clock is ticking down faster than you would like. Calm down and maintain the pace that you have set for yourself. Especially as you get down to the last few minutes of the test, don't let the small numbers on the clock make you panic. As long as you are on track by monitoring your pace, you are guaranteed to have time for each question.

⊘ Don't Rush

It is very easy to make errors when you are in a hurry. Maintaining a fast pace in answering questions is pointless if it makes you miss questions that you would have gotten right otherwise. Test writers like to include distracting information and wrong answers that seem right. Taking a little extra time to avoid careless mistakes can make all the difference in your test score. Find a pace that allows you to be confident in the answers that you select.

⊘ Keep Moving

Panicking will not help you pass the test, so do your best to stay calm and keep moving. Taking deep breaths and going through the answer elimination steps you practiced can help to break through a stress barrier and keep your pace.

Final Notes

The combination of a solid foundation of content knowledge and the confidence that comes from practicing your plan for applying that knowledge is the key to maximizing your performance on test day. As your foundation of content knowledge is built up and strengthened, you'll find that the strategies included in this chapter become more and more effective in helping you quickly sift through the distractions and traps of the test to isolate the correct answer.

Now that you're preparing to move forward into the test content chapters of this book, be sure to keep your goal in mind. As you read, think about how you will be able to apply this information on the test. If you've already seen sample questions for the test and you have an idea of the question format and style, try to come up with questions of your own that you can answer based on what you're reading. This will give you valuable practice applying your knowledge in the same ways you can expect to on test day.

Good luck and good studying!

General Principles of Transport Nursing Practice

Scene Operations Management

Scene-of-Incident Safety Considerations

The transport team must do a 360° assessment of the scene of incident on arrival and determine safety considerations. The team should make note of any gunshots heard, downed power lines, buildings in a state of collapse, leaking fuels/fluids, fire, smoke, broken glass, and other hazards. Transport personnel may need to wait until the site is safe to proceed. The transport nurse should assess the mechanism of injury (accidents) and the need for appropriate PPE (gloves, gown, mask, face guard) and must keep the patient informed of all actions and prevent harm or further injury. The ambulance should be parked off of the roadway if possible or parked at a 45° angle (front wheels out) to shield the work area, making sure not to block access for other emergency vehicles. Parking uphill is safer than downhill, and upwind is safer than downwind. If flares are used to warn other drivers, they should extend at least 300 feet from a collision. Yellow warning lights at the scene are the safest, but excessive lighting may blind other drivers at night.

Environmental Risk Factors

When assessing a patient, it's important to consider that environmental factors may place the patient at an increased risk for harm or may be a factor in disease. There are a number of different types of environmental factors to consider.

Factors	Examples	Effects
Toxic chemicals	Lead, arsenic, muriatic acid, sulfuric acid, ammonia, lime	May result in poisoning (lead, arsenic) or burns (acids, ammonia, lime) through direct exposure or inhalation
Physical objects	Guns, cars, knives, equipment	Accidents, gunshot wounds, stabbings, various injuries (blunt and penetrating)
Biological organisms	Bacteria, fungi, viruses	Infections
Temperature variations	Heat, cold	Burns, dehydration, heat stroke, hyperthermia, hypothermia, frostbite
Ambient noise	Sirens, loud music, traffic noise, work-related noise	Hearing loss/deafness, increased anxiety
Psychosocial	Increased stress	Anxiety, hypertension, suicidal ideation

Hazardous Materials, Exposure, and Absorption

Hazardous materials are any materials that may cause harm to humans or animals by themselves or through interaction with something else. Hazardous materials may be any of the following:

- **Chemical**: Blister agents, blood agents, choking agents, nerve agents, asphyxiants, or irritants that can enter the body through inhalation, absorption, ingestion, or injection
- **Radiological**: Nuclear material and radioactive substances (alpha/beta particles)
- **Physical/Biological**: Infectious wastes, blood and other body fluids, and biotoxins

Almost any material or substance can be classified as hazardous depending on various factors such as its location, amount, and interactions. Exposure occurs when a person/animal comes in contact with the hazardous material, and contamination is the residue resulting from exposure. Absorption is the method by which hazardous material enters the bloodstream. Exposure and contamination may result in an immediate response (blistering, itching, and pain) or a delayed response (nausea, vomiting, cancer, and lung disease).

Classification of Hazardous Waste

The Environmental Protection Agency (EPA) classifies hazardous wastes according to the following characteristics:

- **Ignitable**: Liquids and nonliquids that can ignite and cause fires with flash points of <60 °C (140 °F)
- **Corrosive**: Based on pH (<2 or >12.5) or its ability to corrode steel
- **Reactive**: Wastes that are unstable, may react with water, may result in toxic gases, or may explode
- **Toxic**: Heavy metal compounds that are harmful if ingested or absorbed

Wastes may also be classified as listed wastes. These include wastes from manufacturing and industrial processes. Hazardous wastes are often produced in manufacturing, nuclear power plants (nuclear wastes), and healthcare facilities (needles and materials contaminated with body fluids). Nuclear wastes are classified as mixed waste because they contain a radioactive component as well as a hazardous component. Hazardous wastes can result in disease (such as from needle punctures), injury (from fire and explosions), and death (from toxic exposure and disease).

Hazardous Waste Site Characterization

The purpose of hazardous waste site characterization is to identify hazards and select the appropriate PPE. The team leader is responsible for the assessment, but he or she may request assistance from outside experts, such as chemists. The three steps to hazardous waste site characterization include the following:

1. **Off-site characterization**: Gather information/data before personnel enter the site, including the location, a description of the activities, the duration of the event, terrain information (photographs, maps), habitation/population data, accessibility, paths of least resistance, and properties of any hazardous materials/substances. Conduct the needed interviews and review of records. Perimeter reconnaissance is done with observations, air sampling, and development of a preliminary site map.
2. **On-site survey**: Verify the information gathered from perimeter reconnaissance, survey the area and situation, note potential exposure to hazardous materials (dust, liquid, dead animals, gas) and safety hazards (obstacles, terrain, poisonous plants), and develop a site safety plan. The entry team should have at least four members: two to enter and two for outside support who can enter the site in an emergency.
3. **Ongoing monitoring**: Monitoring should be continuous.

Chemical Hazardous Waste Materials

Types of chemical hazardous waste materials include the following:

- **Blister agents**: Include sulfur mustard (mustard gas) and nitrogen mustard, which are both highly toxic. Exposure by inhalation, contact, or ingestion results in skin (erythema and blistering) and eye irritation and injury to the respiratory system as well as bone marrow suppression and gastrointestinal and neurological damage. The patient should be decontaminated within 1 to 2 minutes by flushing the eyes with water for up to 20 minutes and removing clothing and showering with soap (if available) and water for 20 minutes. Rescuers should use a self-contained breathing apparatus (SCBA), PPE (including eye protection), and chemical-protective gloves.
- **Asphyxiants**: Gas exposure (such as by butane, helium, and propane) lowers oxygen levels and results in suffocation. Patients require oxygen administration and may need CPR. This is especially a risk in confined spaces. Rescuers should use an SCBA.
- **Blood agents**: These include cyanide chloride, hydrogen cyanide, and arsine. Exposure by inhalation or ingestion. They prevent oxygen transfer from blood to cells. The patient may need oxygen and the antidote. Rescuers should use an SCBA.

- **Carcinogens**: Agents such as asbestos, nickel compounds, and ionizing radiation that result in genetic mutation and cancer. There are various types of exposure. Patients must be removed from exposure. The rescuer must wear adequate PPE, and in some cases, he or she should use a mask or SCBA.
- **Choking agents**: Often, a chemical weapon is used (ammonia, chlorine) that is designed to inhibit breathing and incapacitate the person. Exposure is by inhalation, contact, or ingestion (rare). They may be corrosive to the skin and result in fluid in the lungs, leading to suffocation. Patients require supportive treatment and oxygen. Rescuers should use PPE and SCBA for most agents.
- **Convulsants/Nerve agents**: These include hydrazine and strychnine. Exposure may be by inhalation, contact, and ingestion. The severity of convulsions and nervous system impairment is dose related. Patients require supportive treatment. Rescuers need SCBA and protective suits (according to the exposure level of the agent).

Hazard Signs and Symbols

Sign/Symbol	Interpretation
	Flame: Includes flammable, self-heating, or self-reactive materials and gases.
	Corrosion: Includes substances that can cause skin burns, metal corrosion, and eye damage.
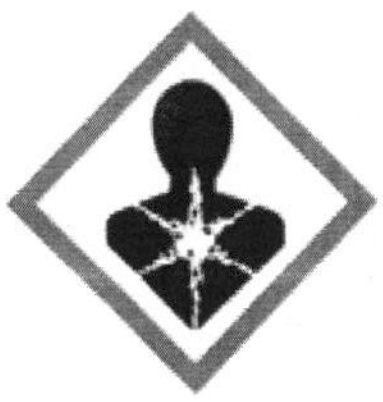	Health hazard: Includes carcinogens, toxic substances, and respiratory irritants.
	Poison: Includes materials, gases, or substances that are extremely toxic and may result in death or severe illness.
	Irritant: Includes materials, gases, or substances that are irritants to the skin, eyes, and/or respiratory tract, are acutely toxic, or have a narcotic effect.

Sign/Symbol	Interpretation
	Biohazard: Includes biological substances, such as body fluids, that pose a threat to humans. Appears on sharps containers that hold contaminated needles.

Emergency Vehicle Operations

Emergency Medical Services (EMS) History

Historically, the **first use of an ambulance** was in the Siege of Málaga in Spain in 1487, when horse-drawn wagons were used to carry the wounded to safety. Military ambulances became more common in Europe throughout the following centuries. Napoleon Bonaparte assigned battlefield vehicles and attendants in 1793. The first ambulance service in the United States was instituted by the US army in 1865 in Cincinnati, followed by an ambulance service in New York just four years later. Hospital-based ambulance services increased in the 1900s, but many hospital ambulance services shut down during World War II, so fire and police departments filled the roles. At this time, there were no laws regarding minimum training for ambulance personnel. Following World War II, the use of ambulance services increased, but the quality was often poor until basic training standards were developed in 1968 along with the 911 emergency system. The EMS Systems Act was passed in 1973, the EMS for Children Act in 1983, and the Trauma Care Systems Planning and Development Act in 1990. In 1991, standards and benchmarks for ambulance services were established by the Commission on Accreditation of Ambulance Services.

EMS Systems

The **National Highway Traffic Safety Administration** (**NHTSA**) is the lead agency for coordinating and promoting evidence-based emergency medical services (EMS) (fire based, third service, and hospital based) and the 911 system. The **public safety answering point** (**PSAP**) is the designated call-receiving site that directs calls to the appropriate emergency services. Each state defines the scope of practice, licensure, and credentialing for prehospital personnel and sets education standards based on national EMS standards. The EMS provider of any level is expected to maintain certification through maintenance of skills and continuing education and should exhibit professional behavior, including working with integrity and empathy, being an effective member of a team, showing respect and tact, maintaining a professional appearance, communicating effectively, and advocating for patients. The provider must be alert to patient safety and recognize that most errors result from skills-based, rules-based, and knowledge-based failures. Error reduction requires the use of decision aids and protocols, asking for assistance when appropriate, questioning assumptions, and making debriefing calls.

Driving Safety

The ambulance driver should stop briefly or slow significantly at intersections because other drivers may not hear or may ignore sirens. The driver should keep the brake covered with the left foot for fast braking and avoid excessive speeds because of the increased risk of accidents, especially on curves. The speed should be adjusted for road and weather conditions and should not be influenced by use of the siren (siren syndrome). Snow and ice should be cleared from the ambulance before driving it. At least one vehicle length should separate the ambulance from other vehicles for every 10 mph of speed. A spotter should always be used when backing up the ambulance because of poor visibility. All personnel in the ambulance should be seated and secured with seat belts or safety harnesses before the ambulance moves. Studies have shown that CPR is most effective if done from a sitting position in an ambulance rather than standing, despite common practice. Patients and gurneys should also be secured.

Lights and Sirens

Lights and sirens should be used together, and they are indicated when going to a scene and when transporting a patient in a serious emergent situation. There are four types of warning lights used on emergency vehicles such as ambulances: rotating lights (resulting in a flashing sensation), fixed flashes (usually red or blue), strobe lights, and LED lights. Red (the most common) and blue lights are generally used to indicate emergency vehicles and can be used to obtain the right-of-way or to block the right-of-way. These colors may be interchangeable, although in some states the color blue is restricted to law enforcement vehicles. Amber lights are warning lights and can be used by all vehicles, but they do not require others to stop. Some emergency vehicle lights change to amber when the vehicle is parked. Green lights are sometimes used to indicate a mobile incident command post, but in some states, green lights may also indicate private security vehicles or volunteer firefighters.

Communications

Transport Team Communication

With the transport team arrival at the scene of an incident, he or she should assess the situation and the need for added resources, such as additional personnel or police, and contact the appropriate authorities to request assistance. When additional personnel arrive or contact is made with medical control or the receiving facility, the transport nurse should self-identify and provide a verbal report of the patient's current condition, including demographic information such as age and gender. The provider should report the patient's chief complaint and provide any history that is pertinent as well as the condition of the patient on arrival and any history of major illnesses. The transport nurse should also report the results of the patient assessment, including the vital signs and any physical/psychological findings, as well as any treatment provided and the patient's response to the treatment. The provider should communicate with law enforcement officers and other responders, such as firefighters, especially regarding safety concerns.

Emergency Medical Services Communication System

Components of an emergency medical services communication system include the base station of a two-way radio system, which is in a fixed location, such as a dispatch center. The base station facilitates communication among a number of hand-held/mobile radios. There is often only one channel per base station, so additional base stations may be installed to add more channels. Radio transmitters/receivers may be vehicular mounted or mobile, although mobile transmitters/receivers may have limited range because they tend to have lower power (1–5 watts) than do base stations (20–50 watts). Typically, the mobile device has a range of 10–15 miles over average terrain, but it is shorter in rugged terrain. The Federal Communications Commission (FCC) controls radio frequencies, and those used for EMS are in the public safety pool.

Communication with Medical Control

The transport team may be in communication with medical control regarding a patient's condition and need for medication. Medical control may be at the receiving facility or at a separate site. Upon receiving an order by phone or radio, the transport nurse should repeat back the order and dosage to ensure that the message was received correctly. When using the radio, the radio must be turned on and the press-to-talk (PTT) button must be pressed before beginning transmission. The provider should address the medical control person by name and give the name of their unit. Transmissions should be brief and to the point, avoiding unnecessary pleasantries, codes, agency-specific terms, profanity, and meaningless phrases, keeping in mind that the airways are public. The transport nurse should give individual digits for long numbers, use "affirmative" and "negative" in place of "yes" and "no," and say "over" when the transmission is finished. Reports should be objective rather than opinion based and should avoid offering a diagnosis. The dispatcher must be notified when the unit leaves the scene.

Phone/cellular communication is similar to radio communication, but transport team should be familiar with important phone numbers (such as medical control, hospitals, trauma centers) or have the numbers prominently posted for access. They should also be aware of dead spots that may prevent communication and should have a backup plan (radio) for when cellular transmission fails.

Radio Operations

Types of Radio Bands

The very high frequency (VHF) high-band frequency modulation (FM), which ranges from 148–174 megahertz (MHz), offers a straight line radio signal. The VHF low-band FM, which ranges from 30–50 MHz, has the greatest range, as it follows the Earth's curvature. With ranges from 118–136 MHz, the VHF amplitude modulation (AM) is generally the band used for radio communication related to aviation. Ultra-high frequency (UHF) radio bands, which range from 403–941 MHz, provide a limited range of communication; they are most effective when used between ground units and base stations. UHF radio bands can be used to communicate between the ground and the air, but only for short distances. Computer-controlled digital communication (800 MHz) provides the ability for multiple organizations to communicate with one another. This radio band offers a higher frequency and less noise than others.

Most Commonly Used Response Codes

When an emergency vehicle responds to a call, the emergency medical personnel need to determine whether the transport status should be categorized as emergent or non-emergent. A code 1, referred to as a cold response in certain agencies, indicates a non-emergent transport whereby no emergency lights or sirens should be used. When an emergency vehicle turns its lights on without utilizing the sirens, the response code is known as a code 2. A code 3, referred to as a hot response in certain agencies, denotes a transport situation of emergent status whereby both emergency lights and sirens should be used.

Simplex vs. Multiplex Radio Communication Systems

A simplex radio communication system is one in which communication can only occur in one direction at a time. For example, one party involved in the communication process can transmit a message to the receiving party. If both parties attempt to transmit messages simultaneously, one of the messages will be blocked. In contrast, a multiplex radio communication system is one in which two or more types of information can be transmitted simultaneously using the same radio frequency. For example, a multiplex system has the ability to transmit electrocardiogram (ECG) data via radio at the same time voice communication is being transmitted via radio.

Patient Handoff

Patient-Related Information to Obtain Prior to Transport

It is essential to gather an accurate description of the diagnosis and the current condition of the patient being transferred. Having correct information about the patient's diagnosis and medical status can assist the transport team in determining the most appropriate medical personnel and medical equipment to have available on the vehicle prior to transport. Additionally, the transport team should attempt to collect as much information as possible about who will accompany the patient on the ride. Finally, the transport team should ascertain whether the patient being transported has a "do not resuscitate" order in effect.

Physical Exam Findings to Share with Receiving Facility

When reporting a patient's condition to a receiving facility, the first component of the physical examination that should be addressed is the patient's ABC status—the functioning of his/her airway, breathing, and circulation. The patient's neurological status should be reported to the receiving facility, and if applicable, his/her Glasgow Coma Scale score should be provided as well. Abnormal findings encountered during a head-to-toe examination of the patient should be emphasized, and general findings from such an assessment should also be addressed. Additionally, the receiving facility should be informed of the patient's electrocardiogram (ECG) rhythm and his/her vital signs.

Effective Communication and Interview Techniques

Effective communication begins with a self-introduction and an introduction of other team members to the patient and family and includes respecting the patient's privacy by shielding the patient from passersby if possible and avoiding loudly repeating any patient information. If possible, the transport nurse should adjust lighting and limit outside distractions such as noise.

If possible, the patient should be **interviewed** alone or should be asked if he or she wants family members present. Verbal and nonverbal responses should be observed during an interview. Information should include not only the patient's facts but also the patient's attitude and concerns. The transport nurse should ask one question at a time in language that the patient understands and avoid providing false reassurances and advice or interrupting. Strategies include the following:

- Ask **open-ended informational questions** (as opposed to yes/no) with "who," "what," "where," "when," and "how," but avoid questions with "why" if possible.
    - Instead of "Why do you continue to use heroin?" ask "Have you tried to quit drug use?"
- Ask brief **clarifying questions**: "How long have you had weakness in your left side?"
- Provide a **list of options**: "Is your headache throbbing, stabbing, or dull?"
- **Rephrase/reflect** to encourage clarification.
    - Patient: "My husband had the same type of fall and died a month later."
    - Nurse: "You're afraid you might die from this fall."

Special Interview Situations

Hostile, Aggressive, or Impaired Patients

Interviewing hostile patients requires a calm response, avoiding negative responses and using reflective statements, such as "I can understand your feelings." The transport nurse should maintain eye contact (50–60% of the time) and try to defuse the situation, but he or she should avoid staring or standing too close and having crossed arms because this may be misinterpreted as threatening behavior. If patients are sexually aggressive, it's important to tell them that the behavior is inappropriate and to ask them to stop. When interviewing patients under the influence of drugs or alcohol, try to ask essential questions such as the type and amount of drug/alcohol ingested. Obtain information from family or friends if necessary. When patients are hearing impaired, the transport nurse should face the person directly, speak slowly and distinctly (but avoid shouting), provide information in writing if possible, use pantomime, and try to reduce environmental noise. Knowledge of the alphabet in sign language can be very useful to communicate with the deaf, especially if a sign-language translator is unavailable.

Elderly Patients

When interviewing elderly patients, the transport nurse should be alert to possible cognitive, hearing, or vision impairments, especially if the patient appears confused upon questioning or his or her answers are inappropriate. They should ask if the patient has eyeglasses or a hearing aid and should obtain them if possible. The patient's family may be able to assist with the interview. If the patient's speech is unclear, he or she may need to put in dentures. When communicating with a pediatric patient, the transport nurse should have the parent or caregiver comfort the child and answer questions, especially if the child is an infant or is very young. The provider should use simple sentences and age-appropriate language and explain to the child what he or she is doing to help alleviate the child's fear. Adolescents should be addressed directly even if a parent or caregiver is providing some information, and, in some cases, the adolescent will provide more information if the parent/caregiver is not present.

Non-English or Limited English-Speaking Patients

The transport nurse should begin an interview with a non-English or limited English-speaking patient first in English. If a patient does not respond verbally and appears confused and/or frightened when questioned, and it is suspected that the patient doesn't speak English, the provider should ask directly if he or she can understand English. When a patient is a non-English speaking or a limited English speaker, the important thing is to communicate. Although children, friends, bystanders, and family are not usually used as translators, in emergent or life-threatening situations, an exception is made. The transport nurse may use signs, gestures, and pantomime to communicate and use simple words or phrases, such as "Pain?" and "OK?" because even non-English speakers may understand a few words. The provider may use a language line if available and the situation permits, and he or she should alert the receiving hospital of the need for a translator as well as providing information about the patient's language. The transport nurse should point to a body part before touching it.

Crew Resource Management

Crew resource management (CRM) encompasses procedures designed to eliminate the risks associated with human error, which often results from inadequate leadership, ineffective teamwork, and poor decision-making. The focus of CRM is on interpersonal skills and improving communication among all crewmembers (rather than technical skills) to improve situational awareness which helps the crew better function as a team, carrying out problem solving and making decisions. CRM may include protocols for dealing with problems as well as checklists to ensure that no steps in a process are overlooked. While CRM was initially developed as part of aviation training, the basic procedures can be applied to virtually all aspects of healthcare. Classroom training is carried out in conjunction with transport simulation for all trasport team members. Topics include the information processing model, strategies to avoid human errors, workload over/underload, stress, fatigue, elements of situational awareness (perceiving, comprehending, and projecting), debriefing, coordinating, communicating, and automation.

Safety and Survival

Navigation

Global Positioning System (GPS)

The Global Positioning System (GPS) is a radio-navigation system operated by the US Air Force, based on satellite technology and utilized with mapping software to provide location information. GPS mapping software can provide address, location, and mapping directions for emergency medical services. GPS tracking devices to help locate places, individuals, and devices/equipment are increasingly present in smart phones, motor vehicles, aircraft, and even toys and shoes. GPS fleet tracking software can be utilized to track the location of a fleet of motor vehicles or aircraft in real time. GPS can also be utilized to determine the shortest route to a destination. However, mapping systems are not always up-to-date regarding changes (such as road closures), so errors can occur. Satellite signal interference may also cause problems, so ground crews should always have backup maps. GPS software should be routinely updated. The TRANSPORT NURSE should be proficient in the use of local facility GPS and communication systems.

Emergency Locator Transmitter (ELT)

An emergency locator transmitter (ELT) is a tracking device that utilizes special frequencies to communicate emergency distress signals to satellites. The primary purpose of such a device is to track down individuals or groups in need of rescue in a timely manner in order to increase the chances of survival. In addition to distress signals, an ELT has the capacity to carry and transmit voice communication to search and rescue teams over an emergency frequency. Additionally, ELT units can be helpful in search and rescue efforts given that position and altitude can be communicated through the device. Considering the crucial nature of the first several hours following the occurrence of an injury or injuries, ELTs are vital components of any transport team.

Night Vision Goggles

Night vision goggles are used for transport team members to improve vision, especially in mountainous terrain and unimproved areas. NVGs comprise the mount (helmet), battery pack, and binocular assembly. The retina of the eye contains cone cells for daylight or high-intensity light vision (photopic vision) and rod cells for low intensity light vision (mesoptic [dawn, dusk, and moonlight]) vision or nighttime vision (scotopic vision). At night, color perception and fine details are lost, and a blind spot impairs central vision. Depth perception changes in low light, and image distortion occurs. Contrasts are often poor, such as between water and landmass; therefore, NVGs should only be utilized after appropriate training and individual fitting. Because exposure to bright lights impairs adaptation to the dark, transport members should wear sunglasses on the day of a night shift when outside, vehicle lighting should be dim blue-green, and uniforms and helmets should be dark. Techniques for NVGs include scanning from side to side, off-center viewing, and distance estimation.

PRE-MISSION PREPARATION

APPARATUS AND EQUIPMENT READINESS

The transport team should ensure that the ambulance is ready for use at all times and that the tires are properly inflated, the gas tank is full, warning devices are working, and engine fluid levels are appropriate. All necessary safety equipment, such as PPE (masks, gowns, gloves, and goggles or face guards) and safety devices (safety vests, road flares, and signs) as well as seat belts and harnesses, should be available and in proper working condition. All equipment in the cab, the compartments, and the rear of the ambulance should be in the proper place, labeled, and secured to prevent shifting during transportation. High-risk situations include going through intersections, inclement weather (especially with poor visibility), careless drivers, highway access, unpaved roads, and driver distractions (conversation, eating, drinking, mobile devices, music, GPS devices, and fatigue). During transportation, all personnel as well as patients should be properly secured with safety equipment.

SECURING EQUIPMENT AND PATIENTS FOR TRANSPORT

Transport nurses are responsible for ensuring that medical equipment and devices are properly secured on the vehicle. It is essential that transport nurses evaluate the security of such items prior to every transport, as the team members and/or the patient may be injured if a piece of unsecured equipment becomes a projectile during transport. Additionally, to prevent injury to the patient, the transport nurse must ensure that the patient is properly restrained; proper restraint includes keeping the patient away from the driver and the vehicle controls. Pediatric patients must be restrained during transport; it is not acceptable for a pediatric patient to be held during transport. As such, they must be restrained in an acceptable car seat that is attached to the stretcher. If physical restraints are required for a combative patient, they must be applied prior to transport. Policies specific to individual transport programs govern the use of physical restraints.

PRE-TRANSPORT EQUIPMENT AND SUPPLY CHECK

A pre-transport check consists of an assessment of the availability of equipment and medical supplies; this assessment should follow a standardized list of equipment and supplies. Equipment and/or supplies that bear expiration dates should have their expirations verified; if any items are past their expiration dates, they should be replaced. Medical equipment that is used in patient care processes should be examined to determine whether it is functioning properly. Prior to each transport encounter, equipment and supplies that are deemed necessary and/or deemed possibly necessary during the transport process should be identified, as certain items that may not be standard need to be acquired before departure. Oxygen and air quantities should be checked prior to transport as well in order to verify that the supply of both gases is sufficient.

TRANSPORT-SPECIFIC PPE

Transport-specific PPE may consist of helmets, fire-resistant clothing, protective footwear, and/or hearing protectors. Helmets may potentially protect transport team members against head injuries. To obtain the greatest benefit from a helmet, it must fit appropriately, be lightweight and comfortable, and its lining must absorb energy. Uniforms that are fire-resistant may protect the team from dangerous skin exposure and tissue damage that can occur during fires resulting from an aircraft accident. Protective footwear such as boots can provide team members with protection from injuries such as punctures and cuts. Earplugs or earmuffs can be worn when transport encounters involve extreme levels of noise; such hearing protection may protect against hearing loss. Universal PPE should be in the appropriate size for an individual:

- **Eye protectors**: Should be worn with risk of splash or spray with body fluids or contact with debris. (Prescription glasses do not take the place of goggles.)
- **Face shields**: Provide protection for face, eyes, nose, and mouth. Preferred to goggles when there is risk of spray or splash of body fluids.
- **Masks**: Protect the nose and mouth from fluids and particles and should be fluid resistant, fit snugly, and have a flexible nosepiece.
- **Respirators** (such as N95, N100): Protect the nose, mouth, and airway passages exposed to hazardous or infectious aerosols, ng bacteria (TB, measles patients*)*.

Rescues in Confined Spaces

A confined space is one in which access is limited and the space is surrounded by walls or structures that are not suitable for habitation. A confined space may occur in a building (such as with a collapse), a silo, a motor vehicle (such as a large vehicle involved in a crash), a cistern or septic tank, or a well. A confined space may pose a risk to the patient and transport personnel because of difficulty moving about and accessing the patient as well as decreased ventilation that may result in the buildup of toxic gases and/or a lack of oxygen. Before entering a confined space, the transport nurse should test the atmosphere and use the correct breathing equipment. This is especially important if the patient is nonresponsive, which is often an indication of poor air quality. The provider should also carefully assess his or her ability to access the patient and the best means of doing so.

Patient Extrication

Extrication involves the removal of forces that are restricting a patient and/or holding him/her back from moving freely. When moving an object or force from a patient, the first step in the process is to remove items around the patient that are confining him/her in a limited space. During the extrication process, it is important to offer emotional support to the patient; one way to offer support is to describe what is being done during the process. Throughout the process, transport team members should always be cognizant of the patient's location in relation to removing other objects and/or forces and do everything possible to protect the patient's safety. Using special extrication equipment, the next step of the process involves generating new openings around the patient and/or expanding openings that already exist in order to facilitate the final removal of the forces.

Extrication from a Motor Vehicle (Car, Truck)

Scene Management

Scene management at the site of an accident that requires vehicle extrication incudes initial evaluation of any hazards at the site (360° evaluation), such as oncoming traffic, fallen wires, spilled fuel, and fire/explosion risk or presence. The scene must be secured (45° parking, police security, flares, and cones) and the transport nurse should don protective equipment as necessary and access the patient to provide life-saving care. The patient must be disentangled from the motor vehicle as much as can be done safely. The patient is prepared for extrication (such as by applying pressure to bleeding sites and placing a cervical collar), removed from the vehicle, and then prepared for ground or air transport and provided emergent treatment. For extrications in difficult terrain, assess the following:

- **Terrain**: Forests, desert, cliff, water, snow
- **Obstacles**: Trees, rocks, light, unavailability of landing sites
- **Methods to be used**: Helicopter extrication, overland carry, or other type of extrication
- **Alternative solutions**: Abort, contact search and rescue
- **Safety issues**: Review all safety concerns

Initial Actions

For vehicle extrication, the vehicle must be stabilized before the transport personnel attempt to enter the vehicle or administer aid to the patient, especially if the vehicle may slide or is on its side and the personnel must access the vehicle from the top because the vehicle may shift and further endanger the patient as well as transport personnel. Transport personnel can access the vehicle through a window, breaking it if necessary, or a door if one is operable (the patient may be able to assist in opening a window or door). The transport team should carry an airway (in case the patient requires ventilation), dressings (to apply pressure if the patient is bleeding), and a rigid cervical collar (to protect against spinal injury or further spinal damage) and should do rapid triage on access to the patient. Oxygen is usually not administered until after the patient is extracted because of the danger of fire, especially if the patient is saturated with fuel, and CPR is not done until the patient is in the supine position on a solid surface. If patients are apneic and pulseless, they must be removed as quickly as possible even with only manual protection of the spine being provided.

Extrication Process

For vehicle extrication, once transport personnel have gained access to the motor vehicle, they should unlock its doors, if possible, to allow others to more easily gain access. The transport personnel should ensure that the engine is turned off, the parking brake is set, and the transmission is set to park. If possible, an emergency response person should disconnect the battery to decrease the risk of fire and explosion. If the patient can be removed, a short backboard should be applied before moving the patient. If the patient is wedged between the seat and the steering wheel, the seat may be slid back manually while rescuers support the patient. If the seat has become dislodged from the track, then the patient should be completely immobilized because this type of mechanical damage can result in severe physical injury. If the patient's legs are trapped, lifting the steering wheel away may also lift the dashboard and help to release the patient.

Cutting a Vehicle

If a patient must be cut from a vehicle (such as when the vehicle is on its side and access must be through a U-shaped flap in the roof), he or she should be warned of the noise and should be covered with a safety blanket (heavy aluminized). In some accidents, air bags may deploy with the movement of the patient or vehicle, resulting in danger to the patient and transport personnel. If the air bags have not deployed, then the battery cables should be disconnected or cut (negative side first) to prevent deployment and personnel should avoid being in front of the path of deployment. Transport personnel should check for side air bags as well as front. The air bags should be deactivated before the steering column is moved (keeping in mind that deactivation can take up to 30 minutes), and care should be taken to avoid cutting or drilling into an air bag.

Seat Belt Pretensioners

Since the 1990s, vehicles have been equipped with seat belt pretensioners on three-point (shoulder harness) systems in the front and often also in the back. The purpose of seat belt pretensioners is to tighten any slack in the belts in an accident, pulling the person back into the seat and in the proper position for deployment of the air bag. Evidence of pretensioners is not always visible, although an accordion sleeve near the buckle end may be an indication. This sleeve compresses if the pretensioner fires. Although an undeployed pretensioner poses less threat to the transport nurse than an undeployed air bag, it can increase the risk of injury to the patient or nurse, so the seat belt should be disconnected or cut immediately on access to the patient. If the patient was not wearing the seat belt on impact and the pretensioner fired, the seat belt will be tightly vertical along pillar B. If the seat belt pretensioner fired while being worn, it will be extended and will not be retractable.

Tool Kit

Although large and heavy pieces of equipment, such as hydraulic rescue tools (including the Jaws of Life, cutters, spreaders, truck jacks, and rams), pneumatic tools, and come-along tools, are often used in vehicle extrication, a tool kit with simple hand tools should also be readily available. They may also be needed to access and safely remove a patient from a vehicle. Tools that may be needed for disassembly include adjustable wrenches, screwdrivers (flat and Phillips), flashlight, penlight, medical scissors, headlamp, pliers, bolt cutters, hammers, axes, crowbars, rescue knives (specially designed to cut through seat belts and clothing), and tin snips. Combination rescue tools are available that can be used for a variety of purposes, such as shutting off gas valves, prying open windows, and cutting through battery cables. Tool belt pouches are available to hold small tools that may be needed during an extrication.

Cribbing and Chocking

Cribbing and chocking are used to raise a vehicle and prevent it from rolling, such as when a patient is caught beneath a vehicle.

- Cribbing consists of 2×4 blocks and wedges and 4×4 blocks and wedges that are used to create crib boxes to hold an air bag. Cribs are usually made of Douglas fir or southern yellow pine, which can hold 500 psi and crush slowly. The cribbing is stacked with a 4-inch overhang (to allow for compression), and it should not exceed 48 inches in height. The crib box is put in place with the air bag on top.
- Chocks are large stepped wedges that are placed in front of or behind wheels to keep them from rolling when the air bag is inflated. As the air bag is slowly inflated, capture cribbing stacks are placed on both sides behind it to hold the vehicle when the air bag is deflated. Once the vehicle is elevated and secured, the air bag is deflated and the crib box is removed to allow room for the extrication of the patient.

Vehicles Powered by Alternative Fuels

Some vehicles are powered by alternative fuels, such as compressed natural gas (CNG) or liquefied natural gas (LNG), so transport personnel should look for CNG/LNG logos, often on the right rear or near the refueling port or the right rear of the cab (semitruck). A "natural gas vehicle" warning may be located near the bottom of the rear doors. CNG tanks may be located behind the cabs in semi-trucks, and some may have additional saddle tanks. The power should be turned off, and the 12-volt battery positive and negative cables should be cut. The emergency shut-off valve should be located and turned off, although each tank can also be turned off manually. Electric vehicles pose the risk of stranded energy. Batteries should always be considered energized with a potential for high-voltage injury. Damaged lithium ion batteries that are leaking or sparking are at risk for thermal runaway (fire). The car battery should be shut down immediately. If the battery is damaged, the vehicle must be relocated at least 50 feet from any combustible material.

Bus Extrication

Before accessing patients involved in a bus crash, the bus must be stabilized, especially if it is on its side or if it is upside down. If the engine is still running, a stop button is often located on the left side of the front panel. Access to the bus may be through the front door if possible. Access may also be through the front windshield (which can be removed through removal of the rubber locking strip that surrounds the window), side windows, the emergency exit door or window, the bathroom window, or an opening cut into the top of the vehicle. Removal of injured patients, usually on stretchers, from inside the vehicle often requires rapid triage and the assistance of multiple EMS and transport personnel. If the vehicle remains upright but patients are completely or partially beneath the vehicle, they should be removed quickly because they may be crushed if the air suspension system deflates.

Aircraft Extrication

Communication is essential if transport personnel are responding to an aircraft crash site because they need to know when the crash occurred, the type and size of the aircraft, the number of passengers and crew, reports of fire or explosion, and whether the aircraft is private, commercial, or military, as well as the status (fire, collapse) of any structure(s) that the aircraft may have impacted. For a small plane with the cabin still reasonably intact, extrication may be similar to a motor vehicle, but severe crashes in which the cabin is destroyed and large airplane crashes pose significantly different problems because passengers may have been thrown about inside or outside of the aircraft and seats and belongings and body parts may block access. Victims may lie in the roadway, so emergency vehicles must proceed with caution. Fire and explosions may be a severe risk, and rescuers may need to wait for fire suppression. Triage may begin outside of the aircraft while the aircraft (or the remains of the aircraft) is secured.

Additional Extrication Considerations

Control Zones

Part of the stabilization of the scene is ensuring that it is secure. An outer perimeter is established to block public and media access, and an inner perimeter is established immediately about the scene of the rescue and the working crew. Three **control zones** are established as follows:

- **Hot (coded red)**: This encompasses the inner perimeter and the crew as well as any area that is dangerous, such as an area contaminated by hazardous material or one in danger of a release of toxins.
- **Warm (coded orange)**: Area for trained personnel in support of those in the hot zone. Decontamination of patients, crew, and equipment is carried out in this zone.
- **Cold (coded yellow)**: This is the staging area and the command post (if necessary, for the emergent situation). No members of the public or media should be allowed in the cold zone.

Zones are usually established by placement of police cars and fire-line tape.

Path of Least Resistance

The path of least resistance is an important concept to understand for rescues, especially if they involve fire and any products of combustion (smoke, heat, gas). Fire's path of least resistance is usually vertical and upward, although fire also spreads horizontally, especially if a vertical path is not available. It's for this reason that if there is a fire on the top floor of a building, the roof is breached to prevent horizontal spread. External factors, such as gusts of wind, can affect the path of least resistance. Water, on the other hand, also flows vertically, but downward and then horizontally if the downward flow is blocked. If the transport nurse is rescuing patients from a building, they will often be found near the path of least resistance, such as near a door or window. Patients should also be transported according to the path of least resistance, that is, the route that is the easiest and safest.

Multistep Rescue Process

The multistep rescue process includes the following 10 steps:

1. **Preparation**: Training, readying equipment, and preparing for different types of rescues
2. **Response**: Using protocols for dispatch; contacting others, such as utility companies, which may have the necessary knowledge or equipment
3. **Situation size-up**: 360° site survey to identify hazards and determine the need for additional personnel or equipment (Determine if the situation is rescuer/equipment intensive.)
4. **Stabilization**: Establishing perimeters and control zones, monitoring hazardous atmosphere, carrying out lockout/tagout of industrial equipment
5. **Access**: Gaining access to the patient and providing emergent care
6. **Disentanglement**: Freeing the patient
7. **Removal**: Continuing critical and life support while assisting the patient to move or carrying the immobilized patient (Rapid extraction if his or her condition is life threatening.)
8. **Transport**: Transporting by various means with decontamination done as needed
9. **Scene security**: Police or others providing protection of the scene, crew, and patients
10. **Post-event analysis**: Reviewing the procedures performed and the problems encountered

Use of Vehicle Parts in a Post-Crash Situation

Following a crash, the seats of the vehicle can be used for many purposes. The seats can provide insulation in shelters, they can offer materials to make sleeping more feasible, they can supply many materials to start fires, and—depending on the color of the seats—they can supply materials to create various signals for search-and-rescue aircraft. The vehicle's tires can be used to create black smoke, which can in turn be used to signal search-and-rescue aircraft. Adding rubber to a fire creates black smoke, which may provide greater contrast and consequently, more chances of creating a successful signal with certain crash site environments. Other parts of the vehicle may be utilized as collection devices for rain water and dew, can function as wind breakers, can be used to support shelters, and can provide shade from the sun.

Role of Clothing in a Survival Situation

Clothing plays an essential role in a survival situation, as it may serve as the only shelter an individual has from the environment. As such, in cold-weather environments, an individual's clothing may be the only barrier he/she has against hypothermia. Warm-weather environments call for clothing that provides adequate sun protection; long-sleeve shirts and pants are ideal for such environments. Head and eye gear should also be worn for protection against warm-weather elements. The most appropriate, effective clothing for transport personnel is clothing that is both comfortable and practical. Clothing that fits tightly should be avoided, as it may affect circulation and restrict movement, which is not ideal in the transport setting. Clothing that offers appropriate ventilation provides the best means of adequately regulating heat as well. Layers are ideal for clothing in the transport setting, as they can be removed or added as needed.

Dangers of Natural Shelters

While natural shelters can provide transport team members with protection from environmental factors, they can also pose dangers. Dead trees and dead tree limbs can pose a threat of injury if they fall during strong winds. Additionally, trees and rocks can have the potential to conduct lightning. In addition to the issue of lightning, transport team members also need to be aware of the potential for dangerous rock slides if they choose to seek shelter around rocks or rock formations. While caves and other areas that offer burrowing potential can provide a great deal of natural shelter from storms, cold climates, and additional environmental factors, they can also be home to potentially dangerous inhabitants such as bears and mountain lions. These dangers do not negate the benefits of natural shelters; they only serve as reminders to transport team members to use extra caution when seeking out such protective spaces.

Using Water During a Survival Situation

Water should be rationed to prolong whatever supply the transport team has in order to help maintain adequate hydration levels. Water should be boiled or purified with a water purification tablet prior to consumption. Failing to purify water can lead to bacterial gastrointestinal issues, which can result in diarrhea and/or vomiting, two causes of rapid dehydration. When a survival situation occurs in a snow-filled environment, it is best to melt the snow, as consuming the snow directly can lead to significant body heat loss. Additionally, water kept in cold weather environments should be kept in open, shallow containers; this can help prevent the liquid from expanding and rupturing the container. If the transport team has instant beverage packets such as hot chocolate and/or instant soup packets on the vehicle, it is ideal to mix the packets with water to gain the benefits of combining a meal with liquid.

Rule of Threes for Outdoor Survival

The rule of threes identifies how long the average person can survive without various life necessities. According to the rule, an average person can survive without oxygen for about three minutes. In extreme weather conditions, an average person can live without shelter from such conditions for three hours. The average person can survive without water for three days; he/she can live without food for three weeks. Once medical issues and safety concerns have been handled, the rule of threes can help a transport team prioritize their duties in a survival situation. The rule establishes that the team should first either seek or build shelter; following the creation of some type of safe shelter, the transport team should build a fire and send out smoke signals for assistance.

Signaling Search-and-Rescue Aircrafts

Smoke, Signal Mirrors, and Flares

When used to signal search-and-rescue aircraft in a post-crash situation, smoke is typically considered the most effective signal method to use during the day. With the addition of certain substances, smoke can be created as either black smoke or white smoke. The choice of which color smoke to use to signal should be determined based on which color provides the greatest contrast with the environment around the crash site. A signal mirror can be used by creating reflections off of shiny metal objects or cans found at the crash site or available on the vehicle. Signal mirrors are most effective on overcast days, which offer the greatest opportunities to cast strong reflections. For nighttime, flares or a flashlight, which can both typically be found on the vehicle, can be used to signal search-and-rescue teams.

Clothing, Whistles, Dyes, and Signal Panels

During the daytime, brightly colored clothing can assist the search-and-rescue aircraft with finding the crash site. Certain materials on the vehicle may be bright enough to help identify the site as well. Whistles can be used when search-and-rescue efforts occur on the ground; they are particularly useful at night or when poor weather conditions exist, as search-and-rescue teams will likely need guidance towards the crash site in such circumstances. If the crash site is located near snow or water, dyes offer a useful material for signaling. Furthermore, signal panels can be laid in a geometric pattern to help clearly mark the crash site.

Using the Battery, Doors, and Vehicle Fuel as a Survival Resource

After a crash, the ambulance's battery can be used to power signal lights, to facilitate communication with search-and-rescue teams by powering communication devices, and to help start fires. The doors of the vehicle can be used in post-crash situations as shelter materials, as devices to help break the wind, and to create geometric patterns to form signal panels to help search-and-rescue aircraft identify the crash site. The vehicle's engine fuel can also be used to start fires, which can in turn be used as smoke to signal search-and-rescue teams.

Transferring a Patient from the Scene to an Ambulance

Different types of **stretchers** and **transfer equipment** may be used for prehospital transfer, including the following:

- **Wheeled**: Stretcher that can be lowered and raised with a wheeled base allowing it to slide into the ambulance.
- **Scoop**: Two- to four-piece stretcher that can be connected and placed under a patient.
- **Transfer sheet**: A heavy plastic sheet can be used with patients up to 800 lb to facilitate transfer.
- **Flexible stretcher**: Lightweight flexible (plastic, rubberized canvas) stretcher with webbing handles on both sides. Can be used to transfer patients around corners and up and down stairs where a wheeled stretcher cannot be used.
- **Stair chair**: Safety chair that can be used to transfer patients in tight spaces and up and down stairs.
- **Folding stretcher**: A stretcher made of lightweight materials that allows folding for compact storage in an ambulance.
- **Basket stretcher** (Stokes basket): Used primarily for rescues in the wilderness or from cliffs.

Patient Positioning

Patient positioning should be according to the possible or probable injury, with safety restraints always securing the patient to the gurney and the gurney to the vehicle.

- **Left-side-lying:** Pregnant patients should be placed in this position to increase circulation to the placenta, and unconscious patients should be placed in this position to prevent aspiration and choking if there is no indication of a spinal injury.
- **Supine** (flat on the back): Patient has a suspected pelvic fracture or neck injury (also requires a cervical collar).
- **Supine** (feet elevated above the heart): This is the position for patients in shock to increase circulation to the heart and brain as the BP falls.
- **Trendelenburg** (the entire stretcher is tilted so that the head is below the feet): Position for patients with a suspected spinal cord injury.

- **Semi-Fowler's** (30-45° position): For patients with chest pain, stroke, and/or shortness of breath and no indication of a spinal cord injury.
- **Fowler's** (upright, 90° position): For patients with severe shortness of breath.

Backboards and Cervical Collars

Backboards were originally designed to transfer patients. However, backboards and cervical collars have been routinely used for emergency rescues for many years without evidence-based studies supporting their use. The premise was that stabilizing the spine and neck would prevent further injury in case a spinal injury had occurred, but spinal injuries are relatively rare, and some studies indicate that these devices do not provide any protection and, in fact, may cause damage. Additionally, cervical collars restrict the airway by 20% or more and may worsen injuries if not properly sized for the patient. Because of these findings, some emergency medical services no longer routinely use backboards but use a vacuum mattress in a scoop basket instead. The American Association of Neurological Surgeons/Congress of Neurological Surgeons (AANS/CNS) 2013 guidelines advise that spinal immobilization using a backboard be reserved for known or suspected spinal cord injury without penetrating injury, although the use of the cervical collar is still recommended until the cervical spine is assessed for injury. Short backboards may be used to support a patient's back in a sitting position.

Emergency Moves

Emergency moves may be needed if the patient and/or transport personnel is in immediate danger from fire, explosives, or other hazards; if the patient requires life-saving treatment, such as cardiopulmonary resuscitation (CPR); or if the patient is in water, such as a pond or lake. Emergency moves include the following:

- **Blanket drag**: Logroll the patient onto a blanket, wrap the patient in the blanket, grasp the blanket near the patient's head while in a squatting position with your back straight, and drag. If there are two rescuers, the other should be positioned at the patient's feet and should be pushing.
- **Clothing drag**: Squat down by the patient's head, securely grasp the clothing near the patient's neck or shoulders (avoid grasping by a T-shirt), and drag the patient.
- **Arm drag**: Squat down by the patient's head. Fold the patient's arms across his or her chest. Grasp the patient under the arms, wrapping your arms about the torso and grasping the patient's wrists to stabilize his or her arms. Drag the patient.

Urgent moves, such as with altered mental status, shock, or breathing difficulties, should also be done as quickly as possible.

Emergency moves can be carried out by one rescuer if no other assistance is available, as follows:

- **Firefighter's drag**: Tie the patient's wrists together with any available material. Straddle the patient and pull the patient's arms over your neck and then crawl forward, dragging him or her beneath you.

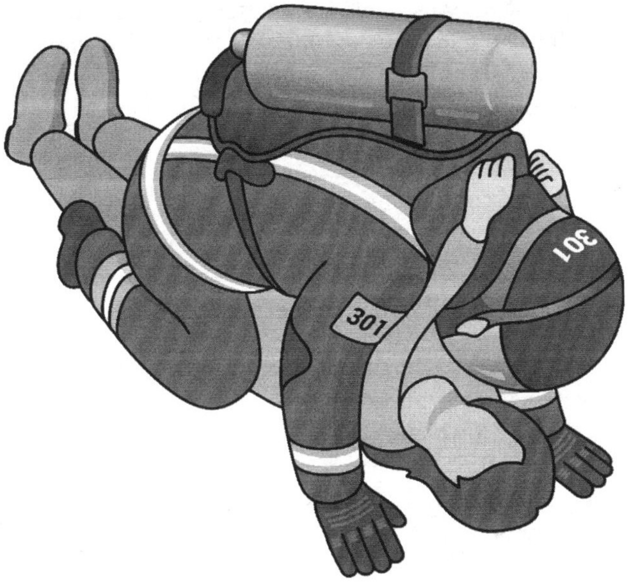

- **Firefighter's carry**: Grasp the patient's knees and pull them together and up. Stand on the patient's feet and reach out and grab one of the patient's arms with one hand. Pull the patient upright, and, as the patient elevates, place your other hand between the patient's legs. Place the patient's arm behind your neck and continue to pull the patient and lift until he or she is draped across your upper back with the arm hanging free. Then grasp the patient's arm that is hanging with the hand that is between the legs to secure the patient.

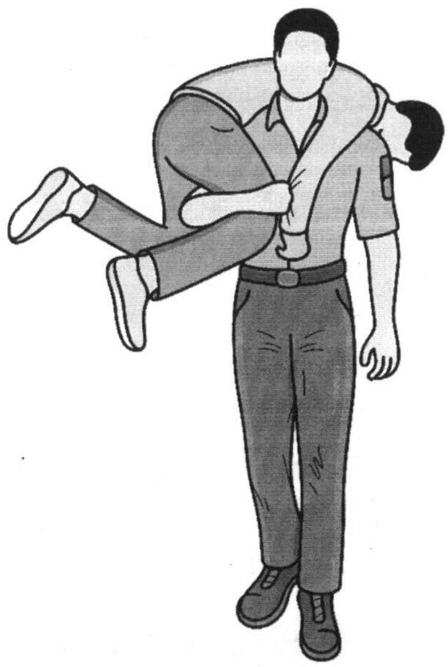

Disaster Management

FEMA IS-700.A NIMS

FEMA IS-700.A outlines the **National Incident Management System (NIMS)**, which, under the direction of the **Federal Emergency Management Agency (FEMA)**, an agency of the U.S. Department of Homeland Security, provides the foundation for collaboration among different governmental and nongovernmental agencies, jurisdictions, and specialties/disciplines in handling large-scale incidents that threaten life, property, and/or the environment. Components of FEMA IS-700.A include the following:

- **Preparedness**: Focuses on planning, procedures and protocols, training and exercises, personnel qualifications/certification, and equipment certification, and it includes the National Response Framework, which establishes protocols and ensures that local jurisdictions retain control while still using a unified approach.
- **Communications and information management**: Systems must be interoperable, reliable, portable, scalable, resilient, and redundant.
- **Resource management**: This includes personnel, equipment, supplies, and facilities, which must be inventoried and categorized using a standardized approach.
- **Command and management**: This includes the Incident Command System (this standardized approach outlines the responsibilities of the incident commander, area command, command staff, and general staff), multiagency coordination systems, and public information.
- **Management and maintenance**: The National Integration Center (NIC) is responsible for NIMS management.
- **Flexibility**: Components are scalable and adaptable to all types of incidents.
- **Standardization**: The NIC develops standards in cooperation with standards development organizations.

ICS-100.B

ICS-100.B, the **Incident Command System** course, meets NIMS requirements for operational personnel and outlines a standardized approach to incident management. ICS is used for any type of major event, planned or otherwise, and large- or small-scale incidents, including natural (disasters), technological (hazmat release), and human-caused (civil disturbance) hazards. ICS outlines the chain of command; the incident commander is in control and orders go through supervisors. Every incident requires an incident action plan, resource management, and processes for reimbursement. The incident commander establishes an incident command post and staging areas (gathering places) as well a base (coordination area for logistic and administrative functions), camps (for sleeping, eating, and sanitary services), helibases, and helispots. Primary features of ICS include common terminology, establishment/transfer of command, chain of command/unity of command, management of objects, incident action planning, modular organization, manageable span of control, comprehensive resource management, incident facilities and locations, integrated communications, information and intelligence management, accountability, and dispatch/deployment.

Chain of Command, Unity of Command and Unified Command

Each organization must establish the **chain of command** for its incident command system. Although these may vary somewhat, an incident commander is ultimately in charge with individuals assigned as incident managers in different areas, such as triage, treatment, transport, security, and liaison.

Unity of command means that each incident commander should have control over personnel assigned to his or her area, and each individual within the chain of command should have a clear understanding of whom to report to at the scene so that communication is efficient and timely.

Unified command means that when multiple agencies are involved from multiple jurisdictions, the chain of command that has been established is recognized and respected even though each agency retains its own authority and accountability and is responsible for carrying out its own duties. A unified command system prevents duplication of effort as well as neglect of important functions.

Incident Action Plan

The purpose of the **incident action plan** is to outline control objectives, resources, and strategies for dealing with an incident. Incident action plans should be updated frequently. Incident action plans may be designed for various types of incidents (terrorist attack, disease outbreak, hurricane) and modified as needed and should include the following:

- Goals and objectives, including expected outcomes
- Strategies and tactics for responding and accomplishing the goals and objectives
- An outline of the chain of command for the incident command system, including the span of control (the number of people reporting to an individual)
- Tasks assigned to each level in the chain of command
- Safety/Health plan for responders to prevent injury/illness and to treat victims as needed
- Communications plan outlining how information will be exchanged, including alternative methods of command if, for example, cell phone towers are out of commission
- Logistics plan regarding the acquisition and use of resources, such as supplies, personnel, and equipment
- Maps and demographic information

Incident Commander

When a multiple-casualty or mass-casualty event occurs, the first lead emergency medical responder on the scene generally assumes the role of incident commander, carries out a rapid assessment of the scene, and calls for additional resources as indicated while another medical responder begins triage. The incident commander should begin to establish a command center in an area that is safe and out of the way of emergency vehicles while awaiting assistance. This first incident commander will relinquish the role when the staffed and/or assigned incident commander arrives to take command and should then report to the person who is assuming the role of staging officer. The incident commander's duties include establishing command, assessing needs, developing a plan, coordinating all activities, delegating responsibilities, ensuring the safety of all personnel and patients, liaising with other agencies, and communicating information.

Triage During Disaster Response

Triage is the process of sorting patients by prioritizing care, treatment, and transportation based on injury severity. One benefit of triage is that it provides prompt medical care to those patients whose lives or limbs are in jeopardy. Triage also directly affects the medical facilities that are available to care for victims of disasters; by sorting patients based on injury severity and identifying those with minor injuries, the burden placed on the receiving hospitals is lessened, as they are not attempting to provide care to patients with only minor injuries. In turn, this benefit affects patients with the most severe injuries by creating more hospital time and personnel to care for those with life-threatening injuries. Triage also helps alleviate some of the burden placed on receiving hospitals when a disaster occurs by distributing casualties among several hospitals rather than burdening only one hospital with all of the victims.

Classification Systems

Victims of disasters are triaged according to their potential for survival absent extraordinary life-saving techniques; they are also triaged according to the severity of their injuries in relation to other victims of the same disaster. Disaster victims are generally classified as: 1) immediate care; 2) delayed care; 3) minor care; or 4) dead. A victim requiring immediate care is a victim whose life can be saved if advanced medical intervention is initiated within one hour. A victim classified as requiring delayed care is one whose condition is not life-threatening and whose condition will not decline if medical attention is not initiated within one hour. Victims requiring minor care are those whose injuries are not severe; they can generally receive care on an outpatient basis in an ambulatory setting, and the care does not need to be provided within a certain amount of time following the occurrence of a disaster.

Advanced Trauma Life Support Protocol

The Advanced Trauma Life Support protocol steps include:

Primary Survey

- Airway with C-spine control
- Breathing (assess oxygenation and ventilation and correct if needed including chest tubes)
- Circulation (assess for and stop bleeding), IVs, response, tissue perfusion
- Disability (GCS, pupils, prevent secondary brain injury)
- Exposure/environmental (assess temp and correct, remove clothing)

Adjuncts (foley, g-tube, hemodynamics/resp monitoring, ABGs, labs, etc.)

Secondary Survey

- History
- Complete Head to toe physical exam

Definitive Treatment

Ongoing Assessment

Simple Triage and Rapid Treatment (START) Plan

According to the Simple Triage and Rapid Treatment (START) approach, if a non-ambulatory disaster victim is not breathing, attempts should be made to restore his/her breathing; if attempts are unsuccessful, the victim should be labeled as deceased. If the victim is breathing, triage personnel should evaluate his/her respiratory rate. If the victim's respiratory rate is greater than 30, he/she should be identified as needing immediate care, as the increased rate may indicate impending shock. If the rate is less than 30, perfusion should be performed, and pulse and circulation should be evaluated during the perfusion process.

According to the Simple Triage and Rapid Treatment (START) approach, perfusion should be performed on a non-ambulatory disaster victim if the victim's respiratory rate is less than 30. Pulse and circulation should be assessed during perfusion. A victim with no pulse should be identified as needing immediate care. If a pulse is detected, consciousness level should be evaluated by asking the victim to follow commands. Victims who are able to follow simple commands should be identified as delayed care victims while those who are not able to follow commands should be identified as immediate care. Circulation is evaluated using a capillary refill test; victims whose refill times are greater than two seconds should be labeled as immediate care, and victims whose refill times are less than two seconds should be evaluated to determine level of consciousness using the simple command test.

Multiple-Casualty Incidents Versus Mass-Casualty Incidents

Multiple-casualty incidents involve more than one person, but different jurisdictions may quantify the total number of persons differently. It usually refers to the following:

- An incident involving at least three patients
- An incident involving only one jurisdiction and only 1–3 agencies (ambulance, fire department, and police)
- An incident requiring triage, but generally only primary triage
- Standards of care are maintained, and all patients not coded black (deceased) are transported for care

Mass-casualty incidents also involve more than one person, but may involve much larger numbers—dozens, hundreds, or thousands.

- Often involves multiple jurisdictions and agencies
- Requires triage but may also involve separate waiting areas for color-coded individuals and secondary triage
- Standards of care may be modified, and patients coded black (expectant) and not expected to live may be left in the field and/or receive delayed care if they are still living after the red- and yellow-coded individuals are transported

Role of the Transportation Officer in a Mass-Casualty Incident

During a mass-casualty event, the transportation officer must maintain constant communication with hospitals and trauma centers, triage officers, police, ground ambulance services, and air medical transport services. The transportation officer controls the flow of patients for treatment and must determine where to route patients in order to prevent a backlog at the receiving facility. They must also coordinate incoming and outgoing ambulances in the transportation staging area. The transportation officer must obtain information about each facility's surge capacity and the number and types of patients the facility is prepared to care for. The transportation officer must also coordinate air medical transport flights and determine, with the triage officer, which patients to transport by air according to their severity of injuries, availability of treatment options, and appropriate levels of care. Speed of transportation and care is often critical in a mass-casualty incident because delays often result in increased death rates.

Role of Triage

In a mass-casualty incident related to terrorism or a disaster, rapid triage and tagging must occur and patients must be sorted according to priority for transportation or field treatment. Because of the large numbers of casualties, triage should begin with the first patient encountered, proceeding from one to another. According to some plans, patients who are alive but expected to die are coded red, but this can result in overtriage, with too many red-coded individuals having to be transported and/or treated, resulting in patients dying during the wait. With other plans, patients expected to die are black-coded as "expectant" and left in the field or left aside until red- and yellow-coded individuals are transported and/or treated. If patients are undertriaged (such as patients who should be coded red being coded yellow instead) this can also result in increased deaths while other patients are waiting for transport or treatment.

Guidance for Increasing Survival Rates in Mass-Casualty Events

Terrorist or other attacks that involve active shooters or improvised explosive devices (IEDs) often result in injuries similar to those encountered in combat situations in which the most common causes of death are extremity hemorrhage, tension pneumothorax, and airway obstruction. The **THREAT acronym** provides guidance for dealing with these situations in the following ways:

- **Threat suppression**: Use of police protection, ballistic vests, concealment, cover, and situational awareness. One concern is that most of the protective gear available to emergency medical personnel is for ballistics rather than explosive devices.
- **Hemorrhage control**: Use of tourniquets (military style) and hemostatic dressings (QuikClot) to control bleeding.
- **Rapid Extrication to safety**: Move patients and personnel out of the danger zone to prevent further injuries.
- **Assessment by medical providers**: Includes provision of a nasopharyngeal airway or upright seating and leaning forward for airway compromise and spinal precautions.
- **Transport to definitive care**: Medical treatment should continue during transport.

Safety Considerations Associated with Active Shooters and Terrorist Bomb Attacks

With **active shooters**, standard protocol has been for emergency response services to wait until the police have removed the threat and secured the area before moving in to care for victims; however, this delay in treatment may result in death, so some authorities are now recommending that emergency response personnel enter the scene with police while wearing appropriate protective equipment, although this does pose some risk, especially with additional shooters or a secondary attack.

With a **terrorist bombing** and improvised explosive devices (IEDs), situational awareness is critical because multiple explosive devices (some undetonated) may be at the scene. IEDs may be inside backpacks, suitcases, and packages left unattended, and in emergency situations innocent people often drop backpacks and packages and run away, making it difficult to tell identify a threat. Additionally, attackers wearing suicide vests or belts may mix in with other victims or people escaping the blast area.

Bomb Threat Standoff Recommendations

Threat	Explosive capacity (lb)	Mandatory evacuation distance (ft)	Preferred evacuation distance (ft)	Shelter-in-place zone (ft)
Pipe bomb	5	70	1200+	71–1199
Suicide bomber	20	110	1700+	111–1699
Suitcase/ Briefcase	50	150	1850+	151–1849
Automobile	500	320	1900+	321–1899
SUV/Van	1000	400	2400+	401–2399
Small truck	4000	640	3800+	641–3799
Container truck	10,000	860	5100+	861–5099
Semitrailer	60,000	1570	9300+	1571–9299

Source: U.S. Department of Homeland Security.

B-NICE Hazardous Material (Hazmat) Incidents Associated with Terrorist Attacks

Category	Response
B—Biological (bacteria, viruses, fungi, toxins)	Inhalation type—evacuate for 80 feet, shut down air-handling systems, wear appropriate PPE and SCBA, and avoid contamination. Visible agent—decontaminate with soap and water. Symptoms may vary but are usually delayed.
N—Nuclear/ Radiological	Inhalation type (most common)—Isolate/Secure the area, avoid smoke/fumes, stay upwind, and use PPE and SCBA. Isolate victims and decontaminate as appropriate. Symptoms are usually delayed.
I—Incendiary	Be on alert for multiple devices and sabotaged fire suppression equipment. Symptoms include burns, pain, and trauma.
C—Chemical	Isolate/Secure the area, decontaminate victims with soap and water, and be on alert for chemical dispersal devices. Approach toward uphill and upwind. Isolate symptomatic patients from others. Symptoms vary but may include burns, blistering, vomiting, breathing difficulty, and neurological damage.
E—Explosives	Be alert for secondary devices, undetonated devices, and secondary hazards (unstable buildings and debris). Remove victims from the area, secure the perimeter, and stage away from the incident area. Decontaminate as necessary. Symptoms include burns, amputations, cuts, and penetrating and blunt trauma.

"All-Hazards" Safety Approach to Mass-Casualty Incidents

The "all-hazards" safety approach to mass-casualty incidents aims to provide plans that can be used to deal with all types of hazards (natural disasters, terrorist attacks, and mass-casualty incidents) as well as encompassing the four components of emergency management: mitigation, preparedness, response, and recovery. Organizations in an area coordinate to develop joint action plans that can be activated in response to incidents, with the chain of command clearly outlined. This approach lowers costs to individual organizations and provides for a faster and more effective response. However, although the basic structure may be the same for responding to all hazards, there are inevitable differences between (for example) a terrorist attack with active shooters and a natural disaster, such as a hurricane, which can be anticipated and mitigated to some degree. For this reason, modifying existing incident action plans to meet the needs of a situation is essential.

Treating Terrorists and Criminals

In mass-casualty incidents, **terrorists and criminals** involved in the incident may be injured and require treatment, and transport personnel may feel conflicted about providing treatment when others have been injured or killed, but it's important to provide treatment to terrorists and criminals the same as any other individuals both because they are in need of help and because their survival may be critical to identifying co-conspirators and to providing reasons for the attack.

However, these individuals may pose risks to emergency medical personnel, so they should be examined while under police guard. The individual's hands should be examined first to check for weapons and detonators and secured (with handcuffs, if possible). Clothes should be examined and removed very carefully in case the person is wearing a suicide device of some type. Emergency medical personnel should also be aware that the individual may be feigning injury or unconsciousness.

Emergency Response Assistance Program Training

The Emergency Response Assistance Program created through the Defense Against Weapons of Mass Destruction Act of 1996 provides training to emergency preparedness personnel from federal, state, and local agencies in how to operate and maintain equipment that serves various purposes. Emergency preparedness personnel learn how to operate equipment that has the capability to detect biological and chemical agents as well as nuclear radiation. Additionally, they are trained to use equipment that can monitor biological and chemical agents and radiation. The program provides emergency response personnel with training on equipment designed to protect the response team members as well as the general public. Furthermore, they receive training on equipment used for decontamination purposes.

Professional Issues

HIPAA

The Health Insurance Portability and Accountability Act (HIPAA) covers three areas related to the protection of patient health information and to the transmission of claims made by healthcare providers. The first area is called the Transaction and Code Set Rule (TCS Rule); this rule set forth national standards by which all electronic healthcare transactions must adhere. To establish consistency, the TCS Rule also developed national identifiers for claims filed by healthcare providers. The TCS Rule does not have much of a direct impact on transport team members, as billing departments are typically responsible for electronic transactions. The second area—the Privacy Rule—established national standards for protecting patient health information and restricting access to protected health information (PHI). The final area is called the Security Rule, which sets forth national guidelines and protocols for healthcare organizations to follow in order to provide appropriate security against unwarranted access to PHI.

Protected Health Information (PHI)

Protected health information (PHI) can be defined as any physical or mental health information that can be used to identify an individual. PHI can include information maintained in any type of record including oral accounts, written documentation, or electronic records. PHI includes information about the past, present, or future physical or mental health of an individual and/or records of care that patient received from a healthcare provider. PHI can also include demographic information about an individual that might render him/her easily identifiable. Finally, records of payment for services from an individual to a healthcare provider can also be considered PHI, as the conclusion can be drawn that the services being paid for provide information about the individual's past, present, or future physical or mental health.

Treatment, Payment, and Operations Exceptions for Exchanging PHI

According to the Treatment, Payment, and Operations (TPO) exceptions, transport team members are able to disclose protected health information (PHI) to other individuals directly involved in the patient's care without first obtaining the patient's consent. Consequently, the transport team may discuss a patient's condition, status, past or present medical conditions, and the like with individuals at the scene, healthcare personnel at the receiving facility, and via radio transmissions without patient consent. The transport team may also exchange PHI for billing and payment purposes without obtaining consent. While the TPO exceptions place less restrictive guidelines on transport team members with regard to the exchange of PHI, the transport team is expected to disclose and receive the least amount of PHI necessary to meet the needs of the situation.

EMTALA

The Emergency Medical Treatment and Active Labor Act (EMTALA) includes the following components:

- Any patient who arrives at an emergency department and requests an examination to determine the presence or absence of an emergency medical condition shall be provided such an examination
- If an emergency medical condition is present, emergency department personnel are required to provide services to stabilize the patient or to arrange for the patient to be transferred to a different facility once he/she is stabilized
- If the patient must be transferred, the transfer facility must have the space and personnel necessary to care for the patient
- In the case of a transfer, the referring facility must provide all necessary documentation to the transfer site
- Qualified personnel, necessary medical equipment, and the most appropriate transport mode must be available in the case of a patient transfer

ACEP Guidelines for Ambulance Diversion

According to the American College of Emergency Physicians (ACEP), Emergency Medical Services (EMS) systems should develop policies that are mutually agreed upon by EMS systems and other agencies regarding diversion. The ACEP believes that such policies should be established to address certain objectives; those objectives include:

- identifying situations where temporary diversion may be required, particularly situations in which hospital resources such as personnel and beds are insufficient;
- designating a primary EMS agency or central communication facility to inform EMS teams and hospitals when a facility is on diversion
- evaluating the facility's diversion status in a regular manner and continuing to provide updates to affected EMS systems and other agencies
- implementing practices that allow for the safe, appropriate, and timely care of patients who enter the system during an active diversion period
- establishing procedures that lower the likelihood of diversions

Informed Consent

Informed consent involves obtaining consent to provide medical treatment to a patient once the patient has been informed of potential risks of the treatment as well as limitations of the treatment. If more than one treatment option is available to a patient, each option and its associated risks and limitations must be outlined for the patient prior to obtaining consent to treat. The fundamental premise of informed consent is that the patient fully comprehends what is being explained to him/her and that he/she subsequently has the competence to either consent to or refuse treatment based on that comprehension. Due to their age, minors are not able to provide informed consent for themselves and, therefore, must have a parent or legal guardian do so. Additionally, the patient must have all his/her faculties intact and be free from any sort of impairment at the time of consent.

Assessing Capacity to Provide Informed Consent

A patient is capable of providing informed consent if his/her faculties are all intact and if the patient is not impaired in any capacity. A patient must be given a chance to provide his/her informed consent for treatment as long as he/she is conscious and coherent to the point of understanding the potential risks and limitations associated with each treatment option as they are presented by the transport team. Examples of patients who may not have all their faculties intact are patients who are mentally ill or intellectually disabled. Examples of patients who would not be able to provide informed consent due to impairment are individuals who are under the influence of alcohol or other drugs and individuals whose senses are weakened due to a medical condition, illness, or other health-related problem.

Abuse and Neglect

Signs of Elder Abuse/Neglect

Common signs of elder abuse and/or neglect can include but are not limited to the following:

- medication overdoses, which can be confirmed through laboratory tests
- medical problems that have not been treated
- bruises and/or cuts that cannot be explained
- indications that the elder patient has been restrained in some way
- inability to easily move extremities due to muscle stiffness
- fractured bones
- indications that the elder patient is not bathed or clean
- bleeding in the vaginal or anal areas that cannot be explained may indicate sexual abuse

Signs of Child Abuse/Neglect

Common signs of child abuse and/or neglect can include but are not limited to the following:

- burns, bruises, or skin lacerations that may resemble the form of an object may indicate abuse
- children who are abused have a tendency to fear all adults, not just the adult(s) who is(are) abusing the child; alternatively, children who are sexually abused may express fear of a particular adult
- children who are abused may express a desire not to return to their homes
- anger, depression, and/or focus difficulties may signify emotional abuse
- an emaciated appearance and/or extreme hunger can indicate neglect
- indications that the child is not bathed or clean
- missing clumps or patches of hair

Signs of Domestic Violence

Common signs of domestic violence can include but are not limited to the following:

- injuries to the patient's head are common in domestic violence cases; such injuries may include broken teeth or fractured jaws, ear drum perforations, and/or broken noses
- bruising throughout the patient's body and/or bruising concentrated in one location on the patient's body
- bite marks determined to be caused by adult teeth

- indications that the patient has been strangled or choked may occur in domestic violence cases; such indications can include ligature marks on the neck, bruising and lacerations or finger marks about the neck, damage to the larynx, and neck vein distention

Documenting Transport Care

Documentation should always include a log of the patient's complaints, the patient's symptoms related to his/her complaints, and the nurse's responses to each complaint. As a means of charting changes in the patient, this component of the documentation process should be recorded at regular intervals throughout transport. Detailed notes should be recorded about the patient's condition prior to receiving treatment as well as response(s) to such treatment. Documentation that outlines the chain of care, including specific names of personnel as well as responsibilities of those individuals, should be provided. Medical histories and medications the patient is currently taking are also valuable pieces of information to document. Suspected drug or alcohol use should be documented; if the patient readily admits to drug or alcohol use, his/her comments should be documented directly and placed in quotes to signify that the comments are the patient's exact words.

Documenting Critical Incidents

For critical incidents that occur either prior to or during transport, any details that are available about the incident should be documented. This should also include information about what was done in response to the incident and who was involved in the response. For critical incidents that occur prior to the patient being transported, documentation should include names of individuals who are able to provide information about the details of the incident, and the information those individuals provide should be documented in quotes to signify that the information is from someone other than the documenter. When critical incidents occur during transport, it is important to document a timeline of events including specific or approximate times. Documentation should also include information about what was done in response to the event and what procedures were followed during the response.

Legal Concepts in Patient Care

Advance Directives

In accordance to Federal and state laws, individuals have the right to self-determination in health care, including the right to make decisions about end of life care through **advance directives** such as living wills and the right to assign a surrogate person to make decisions through a durable power of attorney. Patients should routinely be questioned about an advanced directive as they may present at a healthcare provider without the document. Patients who have indicated that they desire a do-not-resuscitate (DNR) order should not receive resuscitative treatments for terminal illness or conditions in which meaningful recovery cannot occur. Patients and families of those with terminal illnesses should be questioned as to whether the patients are Hospice patients. For those with DNR requests or those withdrawing life support, staff should provide the patient palliative rather than curative measures, such as pain control and/or oxygen, and emotional support to the patient and family. Religious traditions and beliefs about death should be treated with respect.

Important Legal Terms

Important legal terms for the transport nurse to understand include the following:

- **Negligence**: Taking an unreasonable, careless action that could foreseeably cause harm. Failing to exercise due care for others that a prudent, reasonable person would do. Negligence is accidental. Negligence is not an intentional tort, such as trespass or assault. Business errors, miscalculations, and failure to act can be negligent.

- **Contributory negligence**: If a person is injured partially because of his or her own negligence—even if it is slight—then the person who caused the accident does not pay any damages (money) to the injured person. Forty-four states recognize that applying the rule of contributory negligence could lead to unfair acquittal of genuinely negligent defendants, so they now use a comparative negligence test as a more balanced approach. In the 6 states that still have contributory negligence rules, juries tend to ignore it as unfair.
- **Comparative negligence**: A rule used in accident cases to calculate the percentage of responsibility of each person (joint tortfeasors) directly involved in the accident. Damages (money compensation) are awarded based on a complex formula.
- **Assault and battery**: Assault is declaring or threatening an intent to touch a patient inappropriately or to cause physical harm. Battery is the actual act of inappropriate touching.

Ethical Issues

Ethical Principles

Autonomy is the ethical principle that the individual has the right to make decisions about his or her own care. In the case of children or patients with dementia who cannot make autonomous decisions, parents or family members may serve as the legal decision maker. The nurse must keep the patient and/or family fully informed so that they can exercise their autonomy in informed decision-making.

Justice is the ethical principle that relates to the distribution of the limited resources of healthcare benefits to the members of society. These resources must be distributed fairly. This issue may arise if there is only one bed left and two sick patients. Justice comes into play in deciding which patient should stay and which should be transported or otherwise cared for. The decision should be made according to what is best or most just for the patients and not colored by personal bias.

Beneficence is an ethical principle that involves performing actions that are for the purpose of benefitting another person. In the care of a patient, any procedure or treatment should be done with the ultimate goal of benefitting the patient, and any actions that are not beneficial should be reconsidered. As conditions change, procedures need to be continually reevaluated to determine if they are still of benefit.

Nonmaleficence is an ethical principle that means healthcare workers should provide care in a manner that does not cause direct intentional harm to the patient:

- The actual act must be good or morally neutral.
- The intent must be only for a good effect.
- A bad effect cannot serve as the means to get to a good effect.
- A good effect must have more benefit than a bad effect has harm.

Nursing Code of Ethics

There is more interest in the **ethics** involved in healthcare due to technological advances that have made the prolongation of life, organ transplants, prenatal manipulation, and saving of premature infants possible, sometimes with poor outcomes. Couple these with healthcare's limited resources, and **ethical dilemmas** abound. Ethics is the study of **morality** as the value that controls actions. The American Nurses Association Code of Ethics contains nine statements defining **principles** the nurse can use when faced with moral and ethical problems. Nurses must be knowledgeable about the many ethical issues in healthcare and about the field of ethics in general. The nurse must help a patient to reveal their values and morals to the health care team so that the patient, family, and team can resolve moral issues pertaining to the patient's care. As part of the healthcare team, the nurse has a right to express personal values and moral concerns about medical issues.

Culture and Diversity

With respect to patient diversity, the Diversity Practice Model can help transport team members recognize what similarities and differences exist between them and their patients.

- A: Assumption – Transport team members should examine their assumptions about the individual and/or the community of which the individual is a member;
- B: Beliefs or behaviors – Transport team members should identify how their beliefs affect the type of care they provide and how they behave towards their patients;
- C: Communication – the transport team should assess the patient's communication in terms of capability, language, and other senses such as sight and sound;
- D: Diversity – Visible factors, such as skin color and age, should be identified as possible areas of diversity, and factors that cannot be seen, such as socioeconomic status, should also be identified; and
- E: Education and Ethics – Transport team members should learn what makes patients diverse and recognize that diversity affects ethical decisions.

Psychosocial Issues

Conflict Resolution

It is important for all parties involved in conflict resolution to recognize that conflict is natural and normal and that it does not have to be destructive as long as the conflict is handled in an appropriate manner. Additionally, it is essential that all involved parties acknowledge that not everyone shares the same opinions and views about events and issues. For conflict resolution efforts to be successful, everyone involved must be willing to communicate effectively and to listen effectively; listening is just as important as, if not more important than, verbal communication during attempts to resolve conflicts. In order to ensure effective communication and to prevent misunderstandings, it is beneficial to summarize the other party's points and/or to clarify anything that is not clear. All parties involved should work together to come up with a solution to the conflict that is fair and beneficial to each of them.

Facilitating Communication with Patient's Family Prior to Transport

As time permits and within the limitations of patient confidentiality, the transport team should communicate with the patient's family about what will be done to the patient during transport. In addition to discussing patient care with the family prior to transport, the family should be made aware of the logistics surrounding the transport. They should be informed of approximately how long the ride will last, and, if possible, they should be provided with driving directions to the facility where the patient is being transported. It is helpful to explain to the family where they should go upon arriving at the facility as well as how they should locate the transport team and/or the patient once they arrive. Depending on time, family concerns about the patient and his/her condition and/or about the transport procedures should be addressed before the transport team departs with the patient.

Addressing Family Anger, Hostility, and/or Distrust

When a patient's family responds to a crisis with anger, hostility, and/or distrust, the transport team should provide the family with opportunities to voice their feelings. The root cause(s) behind the feelings must be identified in order to develop appropriate responses. It is important to let the family know that their feelings are normal and acceptable. Particularly in cases where a family expresses a lack of trust in the situation, it is important to implement a schedule of updates for the patient's family. Organized, regular updates about the patient may demonstrate the level of professionalism with which the team is handling the situation; ideally, family updates should be provided by the same individual(s) each time, as this can increase the family's level of trust and comfort. Team members can also talk with families about ways to turn their anger into positive energy that may benefit the patient and/or the situation.

Supporting Family Following a Patient Death

Many people cope with death best by having the ability to see their loved one, which is why it may be beneficial for family members to view the patient's body at the scene. Following the death of a transport patient, many family members have a lot of questions; it is important that the transport team or additional healthcare professionals take the time to address all questions posed by the family. While some families have a lot of questions at the time of death, many do not think of their questions until after they have processed the death. Consequently, it is essential that the family understands how and why the patient's death occurred and that the patient received the highest level of clinical care possible. In every situation, compassion and professionalism should be exercised when responding to family members.

Systems Management

Quality Management

Continuous Quality Improvement and Quality Assurance

Continuous quality improvement (CQI) environments are very patient-centered, which is consistent with the direction health care in general has gone. Patients tend to be more involved in many aspects of their health care than they once were many years ago, and CQI programs support the role of the patient and the patient's family. Conversely, quality assurance (QA) programs operate based on a need to meet requirements that are externally mandated by organizations, laws/regulations, and/or agencies. Consequently, while QA activities are performed solely to serve the purpose of fulfilling a particular requirement, CQI environments are not hindered by such requirements, which allows them to focus solely on the needs of patients.

Quality assurance (QA) methodology has traditionally involved the use of evidence that cannot necessarily be supported and data from studies that have been conducted after the fact with little or no structure to them. Conversely, continuous quality improvement (CQI) programs rely on hard, verifiable data rather than opinions or feelings. Unlike QA environments, CQI environments employ a standardized formula for solving problems rather than solving problems and making decisions using a method that does not lead to predictable results.

Clinical and Laboratory Continuing Education

Clinical and laboratory continuing education must include training in critical care issues as they relate to adult, pediatric, and neonatal patients. The education should also provide information that covers emergency care for the trauma patient as well as labor and delivery protocols. Lab tests required for invasive procedures should be readdressed, and information about the pre-hospital experience should be covered. Additionally, the transport team should participate in regular recertification programs from the American Heart Association on the topics of Basic Life Support (BLS), Advanced Cardiac Life Support (ACLS), Pediatric Advanced Life Support (PALS), and Neonatal Resuscitation Program (NRP). Certification in Advanced Trauma Life Support (ATLS) should also be documented. Nursing certifications must be up-to-date if a particular transport team member position description requires the training.

Healthy Work Environment

Cumulative Stress and Traumatic Stress

Cumulative stress, also known as burnout, occurs when an individual lets distress, or bad stress, build up over time. Cumulative stress may be caused by a series of events or occurrences rather than one stressful event. It can cause physical as well as psychological changes in an individual. Oftentimes, cumulative stress results in a feeling of being overwhelmed with one's life. This overwhelmed, out-of-control feeling can lead to other physical symptoms such as anxiety, nervousness, and an inability to concentrate. Severe cases of cumulative stress that are left untreated can lead to depression, substance abuse, and/or loss of interest in life. Conversely, traumatic stress is stress that occurs as a reaction to a specific traumatic event or occurrence such as the unexpected death of a patient during transport. Physical and psychological reactions to traumatic stress do not typically linger in the individual after the event has ended.

Principles of Crisis Intervention Following a Traumatic Event

Crisis intervention approaches are often used to help deal with acute stress that is brought on by a traumatic incident. The four principles that guide this approach are immediacy, proximity, expectancy, and brevity. Immediacy refers to the idea that crisis intervention support services should be provided to transport team members who are experiencing acute stress as soon as possible after the occurrence of the traumatic incident. The principle of proximity suggests that services should be offered as close as possible to the location where the incident occurred. Expectancy is a principle characterized by the need to reassure the transport team member or members dealing with acute stress that they will be able to return to their work activities as soon as the stress is controlled. The principle of brevity suggests that support services should only be offered for the amount of time necessary to get the stressful reaction under control.

Critical Incident Stress Management

Many Critical Incident Stress Management (CISM) programs begin with an education component prior to field deployment. This education involves informing transport team members about stress-inducing factors common in their line of work. The education additionally provides team members with tools to help strengthen their psychological resiliency so that they can most effectively handle stressful incidents in the field. CISM programs also generally incorporate crisis intervention components that are provided at the time of a disaster. These interventions typically involve psychological decompression sessions available immediately following the critical incident; crisis management briefings presented to large groups of people as an opportunity to disseminate consistent information about the event, answer questions, and offer tools to help team members cope with the event; and follow-up interventions such as peer counseling and group discussions provided several hours or even a couple weeks after a critical event.

Fair Work Environment

A fair work environment is one in which ethics and fair treatment are priorities. The fair work environment begins with publishing, disseminating, and posting a code of ethics by which all members of the organization are expected to comply. Managers at all levels must be trained in ethics and should demonstrate unbiased and fair treatment of employees. Management should have an open-door policy or other means for those at all levels to express their concerns or suggestions to better improve the organization. Performance reviews should have the input of those being reviewed and should be equitable, based on objective standards of performance. Criteria for performance, benefits, promotion, salary increases, and disciplinary actions should be clearly stated. Employees should be paid for overtime, allowed breaks, and encouraged to maintain a balance between life and work. Bullying and harassment or anything that results in a hostile environment must not be tolerated, and safety standards must be maintained.

Prevention of Response-Related Injuries

Prevention of response-related injuries includes the following:

- **Infectious diseases**: Use PPE and understand the spread of infectious diseases—air (coughing), direct contact (blood, vomitus, other body fluids), needlestick, contaminated food/equipment, and sexual transmission. Maintain current immunizations.
- **Personal habits**: Obtain adequate sleep, nutrition, and exercise. Avoid excessive alcohol and tobacco.
- **Environmental hazards**: Conduct a 360° assessment. Note traffic hazards, the vehicle's condition, fire, leaking fluids, downed power lines, hazardous materials (look for placards and warning symbols; avoid the area until it is cleared). Use PPE and respirators as indicated.
- **Violence**: Defuse situations, make a safe response (with the assistance of law enforcement), and use restraints if necessary, for dangerous or violent individuals.
- **Collisions**: Drive safely; avoid speeding and driving through stop signs and red lights when possible. Wear seat belts and/or safety harnesses.

Principles of Body Mechanics

Basic principles of body mechanics include the following:

- Avoid reaching overhead or for prolonged periods of time or more than 20 inches away.
- Avoid pulling—push, roll, or slide instead.
- Avoid lifting—push, roll, or slide instead.
- Lift with leg muscles, not with the back.
- Hold weight close to the body rather than at arm's length.
- Flex at the hips and knees, not the waist.
- Carry patients head first upstairs and feet first downstairs.
- Maintain a straight back and avoid twisting.
- Assess weight and recognize limitations in lifting/carrying.
- Get help when necessary, and communicate every step with your partner ("Lift on the count of three").
- Maintain a firm base of support with feet apart (shoulder width) to stabilize your stance.
- Maintain the line of gravity (the imaginary line between your center of gravity and the ground) within the base of support.
- Position yourself close to an object that is to be lifted or carried.
- Lift patients from stable ground.

Moving and Lifting Patients

Techniques for moving patients include the following:

- **Direct ground lift**: Use only for lightweight individuals with no suspected spinal injuries. Three provider line up on one side of the patient, and each kneels on the same knee. The provider at the head places one arm under the patient's neck and shoulder and the other arm under the patient's lower back. The middle provider places his or her arms above and below the patient's waist, and the provider at the patient's feet places his or her arms under the knees and lower legs. On the count of three, they roll the patient onto their knees and toward their chests. On the count of three, they stand and move the patient.
- **Power lift**: Place feet shoulder width apart and pointing slightly outward; tighten the back and abdominal muscles. Squat down as though sitting. Place hands 10 inches apart with the palms upward (power grip) while grasping the stretcher and lift with the upper body becoming vertical before the hips rise.
- **Extremity lift**: Requires two providers. One provider squats at the patient's head and another is at one side by the patient's knees. The provider at the head folds the patient's arms across the chest and grasps the patient by wrapping both arms around the torso under the patient's arms and grasping the patient's wrists. The second provider slides his or her hands beneath the patient's knees and lower legs, and together they stand and lift the patient.
- **Squat lift**: Requires two providers. One provider squats with the back straight and the weak foot slightly forward at the head of patient, and the other provider is in the same position at the patient's feet. Grasp the patient's upper body as for the extremity lift and grasp the patient's feet. Both providers push up with the stronger foot and lift with the upper body becoming vertical before the hips rise.
- **Logroll**: Used to position carrying devices under the patient and for some transfers; it requires two providers positioned on the same side of the patient. Place the patient's arm on the side that he or she is being turned to above his or her head or over the chest. Place the patient's other arm across his or her chest. If on the ground, squat close to the patient. The provider at the patient's head reaches across the patient and grasps his or her shoulders and trunk while the second provider grasps his or her trunk and legs. On the count of three, they turn the patient in one smooth move.

- **Draw-sheet transfer**: Requires four providers with two positioned on one side of the patient and two positioned on the other side but on the opposite side of the bed or stretcher to which the patient will be transferred. The logroll technique is used to place a draw sheet under the patient. Providers on both sides roll the edges of the draw sheet until the edges are close to the patient. On the count of three, they lift the patient slightly and move the patient across to the bed.

Outreach and Community Education

Educating the Public

The transport team can educate the public about transport programs in a number of ways. They can offer presentations to civic groups throughout their community; these presentations can provide an overview about the types of trauma, critical care, and specialty transport services the program has available. Furthermore, they can sponsor health-related programs and offer them to the public on topics such as injury prevention. The team can also educate the public about their program by delivering educational presentations and demonstrations to schools, which serves the dual purposes of promoting health education to students in their local communities as well as marketing the transport program. The media, including newspapers, radio, television, and internet, and printed materials such as flyers and brochures are also effective avenues for getting information to the public about transport programs.

Educating Schools

Transport team members participate in educational opportunities at schools by offering presentations that may include lectures, videos, and transport team personnel demonstrations. Presentations of this sort can offer information such as ways to prevent trauma injuries, what to do when a trauma injury occurs, guidelines for maintaining safety around firearms, how to recognize signs of drug abuse, and tips to prevent drinking and driving. In any presentation delivered in a public education setting, the information presented should be relevant to the age(s) of the audience members, and it should be constructed in a manner that the information can be easily understood by the audience. One powerful way to deliver public education messages is to incorporate information, either directly or indirectly, from patients who have previously utilized transport services.

Resuscitation Principles

Principles of Assessment

Primary Assessment

After surveying the environment for safety issues, the transport nurse should quickly conduct a primary assessment to identify conditions that are life-threatening, as follows:

- **Level of consciousness**: Alert, responsive to verbal stimuli, responsive to painful stimuli, nonresponsive
- **Breathing status**: Normal, abnormal, rate abnormalities (>24 or <8), apnea, choking, normal or abnormal chest movement, chest rise and fall, noisy respirations, use of accessory muscles, tripod position, nasal flaring
- **Circulatory status**: Radial, carotid pulse, pulse abnormalities, major bleeding, skin color (pink, blue [cyanotic], pale), skin temperature, skin moisture, capillary refill, signs of shock

Life-threatening conditions must be treated immediately, as follows:

- **Carotid pulse present with no radial pulse**: Lay the patient flat and elevate his or her feet 8-12 inches.
- **No pulse**: Begin CPR.
- **Shock**: Lay the patient flat, elevate his or her feet 8-12 inches, and administer oxygen at 15 L/min.
- **Bleeding**: Apply pressure to control any bleeding.
- **Abnormal breathing**: Provide oxygen with a nonrebreather mask. If the patient is unresponsive, cyanotic, or in respiratory distress, use a BVM with supplemental oxygen.
- **Unresponsive**: Ensure a patent airway.

Based on the primary assessment, the patient is then classified as stable, potentially unstable, or unstable.

Primary Breathing Assessment

During the primary breathing assessment, the rate and depth of the patient's respirations should be noted. Determining whether the patient's skin appears cyanotic (manifested as a bluish discoloration) is another assessment component. Identifying tracheal positioning should also be part of the assessment. The transport team should note whether the patient's breathing is labored and/or whether any injury exists that may impact breathing capacity. Using muscles other than the diaphragm or the intercostal muscles for breathing should be noted, as that can signal respiratory distress. Flaring of the nostrils can be another indication of respiratory distress, and should be noted if present. The primary breathing assessment should further include an evaluation of whether breath sounds occur bilaterally, whether chest movements are symmetric, and whether abnormal sounds such as crackles or rales are present. Finally, the assessment should incorporate palpation of crepitus, which are crackling or popping sounds that occur under the patient's skin or joints.

Secondary Assessment

The secondary assessment is a head to toe evaluation of a patient. Inspection, palpation, and auscultation provide information about the patient during the evaluation. First, the secondary assessment should include an evaluation of the overall appearance of the patient; this appearance evaluation should include an assessment of the patient in relation to his/her environment. The transport team should observe whether the patient is cognizant of his/her surroundings and how he/she interacts with them. In addition to assessing the patient's general appearance and understanding of his/her environment, the transport team should evaluate the patient's skin; head and neck; eyes, ears, and nose; mouth and throat; thorax, lungs, and cardiovascular functioning; abdomen; genitourinary system; and arms, legs, and back. Skin color and temperature, sensory functioning, cavity drainage, lacerations, injuries, breath and heart sounds, pelvic tenderness, bleeding, and pulses are examples of things the transport team should examine during the secondary assessment.

REASSESSMENT

Reassessment involves ongoing monitoring of the patient at regular intervals to determine changes in his or her condition or trends such as decreasing blood pressure or increasing agitation. Reassessment is done after a secondary assessment. Unstable patients should be reassessed at least every 5 minutes and stable patients every 15 minutes. Reassessment should include reviewing the primary assessment, taking vital signs, repeating the physical examination (including evaluation of mental status), and monitoring the chief complaint and response to interventions. Reassessment findings should be compared to baseline findings. The patient's airway, ventilation, and circulation should be reassessed as well as the patient's degree of pain—stable, better, or worse. Each intervention should be reassessed for effectiveness and the need for modifications of treatment or if new interventions should be determined. If the patient is receiving oxygen, the tank and all of the equipment should be checked to ensure that they are functioning properly.

HISTORY TAKING ON ARRIVAL AT A SCENE

History taking should include the following:

- **Chief complaint**: If the patient is unable to explain, information may be gathered from his or her family, friends, or others who are present. Look for a medical alert bracelet or other such jewelry.
- **Nature of the illness or mechanism of injury**: Reason for calling emergency services, cause of injury, type of illness. Look for environmental clues (fire, drug paraphernalia, motor vehicle accident).
- **Signs and symptoms observed or reported by the patient**: Skin temperature, open wounds, blood pressure abnormalities, pain, or difficulty breathing.
- **Precipitating events**: Falls, accidents, violence, eating, exercising, walking, driving.
- **Pediatric considerations**: Check capillary refill to assess blood flow in infants and children younger than 6. Assess the pulse at the brachial artery (inside of the upper arm) for infants up to 1 year of age and the carotid artery in the neck for children older than 1 year. May need to use distraction to gain trust and alleviate fear. Encourage the parents/caregivers to hold the child if possible and assist in calming the child.
- **Geriatric considerations**: Determine if the patient needs assistive devices, such as hearing aids, eyeglasses, cane, walker, or dentures.

OPQRST METHOD OF HISTORY TAKING

O	Onset	The time that the symptoms associated with this event started.
P	Provocative; palliative. Positioning	That which makes it better; that which makes it worse. The position that the patient is in on arrival and the need to remain in this position or to move him or her.
Q	Quality of discomfort	Burning, stabbing, nagging, crushing, sharp, or dull.
R	Radiation of pain	Area to which the pain moves from the original site.
S	Severity of pain	Based on a 1-to-10 or other appropriate scale.
T	Time	Historical onset, such as earlier, similar events.

SAMPLE METHOD OF HISTORY TAKING

S	Signs and symptoms	Pain, bleeding, shortness of breath, injuries, fever, rash.
A	Allergies	Medications, environmental (foods, insects, plants, animals).
M	Medications	Prescribed, over-the-counter (OTC) vitamins/minerals, birth control and erectile dysfunction medications, herbal preparations, recreational drugs, other people's medications.
P	Past pertinent history	Especially related to the current event.
L	Last oral intake	Foods, fluids, other substances.
E	Events (precipitating)	Occurrence just prior to event.

Taking a History of Sensitive Topics

When asking a patient about sensitive topics, the transport nurse should try to provide as much privacy as possible in an emergent situation in order to maintain confidentiality and protect the patient from reprisals. The transport nurse should ask questions directly in a straightforward and nonjudgmental manner, stressing the need for information in order to help the patient, especially if the patient is reluctant to answer. Sensitive topics include the following:

- **Sexual history**: People who engage in unusual or unhealthy sexual practices, such as sadomasochism, autoerotic asphyxiation, swinging, and prostitution, are often reluctant to admit to those practices. Adolescents may be especially reluctant to admit they are pregnant or have engaged in sexual activity or have had an abortion. Males (especially those older than age 40) should be asked about the use of erectile dysfunction drugs (such as Viagra) because they are a contraindication to some medical treatments.
- **Physical/Sexual abuse and/or violence**: Victims often lie about abuse to defend the abuser or out of shame or fear of further violence.
- **Alcohol/Drug use and abuse**: Patients often underreport the extent of their drinking or drug taking or deny it altogether. Patients may be concerned about legal actions, such as if they have been driving drunk and gotten into an accident.

Special History-Taking Challenges

Special history-taking challenges include the following:

- **Silent patient**: Be patient, sensitive, and alert for nonverbal clues.
- **Talkative patient**: Allow the patient to speak freely for a few minutes and then periodically summarize.
- **Anxious patient**: Be patient, provide reassurance, and explain all procedures.
- **Patient with multiple complaints**: Ask the patient to help prioritize his or her issues.
- **Hostile/angry patient**: Remain calm; respond as appropriate.
- **Intoxicated patient**: Avoid cornering, belittling, or challenging the patient or asking the patient to lower his or her voice or stop swearing. Remain calm and treat the patient with respect.
- **Depressed, crying patient**: Question the severity of the patient's depression; listen and remain supportive and nonjudgmental.
- **Patient with a language barrier**: Use a translator if possible. Use hand gestures. Show the equipment before using it; point to the part of the body where the equipment will be used.
- **Patient with a visual impairment**: Announce one's presence and explain all procedures verbally. Tell the patient before touching him or her.
- **Patient with a hearing impairment**: Determine if the patient has a hearing aid, and obtain it if possible. Speak slowly and clearly, facing the patient for any hearing deficit. If the patient has no hearing, use writing, hand gestures, and demonstrations to communicate.

Labs and Point-of-Care Testing

Blood Glucose Monitoring

Blood glucose monitoring is done with a glucometer. Testing is indicated with a decreased level of consciousness or confusion in a diabetic patient or a decreased level of consciousness with the cause being unknown. The glucometer must be calibrated and tested regularly. Test results from capillary blood tend to be lower than test results on venous blood. The testing procedure is as follows:

- Wipe the site with an alcohol swab. The alcohol must be thoroughly dried before puncture, or it may interfere with the test results.
- Prick the side of the finger pad with a lancet or lancing device rather than the fingertip because the fingertip is more sensitive.

- Express a drop of blood onto the test strip.
- Insert the test strip into the glucometer according to the manufacturer's recommendations.
- Read the test results.
- Dispose of the lancet in a sharps container.

Warming the hand or lowering it may help to ensure adequate blood for the test. Hypoglycemia (low blood sugar/insulin reaction) is a reading of ≤70 mg/dL. Hyperglycemia (high blood sugar) is a reading of ≥160 mg/dL.

Complete Blood Count (CBC)

Total erythrocytes (RBCs) normal values are as follows:

- Males >18 years: 4.5–5.5 million per mm^3
- Females >18 years: 4–5 million per mm^3

Hemoglobin: Carries oxygen; it is decreased in anemia and increased in polycythemia. Normal values:

- Males >18 years: 14–18 g/dL
- Females >18 years: 12–16 g/dL

Hematocrit: Indicates the proportion of RBCs in a liter of blood (usually about 3× the hemoglobin number). Normal values:

- Males >18 years: 45-52%
- Females >18 years: 36-48%

Reticulocyte count (immature RBCs): Measures marrow production and should rise with anemia. Normal values:

- 0.5-1.5% of total RBCs

Leukocytes (WBCs) normal values:

- Normal WBC for adults: 4800–10,000
- Acute infection: 10,000+
- Severe infection: 30,000+
- Viral infection: ≤4000

The differential provides the percentage of each different type of leukocyte. An increase in the WBC count is usually related to an increase in one type and often an increase in immature neutrophils, known as bands, referred to as a "shift to the left," an indication of an infectious process.

i-STAT CHEM 8+

There are many point-of-care testing devices available; the one most commonly used for comprehensive blood analysis is the **i-STAT CHEM 8+,** which includes the following tests plus hemoglobin and hematocrit:

Blood urea nitrogen (BUN)

- Normal values: 7–20 mg/dL
- Measures kidney function
- Increases with kidney disease

Carbon dioxide (CO_2)

- Normal values: 20–29 mmol/L
- Measures acid/base balance
- Measures bicarbonate

Anion gap

- Normal values: 8–16 mEq/L
- Measures sodium (chloride + bicarbonate)
- Helps identify metabolic acidosis

Creatinine

- Normal values: 0.8–1.4 mg/dL
- Measures kidney function
- Increases with kidney disease

Glucose

- Normal values: 70–128 mg/dL
- Measures blood sugar level
- Increase can indicate diabetic ketoacidosis; decrease can indicate an insulin reaction

Serum chloride

- Normal values: 101–111 mmol/L
- Measures electrolyte level
- Increase can indicate metabolic acidosis and respiratory alkalosis; decrease can indicate respiratory acidosis and metabolic alkalosis

Serum sodium

- Normal values: 136–144 mEq/L
- Measures electrolyte level
- Increase can indicate excess sweating, diarrhea, burns, or the use of diuretics; decrease can indicate dehydration, vomiting, and diarrhea

Calcium (ionized)

- Normal values: 4.4–5.4 mg/dL (1.1–1.35 mmol/L)
- Critical values:
    - <2 mg/dL (<0.5 mmol/L) may result in tetany
    - >7 mg/dL (>1.75 mmol/L) may result in coma
- Measures electrolyte level

Review Video: Lab Values
Visit mometrix.com/academy and enter code: 120244

Cardiac Biomarkers

When the heart is damaged, it releases **cardiac biomarkers**, substances that aid in diagnosis. Biomarkers include the following:

- **Creatine kinase (CK) and isoenzyme (MB),** also known as CK-MB, is specific to the heart muscle, and the level increases within 4–8 hours after a heart attack; it peaks at about 24 hours after the heart attach (earlier with thrombolytic therapy), and it remains elevated for 72 hours.
- **Myoglobin (heme protein that transports oxygen)** is found in skeletal and cardiac muscles. The level increases 1–3 hours after a heart attack and peaks within 12 hours. Although an increase is not specific to a heart attack, a failure to increase can be used to rule out an MI.
- **Troponin I** is found only in the heart muscle. Levels increase 3–6 hours after a heart attack, peak in 14–20 hours, and return to normal within 5–7 days.
- **Troponin T** is found in heart and skeletal muscle. Levels increase 3–6 hours after a heart attack, peak in 12–24 hours, and return to normal in 10–15 days.
- **Brain natriuretic peptide (BNP)** is secreted by the ventricular muscle with increased volume and pressure. An increased level indicates heart failure.

Bilirubin, Blood, Glucose, or Protein in Urine

Bilirubin is typically excreted into bile by the liver; consequently, liver disease can be indicated when bilirubin is present in a patient's urine. Bilirubin in urine may also indicate that a patient's gall bladder is not functioning properly. Blood in a patient's urine can be particularly serious, as it can indicate a number of possible medical complications. When a patient's urinalysis reveals blood, the blood can be an indicator of an infection or kidney stones, and it can also be an indicator of trauma or bleeding from organs such as the bladder. The presence of glucose in a patient's urine may indicate diabetes; however, it is important to note that a small number of patients do show glucose upon urinalysis without actually having diabetes. A urinalysis that indicates the presence of protein may be a sign of kidney damage or an infection.

Evaluating Consciousness

The AVPU assessment is a quick assessment done to determine the patient's level of consciousness. This may be one of the first assessments done when initially attending a patient.

AVPU (Alert, Voice, Pain, Unresponsive)			
A	Alert and awake, aware of person, place, time, and condition. Follows commands. Pediatric: active and responds to external stimuli and caregiver.	Yes	No
V	Responds to verbal stimuli, but eyes do not open spontaneously. Pediatric: Responds only when caregiver calls name.	Yes	No
P	Responds to painful stimuli, such as pinching the skin/earlobe, but not verbal. Pediatric: Responds only to painful stimuli, such as pinching nailbed.	Yes	No
U	Unresponsive, does to respond to painful or verbal stimuli. Pediatric: Unresponsive.	Yes	No

Imaging Studies

Chest X-Ray

After ensuring that the film being viewed belongs to the patient in question, a systematic approach should be used to interpret a chest x-ray. Soft tissues should be assessed for the presence of foreign bodies and/or air, and bones should be examined for fractures. The width of the mediastinum, a group of chest structures between the lungs, should be evaluated, and masses on the structures should be documented. The shape and width of the patient's heart should be assessed from the chest x-ray, and any masses visible on the trachea or hilum should be identified as well. The size of the pulmonary arteries should be evaluated, and enlargement should be documented. Assessment of a chest x-ray should also include an examination for conditions such as pleural effusion and thickening or calcification of the pleura. Lung tissue should be examined as well to determine the presence of any abnormal shadowing.

Spinal X-Ray

On a normal spinal x-ray, the vertebrae do not have any abnormalities in terms of size, shape, or appearance. Additionally, a normal spinal x-ray contains no indications of fractures or dislocations. Upon assessment of the soft tissues surrounding the vertebrae, no foreign objects or air are detected in a normal spinal x-ray. Finally, the curvature of the spine appears to be typical. In contrast, abnormal results of a spinal x-ray may reveal the presence of fractures or dislocations as well as the presence of foreign bodies or air in the soft tissues. Conditions that cause abnormal curvature of the spine, such as scoliosis, can generally be seen on a spinal x-ray. Decreased bone density may be detected as well, indicating the presence of a condition such as arthritis or osteoporosis. When a spinal x-ray reveals narrow space between vertebrae, disc disease may be indicated.

Common Types of Spinal X-Rays

Four common types of spinal x-rays provide various pictures of the 33 vertebrae that comprise a patient's spinal column. Cervical spine x-rays provide images of the seven cervical bones, which are located in a patient's neck. The lumbosacral spine x-ray offers a picture of the five bones in a patient's lower back, known as the lumbar vertebrae, as well as the five bones that are fused together at the sacrum, the triangular bone at the base of the spine. While the view of the five bones fused at the sacrum is limited on a lumbosacral spine x-ray, the sacrum/coccyx spine x-ray provides a more detailed view of those five bones. Additionally, the sacrum/coccyx spine x-ray produces an image of the four fused bones of the coccyx, or tailbone. A thoracic spine x-ray produces pictures of the 12 bones of the chest, the thoracic bones.

Pain and Comfort Assessment

PQRST Method of Pain Assessment

The PQRST method is used to obtain a patient's pain history.

- The P represents "provoking factors."
- The Q represents the pain "quality."
- The R represents "region and radiation" of the pain.
- The S represents the pain "severity."
- The T represents "time" in relation to the pain.

Transport team members should assess provoking factors in terms of the pain. The patient should identify whether specific movements or activities make the pain less or more severe. Asking the patient to describe the qualities and characteristics of the pain may provide information about where the pain originates. The patient should be asked to identify the area(s) on his/her body where the pain radiates. Using a scale of 1 to 10, with 10 being most severe, the patient should be asked to categorize his/her level of pain. Finally, the patient should identify what time the pain began and how long the pain has existed.

Managing Pain During Transport

Several techniques can be employed to help patients manage pain during transport. One effective pain management tool is distraction; providing the patient with an opportunity to think of something other than the pain can help alleviate it to an extent. With pediatric patients, security objects such as blankets and stuffed animals can often distract them and take their thoughts off the pain. Simply engaging the patient in everyday conversation can also provide a distraction for him/her, which might help the patient manage the pain. Maintaining the patient in a comfortable position as well as regulating his/her body temperature to a comfortable level are often effective pain management strategies. When clinical processes need to be performed during transport, the patient's pain can often be managed by having such processes explained to him/her. If appropriate and feasible, having a family member accompany the patient can also help the patient deal with his/her pain.

Preparing the Patient for Transport

Indications for Transport

While no universally-accepted guidelines govern indications for patient transport, general indications do exist. The decision about whether a patient should be transported from one facility to another or from a field site to a healthcare facility generally depends on the extent of the patient's injuries or illness. Time and distance also play roles in making the determination whether to transport a patient. Oftentimes, the terrain and the weather dictate whether transport services can be provided to a patient. If the patient is already at a healthcare facility, the decision to move him/her to a different facility is typically based on whether the patient can receive necessary procedures and expert care at the referring facility. Additionally, sometimes patient transport can be indicated if the patient's family requests such a transfer.

ACS Indications for Transporting Patients with Chest Injuries

According to the American College of Surgeons (ACS), patients with chest injuries may be acceptable transport candidates depending on the severity of the injury or injuries they have sustained. Patients who have a widened mediastinum may require transport; the mediastinum is a group of chest structures between the lungs that are enveloped by loose connective tissue. Transport is also indicated when a patient presents with a pulmonary contusion—a bruised lung—as the injury can potentially become quite serious and, in some patients, can lead to death. Additionally, the ACS recommends transport for patients whose chest injuries necessitate ventilation management for a prolonged period of time.

Stabilizing Patients Prior to Transport

According to the Consolidated Omnibus Budget Reconciliation Act (COBRA), the benefits of transferring a patient who is not stabilized need to outweigh the potential risks he/she may incur from a transfer; this must be certified in writing by the transferring physician. Second, prior to transfer, the transferring hospital should treat the patient to the best of its ability in order to decrease potential risks to the patient during transfer. Third, the receiving facility must agree to have the patient transferred to their facility; in agreeing to do so, the receiving facility is acknowledging that it has space and personnel to care for the patient. Fourth, the transferring facility must provide the receiving hospital with all available medical records associated with the patient being transferred. Finally, qualified personnel and transport equipment must be available to facilitate the patient transfer.

Patient Assessment and Management During Transport

While a patient's injuries generally dictate his/her assessment and management, certain principles can be applied to all situations. During transport, transport team members should always maintain a position that allows for efficient management of the patient's airway, breathing, and circulation. Airway equipment and all lines—intravenous (IV), central, and intraosseous—should be easy to access and in proper working order. Tubes and drainage systems should also be in proper working order; additionally, they should be secured in a manner that helps prevent displacement. If any uncertainty exists about whether a cervical spine injury is present, the cervical spine should be immobilized. Combative patients should be restrained appropriately. Medical monitors on the vehicle should be located in positions where the transport team members can easily view them. Finally, wounds and injured limbs should be left exposed during transport in order for the team to continually evaluate such injuries.

Prehospital Index for Trauma Patients

The Prehospital Index (PHI) is a measurement tool used to help triage patients in the field who have experienced some level of trauma. The PHI looks at the patient's systolic blood pressure, pulse and respiratory rates, level of consciousness, and chest and/or abdominal wounds to help determine the level of care the patient requires. For each of the aforementioned parameters of the PHI, a point score is assigned. The PHI is the total of the combined point scores for systolic blood pressure, pulse rate, respirations, consciousness, and penetrating wounds; the PHI can range from zero points to 24 points. If a patient's PHI is three points or less, it indicates minor trauma; major trauma is indicated by a PHI greater than three points.

Lowering Patient's Risk for Heat Loss Prior to Transport

Prior to transport, several measures should be initiated to reduce a patient's risk of heat loss, which can quickly lead to the development of hypothermia. First, the patient should be covered with a blanket to provide insulation. If examinations need to be performed in the field prior to transport, the amount of skin exposure a patient is subjected to needs to be limited. During transport, it is important that the transport team keeps the patient away from metal, as metal has the ability to draw heat away from the patient's body. Finally, oxygen and fluids administered intravenously may be given to the patient to help reduce heat loss.

Airway

Airway Assessment

When assessing a patient's airway, a determination should be made as to whether the airway is patent (characterized by the patient being awake and alert and having the ability to speak), able to be maintained, or not able to be maintained. The patient's level of consciousness should also be evaluated when assessing his/her airway, as the consciousness level can provide an indication of how effectively the airway is functioning. The appearance of the patient's skin should be determined during the airway assessment as well; the presence of ashen, gray or bluish, pale, or blotchy skin should be noted. During the airway assessment, a determination should be made as to the most effective way to position the patient in order to maintain his/her airway. Additionally, sounds of obstruction in the airway should be identified and noted.

Airway Management

Oropharyngeal Airway (OPA)

The oropharyngeal airway (OPA), a blind-insertion airway device, may be inserted to provide better ventilation, but the OPA requires the head tilt/chin lift or modified jaw thrust as well because the device alone does not ensure a patent airway. The OPA is indicated for unconscious patients, patients with no gag reflex, and patients who are apneic (not breathing) and require ventilatory aid. The OPA is often inserted if a patient stops breathing, such as with a cardiac arrest. The OPA is contraindicated in conscious patients and those with a gag reflex. To insert the OPA, perform the following steps:

1. Estimate the length of the OPA by measuring the patient from the angle of the jaw or the tip of the earlobe to the corner of the mouth.
2. Select the correct size.
3. Open the patient's mouth using the cross-finger technique. Suction any secretions.
4. Tilt the head back (if possible). Insert the device with the tip of the OPA pointing upward for adults and downward for children.
5. Rotate the OPA into position for adults.
6. Ensure that the phalanges of the mouthpiece are securely against the patient's mouth.
7. Check to make sure the OPA is patent (open).

Oropharyngeal Airway

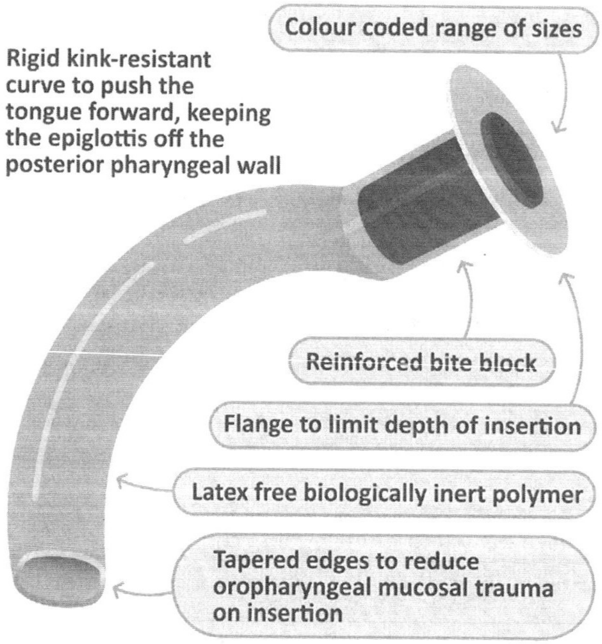

Nasopharyngeal Airway (NPA)

The nasopharyngeal airway (NPA), a blind-insertion airway device, is indicated for unconscious or semiconscious patients who still have a gag reflex or those who cannot tolerate an oropharyngeal airway (OPA), but it should be avoided with severe head injury, risk of basal skull fracture, nasal bleeding, and history of deviated septum or nasal fracture. It's important to use the appropriate size. To insert the NPA, perform the following steps:

1. Choose a size that is slightly smaller in diameter than the patient's nostril.
2. Measure from the tip of the earlobe to the tip of the nose.
3. Lubricate the NPA with water-soluble lubricant and insert it in the larger and most patent (open) nostril. If inserting into the right nostril, insert with the bevel (tip) angled toward the nasal septum (the bony cartilage division between the nostrils). If inserting it into the left nostril, invert the NPA to angle the bevel toward the septum.
4. When the NPA reaches the throat, rotate it 180° into the proper position.

Nasopharyngeal Airway Placement

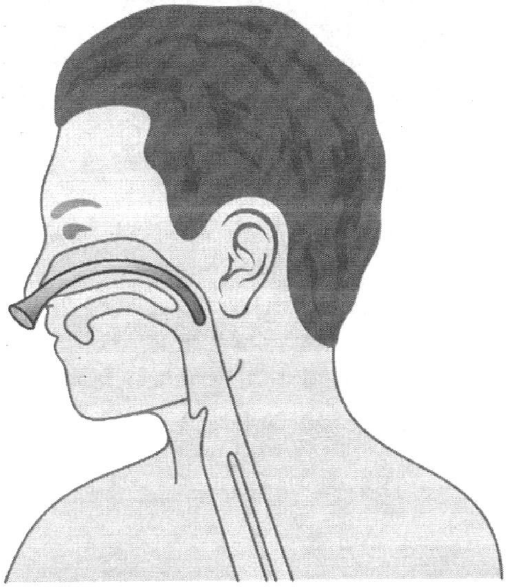

Laryngeal-Mask Airway (LMA)

The laryngeal-mask airway (LMA), a blind-insertion airway device, is an intermediate airway allowing ventilation but not complete respiratory control. The LMA consists of an inflatable cuff (mask) with a connecting tube. It may be used when tracheal intubation can't be done or as a conduit for later blind insertion of an endotracheal tube. The head and neck must be in a neutral position for insertion. If the patient has a gag reflex, then conscious sedation or topical anesthesia (deep oropharyngeal) is required. The LMA is inserted by sliding the airway along the hard palate, using the finger as a guide, into the pharynx, and the ring is inflated to create a seal around the opening to the larynx, allowing ventilation with mild positive pressure. The LMA ProSeal has a modified cuff that extends onto the back of the mask to improve the seal. The CobraPLA (perilaryngeal airway) has a larger pharyngeal cuff and provides a better seal. The LMA is contraindicated in morbid obesity, with obstructions or abnormalities of the oropharynx, and in non-fasting patients because some aspiration is still possible.

Laryngeal Mask Airway

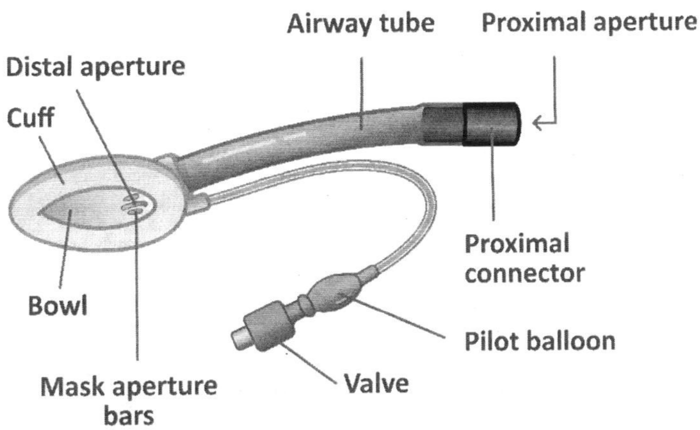

Advantages of an LMA

One of the greatest advantages of using a laryngeal mask airway (LMA) as an airway management tool in a transport setting is that it does not require a great deal of skill or training to effectively use the device.

Additionally, LMAs do not require that the patient's head and neck be moved around much, and they can be inserted with the transport team member positioned either in front of or behind the patient. These advantages make LMAs a particularly good choice in transport settings where the patient may be entrapped and/or difficult to reach, such as motor vehicle accidents. Unlike many other airway management tools, LMAs are available in sizes appropriate for pediatric patients, which is another advantage they offer. Furthermore, LMAs may not irritate patients' throats as much as other methods of intubation can, which is a particularly attractive benefit to patients.

CONTRAINDICATIONS FOR LMA

In order to use a laryngeal mask airway (LMA), the patient must be either unconscious or heavily sedated; consequently, patients who are alert and/or aware are not good candidates for LMAs. Additionally, an LMA does not offer any protection against aspiration of stomach contents; therefore, using an LMA is not advisable with patients who may have full stomachs, as the contents could be sucked into the lungs and cause further medical complications. It is also not advisable to utilize an LMA with patients who exhibit signs of poor pulmonary compliance, with patients who present with problems with their larynx, or with patients who have any kind of abnormalities related to their pharynx.

BAG-VALVE MASK (BVM)

Bag-valve mask (BVM) ventilation equipment used for positive-pressure ventilation (PPV) includes a mask, a ventilator bag, an oxygen reservoir bag, and an attachment for oxygen delivery. The correct mask size is important: The mask should not cover the chin. BVM is contraindicated if the airway is not patent, but it is used for abnormal breathing and for respiratory distress/failure. BVM requires two transport team personnel—one to control the mask and the other to control the bag. Steps are as follows:

1. Position oneself behind the patient's head, place the mask over the patient's nose and mouth, and make a tight seal by holding it in place with the thumbs and index fingers while the other fingers slide under the patient's jaw to lift the chin.
2. Squeeze the bag with inhalations initially for 5 to 10 breaths and then adjust the rate to at least 12 breaths per minute, slowly adjusting the rate and tidal volume delivered.

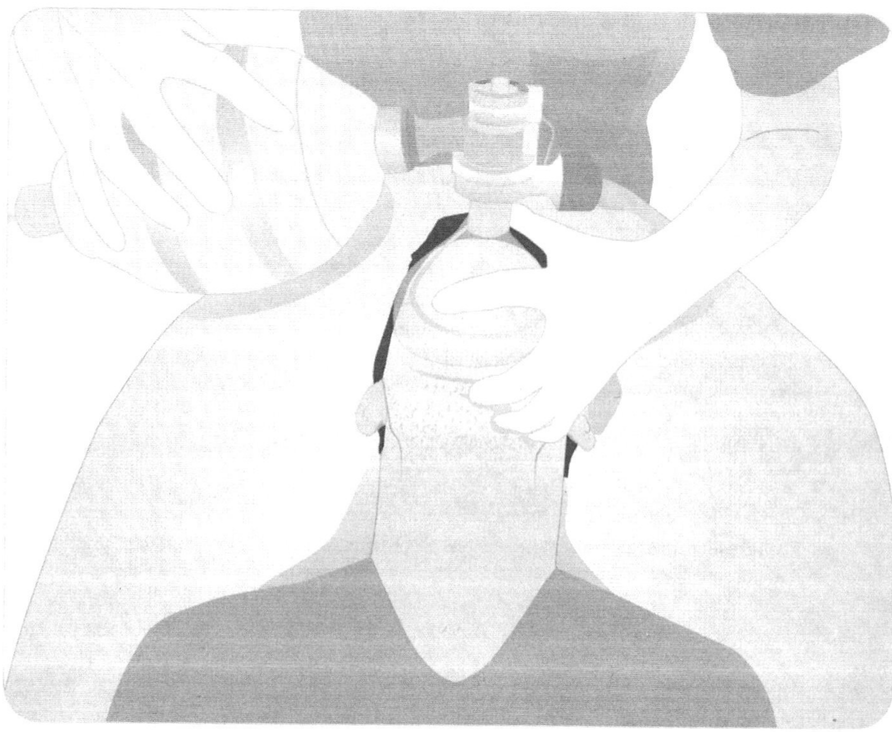

Assessment of lung compliance (the ability to expand and contract) includes observation of chest movement, rate of respirations, and the feel of BVM. Difficult ventilation suggests impaired compliance. Note: The BVM can be used with or without oxygen.

POCKET-MASK VENTILATION

Pocket-mask ventilation is used when administering cardiopulmonary resuscitation (CPR) to a patient who is in cardiac arrest and apneic (not breathing). If two transport personnel are available, one should be positioned at the patient's head to administer pocket-mask ventilation while the other does compressions. If there is only one transport personnel, then that person should be positioned at the patient's side. Administration is as follows:

1. Remove the mask from the container and push the flattened mask to open it.
2. Wipe the patient's face clean with alcohol swab if necessary to remove secretions, vomitus.
3. Do a chin tilt or jaw thrust and place the mask over the patient's nose and mouth, holding it in place with both hands to seal it tightly.
4. Take a deep breath and blow in through the one-way valve, watching the chest rise to ensure that ventilation has occurred.
5. Continue to ventilate the patient at a rate of 30 compressions to 2 ventilations for CPR.
6. Attach supplemental oxygen if available to improve oxygenation.
7. Upon patient recovery or completion of CPR, remove the mask, discard the valve, and disinfect the mask.

Pocket Mask

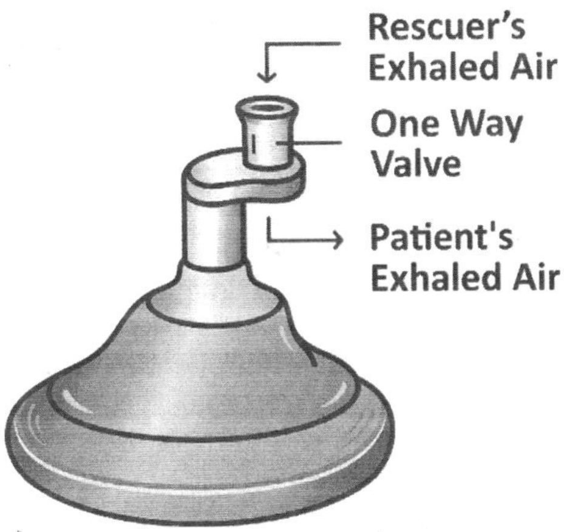

ENDOTRACHEAL INTUBATION AS AIRWAY MANAGEMENT

Apnea, brief pauses in a patient's breathing pattern, and/or respiratory insufficiency, whereby oxygen supply and carbon dioxide removal are inadequate, can be indications for securing an airway via endotracheal intubation. If a patient's upper airway is obstructed, endotracheal intubation is likely necessary as well. Patients with an altered level of consciousness are often intubated with an endotracheal tube in an attempt to protect their airway from potential damage or injury; additionally, patients with other conditions that could potentially compromise their airways are likely to have an endotracheal tube placed as well. Endotracheal intubation is also indicated in patients experiencing increased intracranial pressure, those with hemodynamic instability, and patients presenting with signs of shock.

ORAL INTUBATION

The first step in oral intubation is to position the patient. Those not categorized as trauma patients should have their neck flexed forward with their head extended backward while trauma patients should be in a position of in-line traction. After preoxygenating the patient, the transport team member performing the intubation should open the patient's mouth with one hand while holding a laryngoscope in the other. The laryngoscope blade should be inserted in the right side of the patient's mouth, his/her tongue should be moved to the left, and the blade should be moved toward landmarks. Cricoid pressure should be applied once the epiglottis and vocal cords are displayed. Using the largest tube possible, the tube should pass from the right corner of the patient's mouth through his/her vocal cords. Once the stylet has been removed, the tube cuff can be inflated. After confirming proper positioning, the tube should be secured.

Nasal Intubation

The first steps in nasal intubation are to evaluate nasal patency and anesthetize the patient's nasal passages. Trauma patients should be maintained in a position of in-line traction while those not categorized as trauma patients can either sit upright or lie down with their neck flexed slightly forward and their head extended slightly backward. Oxygen should be supplied to the patient, and the intubation tube should be lubricated. As the transport team member performing the intubation advances the tube into the nasal septum, he/she should listen to the patient's breath sounds coming through the other end of the tube. On inspiration, the tube should be passed quickly into the patient's trachea. Another transport team member assisting with the procedure should apply cricoid pressure to align the glottic opening. After confirming proper positioning, the tube should be secured.

Complications Associated with Nasal Endotracheal Tubes

Paranasal sinusitis, a condition characterized by one or more of the paranasal sinuses becoming infected, can result if the nasal endotracheal tube impedes normal drainage. Sepsis is another illness that can occur while a nasal endotracheal tube is in place. Sepsis is characterized by a bacterial infection in the bloodstream and often occurs in patients with already compromised immune systems or existing medical conditions. The infection can quickly turn fatal without proper treatment. Bacteremia is a condition characterized by bacteria in the bloodstream. Unlike sepsis, bacteremia is generally not serious and often does not require treatment. Another complication that can occur when a nasal endotracheal tube is in place is turbinate damage; turbinates are bony structures on each side of the nose that augment its ability to filter air. Nasal necrosis, death of tissue in the nasal passages, can also occur while a nasal endotracheal tube is in place.

Advantages of Nasal Intubation vs. Oral Intubation

While oral intubation is the most common method of managing a patient's airway, nasal intubation is a fairly simple, well-tolerated procedure that offers advantages over oral intubation. Nasal tubes are easier to secure than oral tubes; consequently, the chance of dislodging an oral tube is greater than the chance of dislodging a nasal one. For patients with an injured neck or jaw, a nasal tube is easier to insert than an oral one. Additionally, nasal intubation is more comfortable for patients who are awake during the procedure; it is also more comfortable when a patient awakens with a nasal tube in place as opposed to an oral tube. Patients with nasal tubes are not able to bite the tube, which can cause added medical complications. Furthermore, nasal intubation allows simultaneous surgery within the oral cavity, if necessary; such surgery is more complicated to perform around an oral tube.

Confirming Tube Placement

Direct observation of the ETT passing through the vocal cords on video laryngoscope is the best confirmation of correct placement. However, there are other techniques that can be assessed together to reliably confirm tube placement. Upon auscultation over the patient's axilla—the armpit—and chest, hearing bilateral breath sounds is suggestive that an oral tube is in the correct location. Additionally, upon auscultation over the patient's epigastrium, which is located along his/her abdominal wall above the belly button, the absence of any gurgling sounds indicates that the oral tube was placed properly. Symmetric movements of the patient's chest wall will also verify placement. In pediatric patients, an appropriate pulse rate, which can be tracked on a cardiac monitor, can imply proper oral tube positioning; improved coloring in pediatric patients is another effective indicator of proper placement. Upon auscultation over the patient's chest, bilateral breath sounds will confirm proper tube placement from a nasal intubation. Symmetric movements of the patient's chest wall will also verify appropriate placement. Accurate nasal tube placement can also be verified by ensuring that the patient cannot speak. All these used in conjunction with general patient assessment and hemodynamic monitoring can help to confirm placement when video laryngoscopy isn't possible.

Rapid Sequence Intubation (RSI)

Rapid sequence intubation (RSI) is performed on patients who need a secure airway in a rapid manner; it involves simultaneous anesthesia and intubation. RSI is indicated in patients with head injuries, as effective airway management is crucial in such situations. Patients who overdose on drugs often require RSI to prevent their airways from becoming compromised as a result of the overdose. Patients presenting with status epilepticus—a condition characterized by the occurrence of a prolonged seizure or two or more seizures that occur in close succession to one another—generally require RSI, as the condition can lead to brain damage or death quite quickly; consequently, it is essential that patients with status epilepticus have a secure airway to maximize their chances for survival. Other indications for RSI include patients who are agitated or combative and those who cannot open their mouths completely, which is a condition referred to as trismus. Two intravenous lines should be in place before RSI and the patient preoxygenated for 3 minutes or more. Sellick's maneuver (pressure applied externally with thumb and index finger to the cricoid) is used to close off the esophagus and prevent aspiration. An induction agent is followed by a muscle relaxant. Sixty seconds after the muscle relaxant, an endotracheal tube is inserted with a laryngoscopy, cuff inflated, secured, and placement verified by capnometer.

Procedure

Once the need for rapid sequence intubation (RSI) has been established, a brief neurological assessment should be performed on the patient. Upon completion of the neurological exam, the patient should be preoxygenated for 2–4 minutes with 100 percent oxygen. During the preoxygenation process, positive pressure ventilation should be avoided. After administering oxygen to the patient, premedications and induction agents should be administered. Cricoid pressure should be applied once the patient loses consciousness, which is indicated by the lack of a lash reflex. A neuromuscular blocking agent should be administered next, and then the patient should be intubated when apnea is detected. At this point, the cuff should be inflated and the patient should receive 100 percent oxygen. After confirming proper placement of the endotracheal tube, cricoid pressure should be released, and the tube should be secured.

Neuromuscular Blocking Agents

The following agents can be used as neuromuscular blocking agents during intubation:

- **Cisatracurium**: Dose is 0.05–0.2 mg/kg
- **Pancuronium**: Dose is 0.07–0.1 mg/kg
- **Rocuronium**: Dose is 0.3–1.2 mg/kg
- **Vecuronium**: Dose is 0.05–0.1 mg/kg

While the onset time for rocuronium is 1–2 minutes, the other three most common neuromuscular blocking agents each have an onset time of 3–5 minutes. With a duration of 60–90 minutes, pancuronium is considered a prolonged blockade. In contrast, the other three agents each last a considerably shorter period of 20–35 minutes.

Induction Agents

Etomidate and Ketamine

Etomidate (pregnancy Category C) is commonly used for induction for rapid sequence intubation (RSI) but has no analgesic properties. Dosage is 0.3 mg/kg IV over 30-60 seconds. Onset of action is 15–45 seconds and duration is 3–12 minutes. Etomidate has few cardiovascular effects, so it is often preferred for cardiac or hypotensive patients. Adverse effects include transient apnea, depression of cortisol level for up to 8 hours, and local pain at injection site. Etomidate is contraindicated for patients <10 and nursing mothers. Geriatric patients may require lower dosages.

Ketamine (pregnancy Category B) may be used for induction for RSI for patients who are hypotensive or having bronchospasms and for babies 3-12 months, children, pregnant women, and adults. Dosage is 1–2 mg/kg IV to a maximum single dose of 500 mg for adults. Onset of action is less than 30 seconds, and duration is only 5–15 minutes although full recovery may take hours. Emergence reactions can include hallucinations, delirium, and disturbing dreams. Contraindications include significant hypertension and drug sensitivity.

Midazolam and Propofol

Midazolam (pregnancy Category D) is a benzodiazepine for rapid sequence intubation (RSI). Dosage is 0.1–0.3 mg/kg per IV push over 2 minutes. Onset of action is 30–60 seconds, and duration is 15–30 minutes. Midazolam does not have analgesic properties but does have anticonvulsive properties, so it is indicated for status epilepticus. Adverse effects include hypotension, so midazolam is usually contraindicated in the presence of shock or hypovolemia. Other adverse effects include respiratory and cardiac arrest.

Propofol (pregnancy Category B) is the most commonly used anesthetic agent for children and adults and can be used as an induction agent for RSI. Propofol reduces airway resistance and is appropriate for patients with bronchospasm. It also has neuro-inhibitory effects, so it can reduce ICP in patients with intracranial pathology. Dosage is 1.5–3.0 mg/kg IV with onset of action within 15–45 seconds and duration 5–10 minutes. Adverse effects include cardiac and respiratory depression and hypotension. Contraindicated in patients with allergies to eggs or soybeans.

Use of Video Laryngoscope During Intubation

The video laryngoscope is a battery-powered laryngoscope with a light source and built in camera, usually near the distal end of the blade to facilitate intubation. It is especially helpful with a difficult airway, allowing indirect viewing of the larynx. Various blades are available, including hyper-angulated, channeled (to guide the endotracheal tube), and the standard Macintosh blade. The blade is inserted into the mouth as with a standard laryngoscope and settled into the vallecula. The epiglottis and vocal cords are viewed through the monitor, which is mounted on the handle. However, the field of vision is closer with the camera than the eye, so the transport nurse should never depend just on the monitor when inserting the ETT. An alternative method of doing a video laryngoscope is to thread an ETT over a fiberoptic scope for intranasal insertion. Once the scope is in the trachea, the ETT is advanced and the scope withdrawn.

Surgical Airways

Indications for Surgical Airway

The establishment of a surgical airway may be indicated in a patient whose airway is inaccessible by alternate means. Patients who suffer trauma around their airway may be difficult to intubate using orotracheal or nasotracheal methods, as trauma can cause anatomy deformities and/or extensive bleeding that can inhibit visualization of the airway. Establishing a surgical airway may also be necessary in patients whose upper airways are entirely obstructed. Foreign objects, mass lesions, and edema—swelling of an organ or tissue as a result of lymph fluid build-up—can all lead to upper airway obstruction. Situations where the establishment of a surgical airway may be counter-indicated include those involving patients younger than 10 years old, those involving patients where the transport team is not able to identify landmarks for puncture purposes, and those involving patients who have either a puncture site infection or a primary injury to their larynx.

Needle Cricothyrotomy

A needle cricothyrotomy is typically performed as a last resort when all other attempts to secure an airway have failed. It is often done as an emergency procedure to manage an airway obstruction until a tracheostomy can be performed. Skin should be prepped with an antiseptic solution and if the situation doesn't permit it, local anesthetic like 1% lidocaine can be given with a 27 g needle. During procedure monitor vitals and respirations. Universal precautions and sterile technique should be used. The patient's head should be placed in a stable, neutral position. With the thumb and middle finger of non-dominant hand, hold tension of skin and trachea in place while using the index finger to feel the thyroid membrane. Using a 10 cc syringe that is half filled with saline and attached to an over the needle IV catheter held in dominant hand, insert the needle midline in the neck at the lowest margin of the thyroid membrane and angle it toward the feet at about a 45 degree angle. While puncturing the skin and underlying tissue, pull back on the syringe while advancing the catheter and needle until air bubbles can be seen. Advance catheter off the needle and rest its hub on the skin (this part of the skill is similar to IV catheter advancement after getting flashback). To confirm placement you can reattach the syringe to the catheter and aspirate, expecting air return. Have the catheter held firmly in place while high pressure oxygen tubing is connected and the catheter is secured in place with sutures.

Rapid Four-Step Cricothyrotomy Technique

The Rapid Four-Step Cricothyrotomy Technique involves palpation, incision, traction, and intubation. First, the patient's cricoid membrane is palpated while his/her trachea is palpated and stabilized. Next, a horizontal incision is made in the patient's cricothyroid membrane using a scalpel held at a 60-degree angle; the incision should be approximately two and a half centimeters (cm) in length. The scalpel should be left in place once the incision has been made. Third, a tracheal hook is placed against the blade of the scalpel and guided down the trachea. In an inferior direction, the tracheal hook's tip should be rotated 90 degrees, and traction should be applied to the cricoid cartilage. At this point, the examiner places his/her hand on the patient's sternum to maintain tracheal traction while the scalpel is removed. Finally, the examiner intubates the patient, and the tracheal hook is removed once correct placement of the tube is confirmed.

Complications of Tracheostomies

Respiratory distress is a common complication of a tracheostomy. Mucus plugs or other forms of tracheostomy (trach) tube obstruction are often the cause of respiratory distress; such obstructions can generally be eliminated through suctioning the trach tube. Given that a tracheostomy opening is made by a surgical incision, the chance of developing an infection around the incision site exists. Pneumothorax, a condition which occurs when air or gas collects outside the patient's lungs, can also be a postoperative complication of a tracheostomy. Signs of the condition may include shortness of breath, cyanosis, and an increased heart rate. Pneumomediastinum, a condition that occurs when air collects in the mediastinum, a group of chest structures between the lungs, is another potential tracheostomy complication. Although rare, bleeding can occur as a complication during the actual procedure.

Suctioning a Tracheostomy

With clean and/or gloved hands, the individual performing the tracheostomy suctioning should pick up the catheter at the end closest to the suction machine; the end that will be placed in the trach tube should not be handled. The catheter should then be attached to the tube on the suction machine, and the machine should be started. Identify how far the catheter should be inserted into the tracheostomy (trach) tube; it should generally be inserted to a point equivalent to the length of the tube plus an additional quarter inch. After identifying the stopping point, the catheter should be advanced into the trach tube. At this point, suction is applied when the individual performing the suctioning places his/her thumb over the catheter's hole while removing it from the trach tube. As the catheter is pulled out, the individual performing the suctioning should roll the tube between his/her thumb and forefinger.

Mechanical Ventilation

Advantages of Mechanical Ventilation

One of the main advantages of using a mechanical ventilator is the consistency it offers across the various aspects required for sufficient ventilation. Mechanical ventilators provide consistent volumes of gas inhaled and exhaled during each cycle of respiration, known as tidal volumes. Furthermore, ventilation rates—or breathing rates—can be maintained in a consistent manner using a mechanical ventilator. Another aspect in which mechanical ventilators offer consistency is the concentration of oxygen they deliver to the patient. Additionally, unlike manual ventilation, which requires healthcare professionals to use their hands during the process of ventilating a patient, mechanical ventilators allow them to utilize their hands for other clinical tasks.

Capnography and End-Tidal CO_2 ($ETCO_2$)

Capnography provides a visual display of end-tidal carbon dioxide ($ETCO_2$/$PETCO_2$) levels in inhalation and exhalation. **Capnography** is recommended to establish the correct placement of an endotracheal tube, to assess the effectiveness of CPR, to evaluate respiratory distress (asthma, COPD, overdose), and to assess the patient's response to treatment. Normal **$ETCO_2$** is 35–45 mmHg. Hypercarbia (a measurement of >45 mmHg) occurs with hypoventilation (overdose, sedation, post-seizure, head trauma, stroke), and hypocarbia (a measurement of <35 mmHg) with hyperventilation (anxiety, bronchospasm, pulmonary edema, decreased cardiac output). $ETCO_2$ levels are less accurate with sidestream measurement used for the nasal cannula and face mask than with the mainstream sensor used with an endotracheal tube, so it's important to keep the sensor close to the mouth and secured.

The normal capnogram is a waveform that represents the varying CO_2 level throughout the breath cycle.

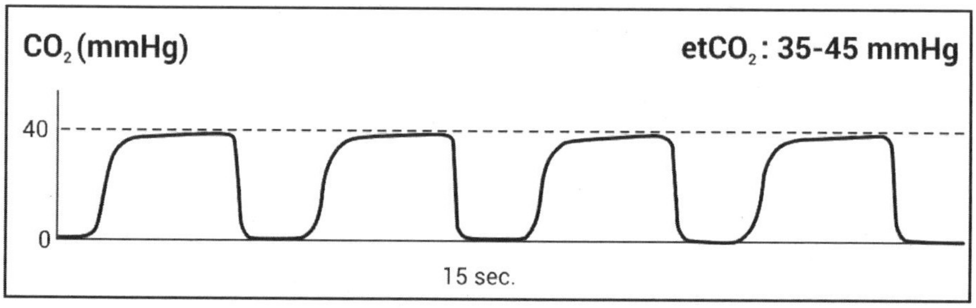

Typical Ventilator Settings

Ventilation settings will vary according to the size and condition of the patient, but typical initial ventilation settings include:

- **Tidal volume**: The maximum is 10 mL/kg of ideal body weight (IBW) if patient has no lung disease but must be kept under 10 mL/kg IBW if lung disease is present.
- **Pressure**: Initially 20–25 cmH_2O and then adjusted to maintain the tidal volume.
- **Respiration rate**: Initially 12-16 bpm although patients with ALI/ARDS need a higher setting of 18-22 bpm.
- **FiO_2**: Initially 100% and the adjusted to a goal of oxygen saturation ≥88% or PaO_2 >55 mmHg.
- **PEEP**: Initially 5 cmH_2O and increased by 2–3 cm every 30–60 minutes.
- **Inspiratory time**: Initially 0.8–1.0 second.
- **I:E ratio**: Initially 1:2 and then adjusted to 1:3 or 1:4 or other settings appropriate for patient.

Ventilation should generally be adjusted to maintain the patient's normal or baseline PCO_2. If oxygenation is inadequate, the FiO_2 and/or PEEP should be increased. If ventilation needs to be increased because of falling CO_2, the respiration rate or tidal volume should be increased.

Modes of Mechanical Ventilation

Modes of ventilation include:

- **Assist control**: The patient receives a preset tidal volume during each inspiration, whether the breath is triggered by the individual or by the ventilator. The mandatory breath occurs at a preset duration of time after the previous inspiration if the patient does not trigger a spontaneous breath. Assist control is the most commonly utilized mode of ventilation.
- **Continuous mandatory ventilation**: The patient receives a preset tidal volume at a preset rate, so the patient cannot trigger ventilation with spontaneous breaths. This mode is commonly used for patient who are paralyzed and during surgery when patients have received muscle relaxants.

- **Pressure support ventilation**: The ventilator delivers a preset level of inspiratory pressure in support of a patient's inspiratory effort. The frequency, duration, and tidal volume are determined by the patient, so the machine should be set with backup settings in the event of apnea if possible.

SIMV Mode

The **synchronized intermittent mandatory ventilation** (SIMV) model of mechanical ventilation is a combination mode in which the ventilator delivers mandatory breaths synchronized with the patient's effort of breathing but allows spontaneous breaths between the mandatory breaths. In the SIMV phase, if a patient triggers a breath at all, the ventilator delivers a preset tidal volume to ensure adequate ventilation. In the mandatory part of the SIMV phase, if the patient does not trigger a breath within the first 90% of the SIMV phase, a mandatory breath is automatically delivered. If the patient breathes spontaneously, the ventilator is not triggered although the ventilator can be set to provide some tidal volume in support of spontaneous breaths that are not adequate. The SIMV mode is often used when weaning a patient from mechanical ventilation.

Non-Invasive Ventilation

Nasal Cannula and Simple Face Mask

A nasal cannula and a simple face mask are two forms of low-flow oxygen delivery systems. A nasal cannula delivers oxygen to the patient through a flexible tube made of plastic that is inserted in his/her nostrils. Oxygen flows through a nasal cannula at the rate of 1–6 liters per minute. Oxygen concentration (FiO_2) using a nasal cannula ranges from about 24–44%. The nasal cannula is the most commonly used low-flow oxygen delivery system. A simple face mask, which covers the patient's nose and mouth, is another low-flow method of administering oxygen therapy. Oxygen can flow through a mask at the rate of 5–8 liters per minute. Using a mask, FiO_2 can reach approximately 60 percent. When administering oxygen via a mask, the minimum flow rate should be five liters per minute to prevent reuptake of carbon dioxide.

Of note, oxygen regulators may have been calibrated for use at regular sea level. If this is the case, the flow rate will change with increasing altitude. So oxygen set to flow at 4 L/min at 8,000 feet will actually be flowing around 5.4 L/min.

Non-Rebreather Mask and Air Entrainment Mask

A non-rebreather mask—one type of high-flow oxygen delivery system—covers the patient's nose and mouth; it also has a reservoir bag attached to it, which receives oxygen from the oxygen source. Oxygen flows through a non-rebreather mask at a rate greater than 10 liters per minute. With a tightly-fit mask and a reservoir bag that inflates properly, oxygen concentration (FiO_2) using a non-rebreather mask can reach 100 percent. As such, non-rebreather masks are appropriate for use in emergencies and with patients in respiratory failure. Air entrainment masks have both variable flow rates and variable FiO_2 levels that can range from 24–50 percent. This method is commonly used for patients whose lungs do not remove an adequate amount of carbon dioxide (CO_2), as it offers the ability to administer oxygen at high rates and to control the FiO_2 level, and the method does not result in CO_2 accumulation.

Utilizing the Recovery Position

The recovery position is used for patients who are unconscious but breathing (such as those with a drug overdose or after a seizure) and have no life-threatening injuries. This position helps to maintain a patent airway and reduces the risk of aspiration from vomitus.

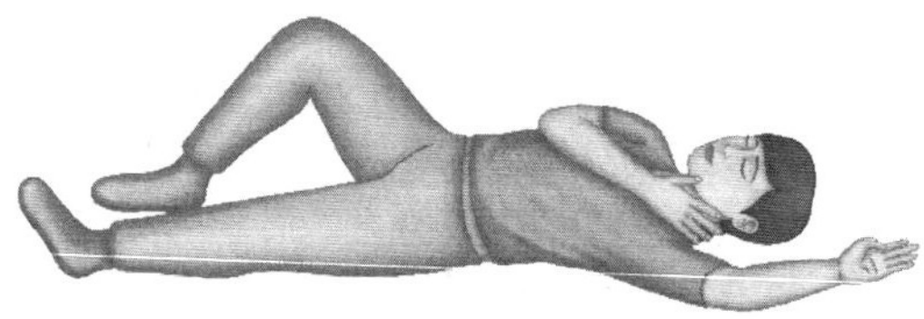	Kneeling beside the patient, lift his or her chin to ensure that the airway is open and place his or her closest arm at a right angle to the body with hand up. Place the patient's farthest arm around his or her neck with the hand touching the opposite cheek. Flex the patient's knee to 90° until the foot is flat on the floor/surface.
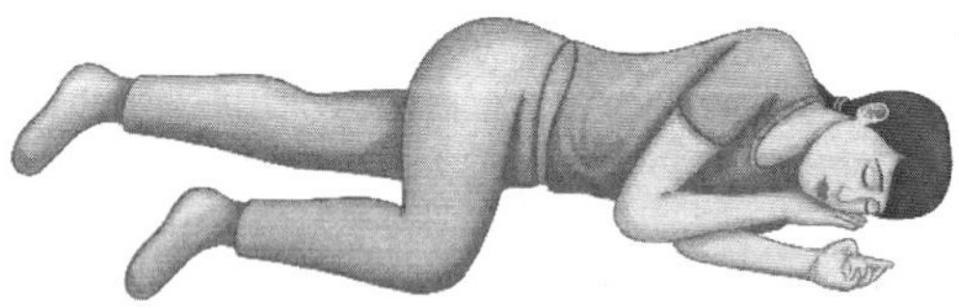	Using the patient's knee as a fulcrum and supporting the farthest arm and shoulder, roll the patient onto his or her side by pulling on the farthest knee. Make sure that the top knee contacts the floor/surface to support the patient's body and that the top hand is under his or her head/neck to keep the neck in a neutral position.

Perfusion

Components of Oxygen Delivery

Rapid Volume Fluid Resuscitation

Rapid volume resuscitation can be accompanied by serious medical complications for the patient if it is not performed correctly. The amount of fluid a patient needs varies from patient to patient; it is dependent upon the volume of fluid loss that has occurred within the blood vessels. During resuscitation efforts, it is particularly important that transport team members carefully monitor the patient's blood pressure, pulse, urinary output, and awareness level. Parameters such as these can indicate when a patient has received a sufficient level of volume resuscitation, and they can also indicate when a patient has received too much fluid during resuscitation efforts. The transport team should also constantly monitor the patient for signs of complications resulting from the rapid volume resuscitation.

Blood Products

Emergency blood product transfusions are usually of plasma and packed red blood cells (PRBCs). Before administration, the transport nurse should check the dates and temperature of the blood supply (generally in a transport cooler). If the blood type was specifically supplied for a patient, the blood type and name should be verified; but for emergency purposes, type O is generally all that is available, as it can be administered to most people without reaction. Indications include hemodynamic instability and acute hypoperfusion with systolic

BP <90 and pulse rate >120 from hemorrhage (traumatic or internal), penetrating chest wound, ruptured aortic aneurysm, or patient-specific hemoglobin (such as less than 7 mg/dL) with ongoing bleeding (such as from GI hemorrhage). Protocols may vary, but generally one unit of plasma and one unit of PRBCs are administered through warmed infusions (to patients 12 or older) and orders sought for additional units. Vital signs, temperature, and patient assessment should be monitored throughout the transfusion, and the receiving facility must be notified of the transfusion.

FFP and Platelets

Fresh frozen plasma (FFP) may be infused to correct hemorrhage or an anticipated large volume blood loss. It can also be used to increase a patient's clotting factor if the patient is deficient. An infused unit of fresh frozen plasma can increase a patient's clotting factor by 2–3% if he/she is average size. Additionally, platelets may be infused in an attempt to increase a patient's clotting factor. They can also be infused to overcome bleeding in a patient with thrombocytopenia, which is a condition characterized by a low platelet count. An infused unit of platelets can increase a patient's platelet count by 5,000 or more if he/she is average size. Patients experiencing hemorrhage, septic shock, or coagulation defects may warrant platelet infusions.

Special Considerations for Fluid Resuscitation

Special considerations for fluid resuscitation include the following:

- **Geriatric patients**: Underlying hypertension may result in shock with systolic BP >100 mmHg. Even small amounts of bleeding may lead to shock, especially if the patient has anemia and is less able to tolerate excessive fluids because of underlying anemia or electrolyte imbalances.
- **Pediatric patients**: Infuse up to 20 mL/kg of warmed isotonic solution, and start a second or third infusion if he or she is nonresponsive to the first infusion. Use continuous infusion for uncontrolled hemorrhage to maintain perfusion en route. It is important to manage temperature control to maintain perfusion. Use an age-specific vital sign chart to monitor vital signs.
- **Pregnant patients**: Shock results in the shunting of maternal blood away from the fetus to the mother's vital organs, so it is critical to maintain the patient's BP as close as possible to normal.

Access Options for Fluid Resuscitation

Intraosseous Needle Placement

Once the need for inserting an intraosseous needle has been determined, the following steps should be taken during the placement of the needle:

- Wearing a mask and sterile gloves, the insertion site should be cleansed.
- Identify and palpate the tibia, the larger of the two leg bones located below the knee.
- Insert the needle in the skin that covers the flat surface of the tibia.
- With the needle at approximately a 10–30-degree angle, advance the needle through the periosteum of the tibia, the tissue that covers the bone.
- Continue advancing the needle into the bone using a twisting motion.
- When the needle is in the marrow cavity of the tibia—the correct location for the needle—a decreased level of resistance will be felt.
- After removing the stylet from the needle, attach intravenous tubing, and secure the needle.

Central Venous Catheter Placement

Following the Seldinger technique for central venous catheter (CVC) insertion, a sharp, hollow needle is used to puncture a blood vessel. Once the needle has punctured the site, a guidewire is advanced through the needle's cavity, and the needle is withdrawn from the site. A flexible tube or cannula that can be used either to remove fluid or to administer medication is then passed over the guidewire, and the guidewire is withdrawn. The cannula can also be used to position a catheter, if necessary. Once the fluid has been withdrawn and/or the medication has been delivered to the patient through the CVC, the cannula is removed, and the procedure is complete.

Reestablishing Circulation

Cardiopulmonary Resuscitation (CPR) for Cardiac Arrest

Cardiac arrest of unknown cause in adults or children is usually treated as though it were ventricular fibrillation or pulseless ventricular tachycardia, but the protocol varies. Cardiopulmonary resuscitation (CPR) involves the following components:

- If a defibrillator is readily available, immediate defibrillation is performed according to protocol with an AED/manual defibrillator (preferred) followed by CPR, beginning with compressions (30:2 compression to ventilation at the rate of 100-120 per minute at least 2 inches deep; two-finger compressions, to one-third of the chest depth for infants and children) for 2 minutes or 5 cycles and repeat defibrillation.
- Repeat cycles of 2 minutes of CPR and defibrillation. (Laypeople may use compression-only CPR.)
- If a defibrillator is not readily available, CPR may begin first. Note that if a BVM is used, the break in compressions should not exceed 10 seconds. If an advanced airway/intubation is in place, ventilation should be at the rate of 8-10 per minute, maintaining oxygen saturation ≥94% but <100% with ventilation between compressions.
- The $ETCO_2$ value should be 10-20 mmHg if chest compressions are adequate, increasing to 35-45 mmHg with the return of spontaneous circulation (ROSC).

Cardioversion vs. Defibrillation

Cardioversion delivers a low energy shock that is synchronized to the QRS. Defibrillation (also called unsynchronized cardioversion) gives a high energy non-synchronized shock anywhere in the cardiac cycle. While both procedures attempt to restore the natural rhythm of the heart, cardioversion is performed on individuals who are not experiencing cardiac arrest, and defibrillation is generally performed as an emergency procedure on patients who are having a heart attack. Both procedures employ electric shock as a method for restarting the heart's rhythm, but cardioversion uses much lower levels of electricity than defibrillation uses. Most cardioversions are conducted to treat atrial flutter, which is a series of stable, regular flutter waves typically ranging from 240–400 beats per minute, or atrial fibrillation, which is a disturbance to the heart's rhythm that begins in the atria. Cardioversion is also used to treat stable ventricular tachycardia. Defibrillation tends to be a more risky procedure because the electrical shock used actually stops the heart altogether in an attempt to restore its normal beating rhythm.

Performing Defibrillation

High quality CPR should be performed as soon as sudden cardiac arrest is recognized and continued until the defibrillator is attached by another team member and ready to use. Interruptions in CPR should be minimized. Airway should be assessed and maintained. Power on the defibrillator. Place one pad on the upper right side of the patient's chest. The area should be right and lateral of the sternum, mid clavicular line. The posterior pad should be placed slightly sub scapular, with the center of the pad about equal with the T7 vertebrae. This is known as anterior posterior (AP) placement and allows for the maximum energy to flow. If AP placement is not possible, place the pad on the left lateral side, midaxillary line, with the bottom of the pad at about the 5th intercostal space. Pads should not be placed on top of pacemakers, body jewelry, or ports. Attach leads to defibrillator pads and charge defibrillator while continuing chest compressions. Stop compression to check rhythm. If VF or pulseless VT, clear patient and then administer shock at 120-200J, according to manufacturer guidelines (for biphasic defibrillators). Unless there is a return of spontaneous circulation (ROSC), immediately resume CPR for 5 cycles. Use epinephrine 1 mg every 3-5 minutes while continuing CPR if pulseless VT or VF persists. After the 5 cycles, about two minutes, check rhythm, clear patient, defibrillate again. If no ROSC, begin CPR cycle again. Continue in this pattern considering causes and treating as able or until ROSC.

Transvenous Pacing

Transvenous pacing may be temporary (most common) or permanent, and is done for hemodynamic instability and arrhythmias, such as BBB, AV block, and bradycardia. Transvenous pacing is often done temporarily if the patient cannot tolerate transcutaneous pacing or needs to be transferred. For transvenous pacing, a pacer is inserted transvenously through the right internal jugular or left subclavian vein into the right atrium or ventricle. (The right internal jugular is preferred for temporary pacing to save the left subclavian for a permanent pacemaker.) The electrode or electrodes of the pacing wire are inserted into an external battery-powered pacing generator. The insertion site should be covered with sterile transparent dressing. The patient must have continuous cardiac monitoring once capture is established. VT due to failure to sense or bradycardia due to failure to capture can occur with pacer wire damage or dislodgement, battery failure, or incorrect settings. The patient should be observed for signs of cardiac tamponade, hematoma, infection, and pneumothorax.

Managing Asystole

Cycles of cardiopulmonary resuscitation (CPR) and rhythm checks lasting two minutes per cycle should be performed on asystole patients who are acceptable resuscitation candidates. Epinephrine can be administered to the asystole patient every 3–5 minutes in an attempt to overcome whatever is preventing the patient's heart from beating. Airway should be assessed and managed. The cause of the asystole should be sought and treated accordingly, if possible. Most common reversible causes include: Hypoxia, hypothermia, hypokalemia (or hyperkalemia), acidosis, thrombosis, toxins, tamponade, tension pneumo. ACLS encourages using end-tidal carbon dioxide measurement and continuous waveform capnography to assess the effectiveness of CPR or detect return of spontaneous circulation. A low end-tidal carbon dioxide level following more than 20 minutes of CPR is the most objective reason to terminate resuscitation for a patient who presents with asystole and has no ROSC. Other determinants that influence decision to terminate resuscitation: long duration of resuscitation with no ROSC, questionable or long length between time of arrest and time of CPR, increased age, and severity of certain comorbidities.

Post-Resuscitation Return of Spontaneous Circulation (ROSC)

If a patient undergoing resuscitation has return of spontaneous circulation (ROSC), his or her ventilation and oxygenation must be supported to maintain the oxygen saturation ≥94% but less than 100% to avoid hyperoxia. Ventilation should be maintained at 10-12 breaths per minute with an $ETCO_2$ value at 35-40 mmHg. Hyperventilation must be avoided. Hypotension (systolic BP <90 mmHg) should be treated with an IV bolus (1-2 L saline) and vasopressor infusion. Treatable causes (the five H's and five T's) should be addressed, and a 12-lead ECG should be used to monitor the patient's condition. If the patient is nonresponsive, therapeutic hypothermia (to 32-34 °C) for 12-24 hours may be considered as a neuroprotective measure. If the patient is responsive and able to follow commands, he or she should be immediately transported to the appropriate receiving facility: the ICU or cardiac cath lab for acute myocardial infarction (AMI) or ST-elevated myocardial infarction (STEMI) for percutaneous coronary intervention (PCI). Note: Brain damage begins within 4-6 minutes of cardiac arrest, and it is irreversible after 8-10 minutes.

Termination of Resuscitation Efforts

Criteria for termination of resuscitation efforts include the following considerations:

- Arrest is cardiac-related and not a condition that may respond to hospital treatment
- Endotracheal intubation was successful and maintained throughout resuscitation efforts
- Standard advanced cardiac life support efforts were used
- Resuscitation efforts maintained for 25 minutes or asystole through four rounds of drugs
- At the time of the decision to terminate, the patient exhibits asystole or an agonal rhythm (the bizarre, ineffective, wide ventricular rhythm associated with dying)
- Official DNR order
- Newborn: No heartbeat detected after 10 minutes of CPR

Note: Older age, quality of life, and time of collapse prior to transport team arrival are not criteria for termination. Generally, resuscitation efforts are continued until arrival at the receiving facility on those patients younger than 18 unless the child has a terminal disease and an advance directive that limits resuscitation efforts. Prior to termination, the transport nurse should have direct communication with medical oversight and consult/advise the family members that are present. Family resistance must be noted and reported. Criteria for withholding resuscitation include DNR status, obvious signs of death (such as rigor mortis/lividity), or conditions that are unsafe for the rescuer.

WITHHOLDING RESUSCITATION ATTEMPTS

Although the goal of emergency medical services is to save lives, it is not always possible or ethical to carry out resuscitation efforts. Withholding resuscitation is justified under the following conditions:

- The patient's condition is not compatible with life (massive injuries, decapitation, crushed chest, severe open head injury with loss of brain tissue), and the patient is not breathing and has no pulse.
- The patient exhibits obvious signs of death, such as rigor mortis or livor mortis, indicating that he or she can no longer be resuscitated.
- The patient has a do-not-resuscitate (DNR) form available, and it is properly signed. Note: The transport provider cannot accept the word of family or friends that the patient does not want to be resuscitated without a DNR order.
- Conditions are unsafe to approach the patient and/or administer resuscitation efforts. This may occur, for example, if there are gunshots heard in the area, if the patient is pinned under a motor vehicle, or if the patient cannot safely be reached in time because of difficult terrain.

ASSESSING OXYGENATION STATUS

A patient's oxygenation status can be assessed using several factors. A pulse oximeter, a non-invasive tool used to measure the amount of oxygen in a patient's blood, may be utilized to monitor the patient's oxygen saturation level (SaO_2). The patient's consciousness level can also be determined to help assess oxygenation status. The tone of the patient's skin as well as the absence or presence of cyanosis—a condition characterized by a bluish skin tone—can also be examined as a means of assessing oxygenation status. Monitoring the patient's airway, breathing, and circulation in addition to his/her pulse are other important components of assessing whether he/she is adequately oxygenated. Finally, monitoring the patient's inhaled and exhaled concentrations of carbon dioxide (CO_2) through capnography provides a helpful indicator of oxygenation status.

PULSE OXIMETRY

Pulse oximetry is a non-invasive technique used to measure the amount of oxygen in a patient's blood. Inaccurate readings may be obtained from patients with inadequate blood flow to their tissue, such as patients experiencing shock or cardiac arrest. The technique may also have limited effectiveness on patients with hypothermia, patients with burns, and those with highly pigmented skin. It may be difficult to obtain exact pulse oximetry values from patients who are not able to maintain a fairly still position as well as from those who have vasoactive drugs in their bloodstream. Additionally, falsely high values typically occur in patients who smoke due to the carbon monoxide in cigarette smoke. A pulse oximeter may also provide inaccurate readings when it is utilized in bright ambient light, as the intensity of the light may lead to abnormally high values.

Always compare pulse oximetry readings to the clinical presentation of the patient.

NORMAL OXYGEN SATURATION

Oxygen saturation values in the range of greater than or equal to 95 % are generally considered normal. However, for some patients, like those COPD, normal saturations may be 88-92%. While 97–99 % saturation can be considered normal values for most patients, some patients may become extremely sick if their pulse oximetry values go above 97 %. The best way to determine a patient's target oxygen saturation is to know their history and normal resting oxygen saturation, but this is not always possible. In the absence of this knowledge and signs of COPD, in an adult patient, as a general rule, patients with oxygen saturation levels below 90 % are in need of ventilation; typically, ventilation with oxygen saturation at a level below 90 % can be performed with a bag-valve-mask device. The most effective way to determine whether a patient is improving as a result of oxygen delivery is simply to compare pre- and post-pulse oximetry values.

Portable Oxygen Cylinders

Two commonly used sizes of portable oxygen cylinders are D tanks (M15; 350 L) and E tanks (M24; 625 L). The transport nurse should use protective equipment (goggles, gloves). The cylinder should be placed upright. A label over the holes on the top of the cylinder indicates that the cylinder is full. Remove the label, leaving the washers in place unless the washers are built into the regulator. Face the opening of the tank away and use the key to crack the cylinder by letting out a small amount of oxygen. Apply the regulator and slide it into place. Tighten and then open the cylinder to check for pressure (there should be at least 200 psi). Close the cylinder, attach the oxygen tubing to the regulator, set the oxygen flow to the correct number of liters, and then open the cylinder and administer oxygen to the patient. When discontinuing use of the cylinder, turn off the cylinder, remove the oxygen tubing, turn the oxygen flow setting up to bleed air from the regulator, and remove the regulator.

Vasopressors

Phenylephrine

Phenylephrine hydrochloride, a vasoconstrictor/alpha adrenergic agent (pregnancy Category C), treats hypotension (including drug-induced). IV administration has immediate onset and 15-20-minute duration. IM/SC administration has 10-15 minute onset and 0.5-2-hour duration. Dosage:

Mild to moderate hypotension: Adult— IV: 0.1-0.5 mg and repeat in 10–15 minutes as needed; 1–10 mg IM/SC: first dose of ≤5 mg and repeat in 1–2 hours if needed. Pediatric—0.1 mg/kg. IM/SC and repeat in 1–2 hours if needed.

Severe hypotension/shock: Adult—10 mg in 250-500 mL D_5W or NS. Initially at 100-180 mcg/minute and decreased to 40-60 mcg/minute after BP stabilizes.

Paroxysmal SVT: Adult—Initially 0.5mg rapid IV infusion with increase in 0.1–0.2 mg dosages to maximum single dose of 1 mg.

Monitor ECG, vital signs, urinary output, and circulation to limbs (color, temperature). Follow protocol or for patients with history of hypertension, maintain BP at 30-40 mmHg below baseline, and for patients with no history of hypertension, maintain systolic BP at 80-100 mmHg.

Norepinephrine

Norepinephrine bitartrate (Levophed) is a vasopressor/direct-acting adrenergic agent (pregnancy Category C) used to treat acute hypotension, especially hypotension associated with cardiogenic or septic shock. The drug should only be administered intravenously in D_5W or D_5NS solution, usually through a central venous catheter or large vein. The initial dose is 8–12 mcg/min and it can then be titrated to an average maintenance dose of 2–4 mcg/min. For patients with history of hypertension, maintain BP at 40 mmHg below baseline, and for patients with no history of hypertension, maintain systolic BP at 80–100 mmHg. The patient should have continuous monitoring with vital signs assessed every 2 minutes until stable and then every 5 minutes. Monitor ECG, vital signs, urinary output, and circulation to limbs (color, temperature). Monitor site for signs of extravasation or blanching, which is treated by stopping the infusion, aspirating (but not flushing) IV, removing IV, elevating extremity and then injecting area with phentolamine diluted in 10–15 mL NS, to prevent tissue necrosis.

Dopamine

Dopamine, a vasopressor/adrenergic agonist (pregnancy Category C), is used to treat hemodynamic instability caused by shock or heart failure in adults and children. It is administered intravenously in D_5W, NS, D_5W in NS, 0.45% saline, or Lactated Ringer's through a central line or large vein to prevent extravasation. Dosage for adults and children initially is 2–5 mcg/kg/min. The drug is titrated by 1–4 mcg/kg/min every 10–30 minutes. If the patient is severely ill, the maximum initial dosage of 5 mcg/kg/min should be used and titrated by adding 5–10 mcg/kg/min to a maximum of 20–50 mcg/kg/min. If the patient has vascular occlusive disease, the initial dosage should begin with 1 mcg/kg/min. Monitor ECG, vital signs, urinary output, and circulation to limbs (color, temperature). Avoid administering a bolus of the drug. Monitor site for signs of extravasation or blanching, which is treated by stopping infusion and infiltrating area with phentolamine diluted in 10–15 mL NS, to prevent tissue necrosis.

Shock Resuscitation and Management

There are a number of different types of shock, but there are general characteristics that they have in common. In all types of shock, there is a marked decrease in tissue perfusion related to hypotension, so that there is insufficient oxygen delivered to the tissues and, in turn, inadequate removal of cellular waste products, causing injury to tissue:

- Hypotension (systolic below 90 mmHg). This may be somewhat higher (110 mmHg) in those who are initially hypertensive.
- Decreased urinary output (<0.5 mL/kg/hr), especially marked in hypovolemic shock
- Metabolic acidosis.
- Hypoxemia <90 mmHg for children and adults birth-50; <80 mmHg for those 51–70 and <70 for those over 70.
- Peripheral/cutaneous vasoconstriction/vasodilation resulting in cool, clammy skin.
- Alterations in level of consciousness.

	Distributive	Cardiogenic	Hypovolemic
Preload	↓(sometimes stays same)	↑	↓
Cardiac Output	↑	↓	↓
SVR	↓	↑	↑

Hypovolemic Shock

Hypovolemic shock occurs when the total circulating volume of fluid decreases, leading to a fall in venous return that in turn causes a decrease in ventricular filling and preload, indicated by ↓ in right atrial pressure (RAP) and pulmonary artery occlusion pressure (PAOP). This results in a decrease in stroke volume and cardiac output. This in turn causes generalized arterial vasoconstriction, increasing afterload (↑ systemic vascular resistance), causing decreased tissue perfusion.

Symptoms	Treatment
• Anxiety • Pallor • Cool and clammy skin • Delayed capillary refill • Cyanosis • Hypotension • Increasing respirations • Weak, thready pulse	• Treatment is aimed at identifying and treating the cause of fluid loss and reestablishing an adequate intravascular volume of fluid through administration of blood, blood products, autotransfusion, colloids (such as plasma protein fraction), and/or crystalloids (such as normal saline). • Oxygen may be given and intubation and ventilation may be necessary. • Medications may include vasopressors, such as dopamine.

Obstructive Shock

Obstructive shock occurs when venous return to the heart (preload) is impeded because of some type of obstruction or direct compression of the heart. Common causes include:

- Pulmonary embolism: Hypotension (SBP <90 mmHg), tachypnea, tachycardia, and cough. Treatment is anticoagulation or thrombolysis.
- Pneumothorax (often associated with fractured rib): Onset is rapid with pallor, hypotension, tachycardia, impaired peripheral circulation, tachypnea, and chest pain decreased or absent breath sounds on affected side. Tracheal deviation is a late indication. Treatment is needle thoracostomy (14 gauge, 3.25 inch) followed by chest tube insertion.
- Pericardial tamponade: Beck's triad (hypotension, muffled heart sounds, and JVD), ECG changes (slow or varying QRS), or tachycardia. Percutaneous drainage under ultrasound guidance may relieve severe symptoms, but patient may require immediate surgical intervention.

In all cases, provide oxygen to maintain oxygen saturation of at least 94%, start an IV line, monitor ECG, keep warm, lie flat or in position of comfort, and transport rapidly.

Distributive Shock

Distributive shock occurs with adequate blood volume but inadequate intravascular volume because of arterial/venous dilation that results in decreased vascular tone and hypoperfusion of internal organs. Cardiac output may be normal or blood may pool, decreasing cardiac output. Distributive shock may result from anaphylactic shock, septic shock, neurogenic shock, and drug ingestions.

Symptoms	Treatment
• Hypotension (systolic <90 mmHg or <40 mmHg from normal), tachypnea, tachycardia (>90) (may be lower if patient receiving β-blockers. • Skin initially warm, later hypoperfused. • Hyper- or hypothermia (>38 °C or <36 °C). • Hypoxemia. • Alterations in mentation. • Decreased Urinary output. • Symptoms related to underlying cause.	Treating underlying cause and stabilizing hemodynamics: • Septic shock or anaphylactic therapy and monitoring as indicated. • Oxygen with endotracheal intubation if necessary. • Rapid fluid administration at 0.25-0.5L NS or isotonic crystalloid every 5-10 minutes as needed to 2-3 L. • Inotropic agents (dopamine, dobutamine, norepinephrine) if necessary.

Cardiogenic Shock

Cardiogenic shock in adults most often is secondary to myocardial infarction damage that reduces the contractibility of the ventricles, interfering with the pumping mechanism of the heart, decreasing oxygen perfusion. Cardiogenic shock has 3 characteristics: Increased preload, increased afterload, and decreased contractibility. Together these result in a decreased cardiac output and an increase in systemic vascular resistance (SVR) to compensate and protect vital organs. This results in an increase of afterload in the left ventricle with increased need for oxygen. As the cardiac output continues to decrease, tissue perfusion decreases, coronary artery perfusion decreases, fluid backs up and the left ventricle fails to adequately pump the blood, resulting in pulmonary edema and right ventricular failure. Decreasing oxygen consumption is a major initial goal of cardiogenic shock.

Symptoms	Treatment
• Hypotension with systolic BP <90 mmHg • Tachycardia > 100 beats/min with weak thready pulse and dysrhythmias • Decreased heart sounds • Chest pain • Tachypnea and basilar rales • Cool, moist skin, pallor	• IV fluids • Inotropic agents • Antidysrhythmics • IABP or left ventricular assist device

Anaphylactic Shock

Anaphylaxis syndrome may present with a few symptoms or a wide range that encompasses cardiopulmonary, dermatological, and gastrointestinal responses.

Symptoms	Treatments
Symptoms may recur after the initial treatment (biphasic anaphylaxis), so careful monitoring is essential: • Sudden onset of weakness, dizziness, confusion. • Severe generalized edema and angioedema. Lips and tongue may swell. • Urticaria • Increased permeability of vascular system and loss of vascular tone. • Severe hypotension leading to shock. • Laryngospasm/bronchospasm with obstruction of airway causing dyspnea and wheezing. • Nausea, vomiting, and diarrhea. • Seizures, coma and death.	• Establish patent airway and intubate if necessary for ventilation. • Provide oxygen at 100% high flow. • Monitor VS. • Administer epinephrine (Epi-pen® or solution). • Albuterol per nebulizer for bronchospasm. • Intravenous fluids to provide bolus of fluids for hypotension. • Diphenhydramine if shock persists. • Methylprednisolone if no response to other drugs.

Complications of Shock

Complications of shock include the following:

- **Acute respiratory distress syndrome (ARDS)**: Damage to the vascular endothelium and an increase in the permeability of the alveolar-capillary membrane when damage to the lung results from toxic substances (e.g., gastric fluids, bacteria, chemicals, toxins emitted by neutrophils as part of the inflammatory-mediated response). These substances reduce surfactant and cause pulmonary edema as the alveoli fill with blood and protein-rich fluid and then collapse (atelectasis). This decrease in surfactant also leads to decreased lung compliance (sometimes referred to as stiffening). Hypoxemia and tachypnea increase as the body tries to compensate to maintain a normal $PaCO_2$. Symptoms occur within 72 (usually 24-48) hours of serious injury. Untreated, this condition results in respiratory failure, multiorgan failure, and a mortality rate of 5-30%. (PEEP is used for ventilation.)
- **Acute renal failure**: The renal tubules are damaged, and the kidneys are unable to filter out the waste products of metabolism.

- **Multiple-organ failure/dysfunction syndrome (MOFS/MODS)**: MOFS/MODS is a progressive deterioration and failure of two or more organ systems with mortality rates of 45-50% with two organ systems involved and up to 80-100% if there are three or more systems failing. Trauma patients and those with severe conditions, such as shock, are particularly vulnerable, especially in those >65 years old.

Acid-Base Imbalances

Arterial Blood Gases

Arterial blood gas studies evaluate the acidity, oxygen content, and amount of carbon dioxide (CO_2) in a patient's blood. The analysis is generally performed to evaluate respiratory diseases and other conditions that affect the functioning of a patient's pulmonary system. Kidney functioning can also be assessed through the acid-base component of an arterial blood gas study. Additionally, the analysis can provide information about how a patient is responding to oxygen therapy. Patients who sustain traumatic injuries, particularly injuries that likely affect their breathing such as head and neck trauma, also tend to have abnormal results on arterial blood gas studies. When drawing an ABG for point of care testing, determine the best arm to take the specimen from (if possible perform the Allen test and assess for AV grafts and other implanted devices). Using universal precautions, prepare site with solution per protocol (usually chlorhexidine). Palpate the radial artery with index and middle finger then locate the radial artery. Puncture skin with needle bevel at 45 degrees. The needle should fill with brightly colored red blood rapidly. After sample has been collected, remove needle and hold pressure for 3 minutes or longer until bleeding is stopped, consider longer for patients on anticoagulants. Immediately perform point of care testing on sample or place on ice. Reassess neuro status of extremity used and make sure there is no further bleeding at site of puncture.

Normal Values

The partial pressure of a gas is the pressure that is exerted by each gas in a mixture of gases, proportional to its concentration, based on total atmospheric pressure of 760 mmHg at sea level. Normal values include the following:

1. Acidity/alkalinity (pH): 7.35–7.45
2. Partial pressure of carbon dioxide ($PaCO_2$): 35–45 mmHg
3. Partial pressure of oxygen (PaO_2): 80 mmHg
4. Bicarbonate concentration (HCO_3): 22–26 mEq/L (a lower level is a base deficit, and a higher level is a base excess)
5. Oxygen saturation (SaO_2): ≥95%

The relationship between these elements, particularly the $PaCO_2$ and the PaO_2, indicates the respiratory status. For example, $PaCO_2$ >55 and PaO_2 <60 in a patient previously in good health indicates respiratory failure. There are many issues to consider. Ventilator management may require a higher $PaCO_2$ to prevent barotrauma and a lower PaO_2 to reduce oxygen toxicity.

Specific Acid/Base Imbalances

Respiratory acidosis: Hypoventilation (decreased breathing or inadequate mechanical ventilation) retains carbon dioxide and increases acid, which decreases the pH (acidity) to less than 7.35 (more acidic). The kidneys retain bicarbonate to compensate.

- **Causes**: COPD, pneumonia, muscle weakness, sedative/barbiturate overdose, obesity, muscle weakness (Guillain-Barré syndrome).
- **Symptoms**: Drowsiness, dizziness, headache, confusion, seizures, flushing, and low BP, tachypnea (tachy- = rapid; -pnea = breathing), tachycardia, and ventricular fibrillation.
- **Treatment**: Improved ventilation and bronchodilators.

Respiratory alkalosis: Hyperventilation (increased breathing) exhales more carbon dioxide and decreases acid, which increases the pH to greater than 7.45 (more alkalotic). The kidneys excrete increased bicarbonate to compensate.

- **Causes**: Hypoxia (low oxygen), brain injury, acetylsalicylic acid (ASA, i.e., aspirin) overdose, pulmonary embolism (clot), and septicemia.
- **Symptoms**: Confusion, lethargy, tachycardia, arrhythmia (irregular pulse), epigastric pain, nausea, and vomiting.
- **Treatment**: Identify and treat the underlying cause, and provide oxygen.

Metabolic acidosis: The kidneys excrete less acid, causing acid retention which decreases the pH, or the body excretes excess bicarbonate (through diarrhea), also decreasing the pH. Hyperventilation occurs in order to exhale additional carbon dioxide and acid to compensate.

- **Causes**: Diarrhea (it causes a loss of sodium bicarbonate), starvation, kidney disease, liver failure, excessive alcohol, shock, severe dehydration, and diabetic ketoacidosis (it causes acidic ketone bodies to build up).
- **Symptoms**: Headache, confusion, abnormal pulse, nausea, vomiting, diarrhea, and low BP.
- **Treatment**: Identify and treat the underlying cause. Bicarbonate is rarely administered, but it may be indicated in severe cases.

Metabolic alkalosis: Vomiting excretes excessive acid and/or the kidneys retain salt and potassium to compensate for vomiting, but in doing so, excrete more hydrogen ions (acid). This increases the body's pH, and hypoventilation occurs to retain carbon dioxide and acid.

- **Causes**: Excessive prolonged vomiting, low potassium level, advanced kidney failure.
- **Symptoms**: Confusion, anxiety, tremors, muscle cramping, seizures, tachycardia (rapid pulse), nausea, and vomiting.
- **Treatment**: Patient may respond to 0.9% IV saline (50-100 mL/hr.), but the underlying cause must be identified and treated. Some patients may require hemodialysis.

Review Video: Blood Gases
Visit mometrix.com/academy and enter code: 611909

Trauma

Principles of Management

Primary Assessment of a Trauma Patient

During the primary assessment of a trauma patient (which should be performed rapidly), the airway and cervical spine should be stabilized first. Following stabilization of the airway and cervical spine, the patient's breathing and ventilation should be assessed. Upon assessing breathing and ventilation, circulation should be evaluated, and any active hemorrhaging should be controlled with direct pressure. Fourth, the patient's neurological state should be assessed to determine any decrease in cognitive functioning. Finally, the patient should be undressed in order to identify and treat any previously missed trauma sites and/or injuries.

Secondary Assessment of a Trauma Patient

The secondary assessment of a trauma patient involves an extensive visual scan of the patient to identify all sustained injuries; consequently, it is most beneficial for the patient to be completely undressed prior to this scan. If it is not feasible for the patient to be fully disrobed, the patient's chest and abdomen should at least be exposed. Restrictive attire such as belts should be removed or cut off. To prevent cold-related emergencies in trauma patients, areas of the patient's body that are not being examined should be covered with blankets. The purpose of the secondary assessment is to reveal injuries; the transport team does not treat specific injuries during this process. To avoid losing valuable time that could be spent treating injuries, it is imperative that the secondary assessment be performed in a quick manner. Inspection, auscultation, palpation, and history taking are essential components of the secondary assessment.

Trauma Score

The Trauma Score is an index that rates physiological characteristics of patients. These characteristics include: 1) systolic blood pressure; 2) respiratory rate; 3) respiratory expansion; 4) capillary refill; and 5) score on the Glasgow Coma Scale. The original Trauma Scale has been revised to include characteristics one, two, and five described above—systolic blood pressure, respiratory rate, and Glasgow Coma Scale score. The Glasgow Coma Scale rates patients in terms of eye response, verbal response, and motor response. Patients are given a score between 3 and 15, where a score of 3–8 indicates severe brain injury, 9–12 indicates moderate brain injury, and 13–15 indicates mild injury. The three parameters of the Revised Trauma Score combined offer a means of predicting patient survival. A higher Revised Trauma Score correlates with a higher probability of survival.

Mechanisms of Injury

Blunt Trauma

Blunt trauma can be the result of a variety of accidents/injuries:

- **Motor vehicle crashes**: Result in 30–40% of accidental deaths and half of closed-head and spinal cord injuries with injuries usually more serious with ejection, lateral (T-bone) impacts, and unrestrained patients, although lap belts increase the risk of abdominal injury (bowel injury in children). Shoulder belts may cause vascular injuries. Injuries include crush (compression), shear (tearing), and burst (rupture from sudden increase in pressure). The risk of death increases if another vehicle occupant dies. Most frontal collisions result in injuries from impact with the steering wheel, dashboard, windshield, or floorboards. More severe injuries occur at speeds of >25 mph.
- **Motorcycle crashes**: Approximately 75% of deaths are from head injuries, but injuries to the spine, pelvis, and extremities, including limb loss, are common.

- **Pedestrian and motor vehicle impacts**: Often results in Waddell's triad (tibiofibular or femur fracture, trunk injury, and head/face injury). Small children are often run over, and adults are thrown over the car by the impact. Intra-abdominal injury and pelvic fractures may occur from fender contact with the hips.
- **Falls**: The most common cause of accidental death in geriatric patients is by falling. Anticoagulants increase the risk of injury with falls. The degree of injury depends on the patient's weight and the fall distance. Injuries are most severe with a fall distance of >20 feet for adults and >10 feet for children. A three-story fall results in 50% mortality; the mortality is almost 100% for five-story falls. Horizontal landings cause fewer injuries (hand, wrist, head/face, and abdominal) than feet-first landings, which often result in fractures of the heel, leg, pelvis, and/or vertebrae.
- **Sports injuries/play**: Injuries vary depending on the type of injury but can include head injuries, musculoskeletal injuries, and abdominal injuries. Helmet or knee contact to the flank area may cause kidney injury. The most common injuries are strains, sprains, and knee injuries.
- **Assaults**: Assaults are most common in young males and include facial and head injuries. Severe torso injuries may occur with kicking/stomping. If the patient is intoxicated and has altered consciousness, then he or she is treated as having a head injury. Assaults include domestic violence and child abuse, with distinctive patterns of injury.

Penetrating Trauma

Penetrating traumas are most often the result of violence, such as gunshot wounds and puncture wounds.

- **Gunshot wounds**: Solid organs (brain, liver, spleen) often suffer more damage than more elastic tissues (fat, lungs). If a bullet is not deformed after entering the tissue, it tends to tumble (180°), creating a tunnel of injury (permanent cavity) and damage to the surrounding tissue (temporary cavity). If the bullet is deformed, it causes more severe localized tissue damage. Bullets usually have a straight trajectory, but they may be deflected if they strike bone. Shotgun blasts within 15 feet cause more damage than other gunshot wounds, but they are usually less severe at a distance.
- Puncture wounds:
    - *Stab:* Includes hand-driven objects (knives, glass shards, ice picks, or pieces of metal/wood). Surface puncture wounds are often small, but their depth varies according to the instrument used, which should be removed surgically.
    - *Slash:* These are usually long but not deep lacerations.
    - *Impalement:* This usually results from objects larger than a knife, often from a fall onto an object, but it can include arrows and nails from pneumatic tools.

Motor Vehicle Crashes

If a driver is not wearing a safety restraint during a motor vehicle crash, head and facial injuries are likely to occur. Additionally, the larynx, sternum, patella, femur, and clavicle are structures that often fracture during a crash when a driver is unrestrained. Cardiac contusion and organ or blood vessel laceration also occur frequently in crashes involving unrestrained drivers. If a driver is wearing a safety restraint when a motor vehicle crash occurs, he/she will likely sustain injuries either from the lap restraint or from the shoulder restraint. Injuries that are often caused by a lap restraint include injuries to the pelvis, spleen, liver, and/or pancreas. Injuries frequently sustained from a shoulder restraint include cervical fractures and injuries to the mitral valve or diaphragm. The mitral valve and diaphragm often rupture as a result of injury sustained from a shoulder restraint during a motor vehicle crash.

Arterial and Venous Injuries

Arterial injuries are characterized by abundant hemorrhaging from open wounds. Venous injuries also have the capacity to produce hemorrhaging from open or closed wounds; however, bleeding from venous injuries is not as plentiful as it is with arterial injuries. Edema—swelling of an organ or tissue as a result of a build-up of lymph fluid—is present in venous injuries. The temperature of the injured area can also help differentiate an arterial injury from a venous one. The site of an arterial injury will be cool in temperature while a venous injury site may either be cool or warm. It is common to see poor capillary filling associated with arterial injuries; capillary filling tends to be good following a venous injury. Both types of injuries may be accompanied by a diminished pulse, but a patient with an arterial injury may also lack a pulse altogether.

Hemostasis

Identifying Type and Source of Bleeding

Any type of trauma can induce bleeding, internal or external. Identifying the type and source of bleeding is critical in managing the bleed.

- **Arterial**: Bright-red spurting blood that is difficult to control; lessens as the BP falls
- **Venous**: Dark-red blood flowing in a steady stream; may be copious, but is easier to control than an arterial bleed
- **Capillary**: Oozing; usually clots spontaneously
- **Internal**: Usually evidenced by increasing signs of shock or discolored swollen, painful tissue, guarding, coughing up blood, or rectal bleeding. Long-bone fractures (femur) and pelvic fractures may result in severe blood loss.

Interventions: Using standard precautions and PPE as indicated, apply sterile gauze dressing and pressure with the fingertips if it is a small bleed or apply direct hand pressure if it is more copious. As dressings saturate, add new dressings but don't remove the old ones. A tourniquet may be needed if the bleeding is uncontrolled. Maintain the patient in the shock position, especially with an arterial bleed or severe blood loss, and keep him or her warm. Avoid giving food or fluids, and transport immediately for severe bleeding. Severity relates to the rate of blood loss volume and the age and health of patient. The blood volume is less with pediatric patients. Moving the injured area, a change in body temperature, medications, and the removal of bandages may impair clotting.

Wound Dressing Selection

The location of the wound—whether it is located superficially or whether it has become a full thickness or cavity wound—should be considered prior to selecting a dressing. Next, a description of the wound should be determined. A necrotic wound is comprised of dead tissue and is often characterized by a black, leathery appearance. A sloughy wound is one characterized by a thick yellow layer covering the wound, while a granulating wound may be characterized by a bright red color; a granulating wound may appear to be shiny, and it may bleed easily. Characteristics of the wound including factors such as whether it is dry or moist and whether it is painful should also be taken into consideration before dressing a wound. The wound's bacterial profile—whether it is sterile, infected, or infected with the potential to cross-infect—is also an important attribute to consider when selecting a dressing.

Controlling Visible Hemorrhage

Many types of hemorrhage exist, but hemorrhage in the general sense means severe bleeding or significant loss of blood. When the source of a patient's blood loss can be visualized, there are ways to control the hemorrhage. First and foremost, the patient's airway, breathing, and circulation should be assessed. Once those have been evaluated, the hemorrhage site should be freed from constrictive clothing or attire of any kind so that the site is exposed. In cases of minor bleeding, direct pressure should be applied to the injury site to stop the bleeding, the site should be cleansed with soap and water, and a sterile dressing should be applied. In cases of serious hemorrhage, the risks of causing further damage to an injured site should be considered against the possible benefits of applying direct pressure to the area.

Tourniquets

Tourniquets are recommended as life-saving devices for uncontrolled arterial hemorrhage of the extremities that cannot be controlled with pressure or other means. The types of trauma tourniquets that are recommended were developed by the military but are now in common use for emergency care. The Combat Application Tourniquet (CAT) and the SOF Tactical Tourniquet (SOF-T) are adjustable bands with a windlass stick to tighten and a windlass clip and strap. The tourniquet is applied about 2 inches above the wound or above the knee for lower leg wounds and above the elbow for lower arm wounds. After the tourniquet is applied, the windlass is twisted to tighten until the distal pulse disappears and bleeding slows considerably or stops. Once bleeding is controlled, the windlass is secured. The tourniquet should be kept open to the field of vision so it is constantly monitored. If no tourniquet is available, a BP cuff can be applied and inflated.

Trauma Triad

The trauma triad is a leading cause of death in trauma patients, usually resulting from tissue injury and severe bleeding:

- **Hypothermia**: Normal temperature 35.6–37.0 °C. Trauma hypothermia—mild (34–36 °C), moderate (32–34 °C), and severe (<32 °C). Can result in decreased cardiac output and myocardial ischemia, decreased response to epinephrine, hypoxia, and arrhythmias. With bleeding, clotting is impaired; with infection, reduces WBCs and increases risk of infection/sepsis. May be exacerbated by alcohol intoxication, older age, chronic disease, and administration of cool IV fluids/blood products.
- **Acidosis**: Occurs with pH <7.35 (normal is 7.35-7.45). May be metabolic or respiratory in nature, or a combination. May result in decreased cardiac output and response to epinephrine, hyperventilation, respiratory fatigue, decreased mental status, coma, and impaired coagulation. May result from poor tissue perfusion, excessive resuscitation with crystalloids.
- **Coagulopathy**: May be dilutional from fluid resuscitation with fluids or blood products that lack lost clotting factors. May also result from pre-existing anticoagulation (warfarin, heparin) or over-activation of coagulation system.

Immobilization

Pelvic Fractures

Patients with pelvic fractures are at risk for significant blood loss and hypovolemia. Pelvic fractures should be suspected with high impact injuries, such as falls from a high place or pedestrian-motor vehicle accidents. Patients may complain of abdominal or back pain, pain in the pelvic area, and/or numbness and tingling of the lower extremities. Excessive palpation or manipulation should be avoided and the pelvis should be stabilized with a circumferential pressure device (remove items from pockets first):

- Sheet wrap: A draw sheet is folded horizontally and made about 1 foot wide, placed beneath the patient, wrapped tightly around the pelvic area, and secured with clamps or other means.
- T-POD: Slide the belt under patient and around patient, adjust size to leave a 6 inch space between belt ends. Attach the velcro pulley system to each side of belt, then adjust pull-tabs to increase circumferential pressure. Finally, secure compression.
- SAM pelvic sling: Place belt under hips and wrap around. Fasten belt snugly, and secure.

Traction Splints for Femur Fractures

Traction splints are applied to mid-shaft fractures of the femur (if no other leg fracture, severe injury, or pelvic fractures are present) to stabilize bone ends, reduce bleeding and relieve discomfort. At least 2 people are usually needed when applying the traction splint and constant communication is necessary. Procedure:

- Stabilize leg and apply gentle steady manual traction.
- Check motor function (move toes), sensation, and distal pulse.
- Apply ankle hitch.
- Position traction device (the Hare device is placed under the leg and the Sagar to the medial aspect of the leg) and secure proximal and then distal straps.
- Attach ankle hitch to the device.
- Apply traction slowly (maximum 10% of body weight or 15 pounds for Sagar), using the uninjured leg as a guide to length if leg distorted.

- Reassess distal circulation.
- Place patient on backboard and secure traction device to the backboard.

If incorrectly applied, the traction splint can increase bleeding, damage nerves and soft tissue, and increase the risk of compartment syndrome.

SPINAL IMMOBILIZATION

To prevent interference with x-rays, jewelry should be removed from a patient prior to performing a spinal immobilization. Additionally, any sharp debris such as glass that is present on the patient should be removed as a means of preventing further injury. Once jewelry and sharp debris have been removed, the patient should be placed in a cervical collar; it is important that the patient's spine remain stabilized during this component of the immobilization procedure. When the cervical collar is in place, the patient should be transferred onto a backboard. As soon as the patient is centered on the backboard, blanket rolls or blocks should be placed so that the patient's spine is laterally stabilized. The patient's head should then be secured with straps to the board; finally, the patient's chest, hips, and knees should also be secured to the backboard with straps.

STABILIZING THE CERVICAL SPINE

A patient is especially at risk for injury of the cervical spine in motor vehicle accidents that involve blunt impact with the windshield or ejection and high-speed motorcycle crashes as well as other types of direct facial, head, and neck injuries. If the patient has a suspected C1 or C2 injury or cervical compression fractures based on neurological assessment, a rigid cervical collar should be applied to limit motion. However, the cervical collar alone will not prevent flexion/extension movement, so it must be used in conjunction with a cervical immobilization device, which has restraining straps for the patient's forehead and chin. The cervical immobilization device is secured to a short or long spinal board. If the patient has difficulty breathing after cervical immobilization, the patient may require intubation and ventilation. If the patient is wearing a helmet and shoulder pads, they should be left in place until the patient arrives at the receiving facility unless they must be removed to secure the airway or better immobilize the head.

ISSUES OF TRANSPORT MODE AND DESTINATION

Issues that arise surrounding transport modes and destination when handling trauma include:

- Patient's triage status and duration of time needed for transport
- Distance from receiving institution
- Patient's need for specialized equipment or medical specialists and availability in ambulance and at receiving institution
- Airlift vs ambulance transport for critically ill
- Low acuity patient's insistence on transport to hospital when transport is deemed unnecessary
- Patient refusal to be transported to hospital
- Patient incompetent to make decisions about transport or unconscious and unable to make decisions
- Use of lights or sirens continuously, intermittently, or not at all (Lights-only may be used to minimize patient's anxiety and to reduce distractions for the transport team. Sirens may be used intermittently at intersections and when traffic congestion is slowing progress.)
- Patient dies prior to transportation
- Patient dies en route (Regulations may vary by state and jurisdiction but may require the ambulance to wait for the medical examiner.)

Neurologic

NEUROLOGICAL SYSTEM

The neurological (nervous) system consists of the **central nervous system (CNS)**, which contains the brain, spinal cord and nerves, and the **peripheral nervous system (PNS)**, which contains the sensory neurons, ganglia (nerve clusters), and nerves connecting to the CNS. The brain consists of the **cerebrum** (frontal, temporal, parietal, and occipital lobes); the **cerebellum**; and the **brain stem**, which is continuous with the spinal cord. The PNS is divided into the **autonomic nervous system (ANS)** and the **somatic nervous system (SoNS)**. The autonomic nervous system controls the body's organs and maintains homeostasis (balance). Functions of the ANS include control of the heart rate and function, respiration, digestion, sexual arousal, and other systems. The SoNS comprises cranial and spinal nerves that connect the CNS to the skeletal muscles and skin. The SoNS is the voluntarily controlled component of the PNS, and it receives and responds to external sensory stimuli from the skin and sensory organs.

Review Video: Brain Anatomy
Visit mometrix.com/academy and enter code: 222476

Review Video: Somatic Nervous System
Visit mometrix.com/academy and enter code: 100382

Anatomy of the Brain and Spinal Cord

The brain is protected by the skull and the meninges, the three layers of lining: the dura mater, arachnoid mater, and the pia mater. Brain tissue is comprised of gray matter (neurons [nerve cells]) and white matter (covered nerve pathways that conduct messages). The main part of the brain is the cerebrum, which is comprised of two hemispheres that contain the frontal parietal, temporal, and occipital lobes. The cerebrum controls higher brain functions, including thought, speech, vision, hearing, and action. The cerebellum lies in the back of the brain below the cerebrum and controls the equilibrium and coordination. The brain stem controls involuntary functions, such as respirations, heart rate, temperature control, and nerve transmission. The brain stem is continuous with the spinal cord, which is also protected by the meninges and the vertebrae (cervical, thoracic, and lumbar). Cerebrospinal fluid circulates within the subarachnoid space of the brain and the spinal cord.

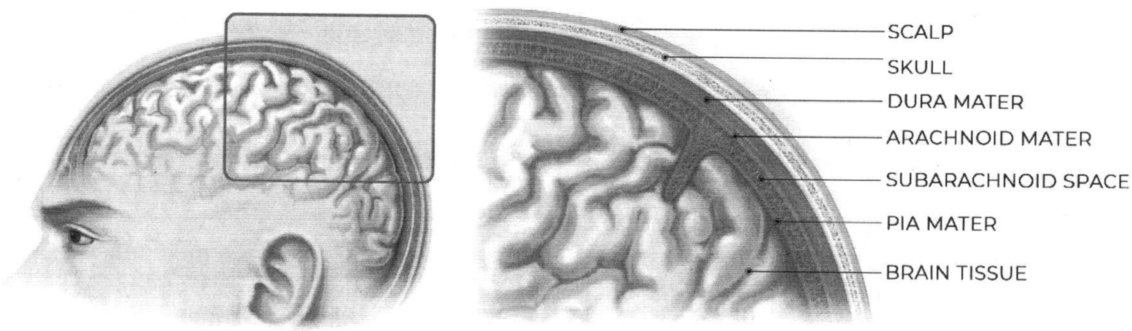

Neurologic Assessment

Mental Status

When assessing a patient's mental status, note:

- Level of consciousness: AVPU assessment.
- Posture and behavior: Abnormal findings include restlessness, agitation, bizarre posturing, catatonia (immobility), and tics or other abnormal movements.
- Dress, grooming and hygiene: Kempt/unkempt, clean/dirty.
- Facial expressions: May vary widely (anxious, depressed, angry, sad, elated, fearful). Note whether expressions seem appropriate to situation/words.

- Speech/Language: Quantity, appropriate/inappropriate, rate, fluency. Note aphasia (inability to speak and/or understand words), dysphonia (abnormal voice/difficulty speaking), or dysarthria (difficulty speaking words).
- Mood: Nature and duration of current mood. Suicidal ideation.
- Thoughts/Perceptions: Note logic, relevance, and organization of thoughts and abnormal findings, such as thought blocking (sudden period of silence in the middle of sentence while speaking), flight of ideas (racing thoughts), incoherence, confabulation (producing distorted memories), loose association (responses not connected to questions or one sentence not connected to next), or transference (redirecting emotions to a substitute). Note homicidal or suicidal thoughts, obsessions, compulsions, delusions, illusions, and hallucinations.
- Judgment: Note insight, ability to make decisions, plan.

Stages of Consciousness

While there may be some motor skill deficiencies and/or confusion with an **alert patient**, he/she is still able to respond well to questions and is able to actively participate in a mental status examination. A **lethargic patient** generally displays characteristics of being drowsy; he/she may also appear to actually be asleep. While a lethargic patient may appear drowsy or asleep, he/she can be awakened relatively easily and can respond to questions in a reasonable manner. An **obtunded patient** is not awakened as easily as a lethargic patient, and he/she does not respond well to questions. The obtunded patient may participate in a mental status examination by responding to questions, but his/her responses tend to be difficult to understand, and the responses are typically not provided in the form of complete sentences.

Levels of the Unconscious State

The two levels of the unconscious state are stuporous and comatose. A **stuporous patient** is one who exhibits an extremely small degree of awareness without being able to communicate in a clear, appropriate manner. The stuporous patient often utters inappropriate words and/or moans in an incomprehensible fashion. A patient can either be in a light stuporous state or a deep stupor. A patient in a light stupor is generally able to respond to pain by moving his/her extremities in an attempt to protect against the source of the pain. However, a patient in a deep stupor typically does not display this protection response and often does not respond to pain at all. **Coma** is the ultimate state of unconsciousness in which a patient displays no signs of alertness. The comatose patient cannot be awakened with stimulation and does not respond to painful stimuli.

Cranial Nerve Assessment

Cranial Nerves I, II, and III

Cranial nerve I, the olfactory nerve, controls a person's sense of smell. Cranial nerve I can be evaluated by asking a patient to identify a familiar smell such as an orange. Cranial nerve II, the optic nerve, controls the visual field and sharpness of vision. Cranial nerve II can be evaluated by holding a certain number of fingers in front of a patient and asking him/her to identify the number of fingers. The optic nerve can also be assessed by moving an object along the patient's peripheral area and asking him/her to identify when the object comes into his/her line of vision. Cranial nerve III is the oculomotor nerve, which controls the pupil's reaction to stimuli. This nerve can be evaluated by shining a light in the patient's eye and observing the response of the pupil. A healthy, normal pupil will promptly constrict when it encounters direct light.

Cranial Nerves IV, V, and VI

Cranial nerve IV, the trochlear nerve, is partially responsible for eye movement. Cranial nerve IV can be evaluated by asking a patient to follow another person's finger as it moves using only his/her eyes and not moving his/her head. Cranial nerve V, the trigeminal nerve, controls facial sensation and pain. Cranial nerve V can be evaluated by touching a patient's face to monitor for a response. Cranial nerve VI is the abducens nerve, which controls ocular motor function. This nerve can be evaluated by examining a patient's lateral eye movements.

CRANIAL NERVES VII, VIII, AND IX

Cranial nerve VII, the facial nerve, is responsible for motor functions in the patient's face. Cranial nerve VII can be evaluated by asking a patient to perform various facial movements and/or to make certain expressions. Cranial nerve VIII is the acoustic nerve; it is responsible for hearing and balance. The hearing component can be evaluated by making a noise such as a finger snap near a patient's ear and monitoring for a response. The balance component can be evaluated by performing Rhomberg's test. Rhomberg's test is conducted by having the patient stand with his/her eyes open, hands at his/her sides, and feet together; next, the patient stands in this position with his/her eyes closed for one minute to monitor whether he/she falls. Cranial nerve IX is the glossopharyngeal nerve, which controls swallowing and taste. This nerve can be evaluated by using a tongue depressor to test the patient's gag reflex.

CRANIAL NERVES X, XI, AND XII

Cranial nerve X, the vagus nerve, is partially responsible for tasks such as heart rate. Cranial nerve X can be evaluated by monitoring a patient's heart rate and/or his/her blood pressure, which may both be lowered if the vagus nerve is activated. Cranial nerve XI, the spinal accessory nerve, controls neck movement. Having a patient shrug his/her shoulders up and down is a good way to evaluate how cranial nerve XI is performing. Cranial nerve XII is the hypoglossal nerve, which controls tongue movements. The hypoglossal nerve can be evaluated by having a patient stick out his/her tongue and press against a tongue depressor to resist it; this provides an effective measure of tongue strength.

GLASGOW COMA SCALE

The Glasgow coma scale (GCS) measures the depth and duration of coma or impaired level of consciousness and is used for post-operative assessment. The GCS measures three parameters: Best eye response, best verbal response, and best motor response, with a total possible score that ranges from 3–15:

Eye opening	4: Spontaneous. 3: To verbal stimuli. 2: To pain (not of face). 1: No response.
Verbal	5: Oriented. 4: Conversation confused, but can answer questions. 3: Uses inappropriate words. 2: Speech incomprehensible. 1: No response.
Motor	6: Moves on command. 5: Moves purposefully respond pain. 4: Withdraws in response to pain. 3: Decorticate posturing (flexion) in response to pain. 2: Decerebrate posturing (extension) in response to pain. 1: No response.

Injuries/conditions are classified according to the total score: 3-8 Coma; ≤ 8 Severe head injury; 9-12 Moderate head injury; 13-15 Mild head injury.

CHEYNE-STOKES RESPIRATIONS

Often seen in patients who sustain significant head injuries, Cheyne-Stokes respiration is a pattern of abnormal breathing. The pattern is characterized by periods of shallow breathing alternating with periods of deep breathing. While the pattern involves a change in the volume of inspiration, the rate of respiration tends to remain fairly regular. Many patients who sustain significant head injuries develop increased intracranial pressure as well, and the Cheyne-Stokes pattern is frequently the first pattern of abnormal breathing to appear in such cases. The abnormal pattern is a result of a malfunction in the respiratory center of the brain.

Reflex Responses

Primitive, Superficial, and Deep

There are three categories of reflex responses:

- **Primitive reflexes** are typically present only in infants; adults who exhibit primitive reflexes have typically suffered from stroke or some type of damage to the brain. Primitive reflexes include such reflexes as grasping, which occurs when an infant closes his/her hand around an adult's finger, and rooting, which is characterized by an infant turning his/her head and making a sucking motion in response to cheek stroking.
- **Superficial reflexes** include the abdominal, anal, conjunctival, corneal, cremasteric, and plantar reflexes. When assessed, superficial reflexes can support or refute the functioning of cutaneous innervation as well as the motor functioning of the corresponding part of the reflex being assessed.
- **Deep tendon reflexes**, which include the ankle, biceps, brachioradialis, patellar, and triceps, are reflexes of the tendons that attach the muscles located next to bones to the bones themselves.

Assessing Superficial Reflexes

When the **abdominal reflex** is tested by stimulating the skin covering the abdomen, the muscles of the abdominal wall should contract. Irritating a patient's perianal skin, the skin around the opening of the rectum, will cause the anal sphincter to contract if the **anal reflex** is intact. A patient's eyelid will close when the conjunctiva is touched if his/her **conjunctival reflex** is working. Additionally, a patient will blink when the cornea is stimulated if his/her **corneal reflex** is intact; this reflex is also known as the blink reflex. The **cremasteric reflex** is specific to males; when this reflex is functioning, the cremaster muscle will contract and pull up the patient's scrotum and testis upon stimulation of the front and inner thigh. The **plantar reflex** can be tested by stroking the outer surface of the soles of a patient's feet, which should cause his/her toes to flex.

Assessing Deep Tendon Reflexes

The **biceps reflex** can be observed when the examiner places his/her thumb over the patient's biceps tendon at the elbow, strikes his/her thumb with a reflex hammer, and watches for movement in the patient's arm. The **triceps reflex** can be observed when the examiner holds the patient's upper arm in one hand and strikes the triceps tendon, located on the back side of the arm just above the elbow, with a reflex hammer. With the patient's lower arm hanging in a relaxed position, it should swing away from the patient's body in response to the hammer strikes. With the patient's arm resting in his/her lap, the **brachioradialis reflex** can be observed by striking the brachioradialis tendon, located in approximately the middle of the superior side of the patient's lower arm, with a reflex hammer.

The **ankle reflex**, which is sometimes referred to as the Achilles reflex, can be observed by holding the patient's foot in a dorsiflexed position, in which the foot is bent backwards towards the patient, and tapping the Achilles tendon, which connects the heel bone and the calf muscle, with a reflex hammer. The **patellar reflex**, which is also known as the knee jerk reflex, is best observed while the patient is in a seated position with his/her legs hanging over the edge of the examining surface. When the patellar tendon, located just at the bottom of the kneecap on the front side of the patient's knee, is struck with a reflex hammer, the patient's lower leg should extend outward at the knee, making a small kicking motion.

Assessing Gross Motor Skills

Gross motor skills are skills typically acquired during infancy and early childhood that involve an individual's large muscle groups; tasks involving gross motor skills typically require the patient's body to move in a coordinated manner. A number of activities can determine a patient's gross motor skills functioning; examples of such activities include walking, balancing on one leg, and jumping or hopping. Contrary to fine motor skills, gross motor skills do not decline when a patient is presented with a stressful situation; gross motor skill functioning has actually been found to improve when a patient encounters stress.

ASSESSING FINE MOTOR SKILLS

Fine motor skills are skills that generally require eye-hand coordination, as they are skills that involve smaller muscle groups. Activities that involve hand-eye coordination can help determine a patient's fine motor skills functioning; examples of such activities include having a patient pick up a small object in one hand and transfer the object to the opposite hand, writing a series of words on paper, and threading beads onto a string. Other activities that utilize a patient's smaller muscle groups and subsequently test his/her fine motor skills include whistling, making facial expressions, and articulating specific words.

CONCUSSIONS

A concussion is a brain injury in which structural damage is not apparent but neurological functioning is impaired. Patients may experience a brief loss of consciousness after a head injury and may experience confusion and even bizarre behavior (if the frontal lobe is affected). Other symptoms include severe headache, somnolence, dizziness, lack of coordination, confusion, disorientation, inappropriate emotional response, nausea, and vomiting. Symptoms are usually transient (lasting from minutes to hours), but up to 50% may have recurrent symptoms (such as difficulty concentrating, headaches, and dizziness) for months. The **American Academy of Neurology classifies concussions** as follows:

- **Grade 1**: Transient confusion without loss of consciousness, with symptoms resolving in <15 minutes
- **Grade 2**: Transient confusion without loss of consciousness, with symptoms resolving in >15 minutes
- **Grade 3**: Any loss of consciousness of any duration

Interventions: Provide supportive care and reassurance, monitor vital signs and neurological status for signs of increasing intracranial pressure that may indicate more severe injury, and elevate the patient's head.

BRAIN INJURIES, THE COUP/CONTRECOUP PATTERN, AND POSTURING

Primary brain injuries are those that result from the original trauma and include direct damage to brain tissue, such as may occur with a gunshot wound. **Secondary brain injuries** result from the effects of the primary injury, such as increasing intracranial pressure, ischemia (most common), hemorrhage, edema, and brain herniation.

Coup/Contrecoup injuries are common in motor vehicle accidents and shaken baby syndrome. With acceleration/deceleration and contact injuries where the head hits a fixed object (such as a windshield) and snaps back from the impact, coup (on the side of impact) and contrecoup (on the opposite side) contusions may both occur.

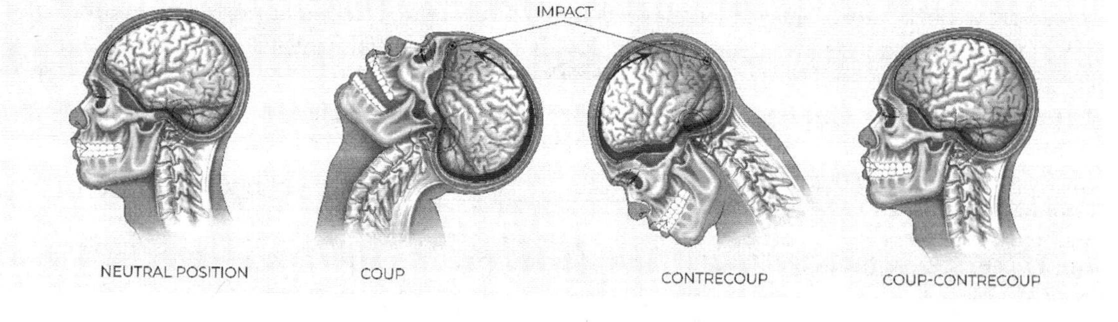

Decerebrate (extension) posturing (with the body stiff, legs straight, feet extended, arms straight, and the head/neck arched back) is associated with severe midbrain damage. **Decorticate (flexion) posturing** (with the body stiff, legs straight, and hands clenched on the chest) is associated with damage to the pathway connecting the brain and spinal cord and may include damage to the cerebral cortex, white matter, or basal ganglia.

Decerebrate Posturing

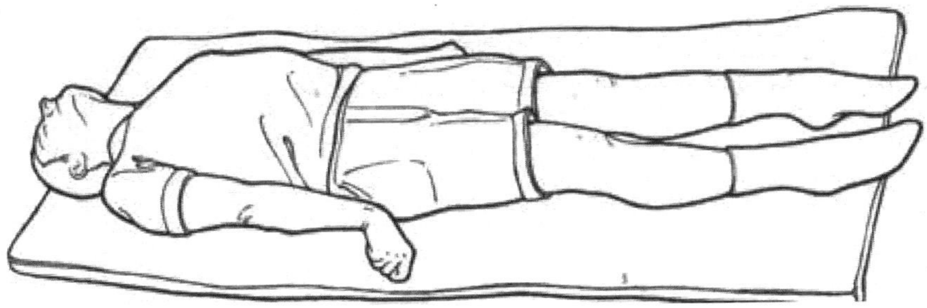

Decorticate Posturing

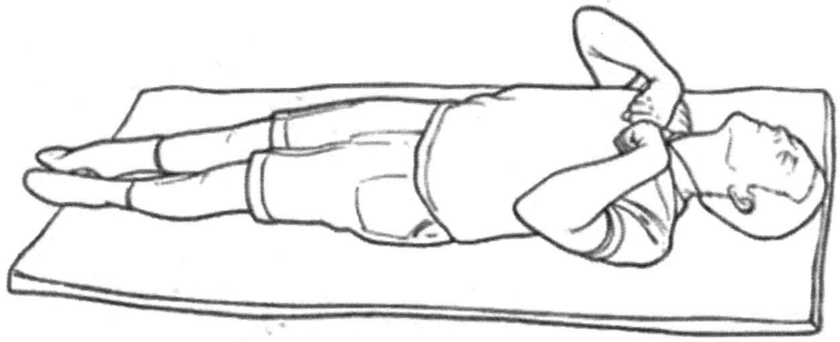

Cerebral Edema and Increased Intracranial Pressure

Head injuries that occur at the time of trauma include fractures, contusions, hematomas, and diffuse cerebral and vascular injury. These injuries may result in hypoxia, increased intracranial pressure, and cerebral edema. Open injuries may result in infection. Patients often suffer initial hypertension, which increases intracranial pressure, decreasing perfusion. Often the primary problem with head trauma is a significant increase in swelling, which also interferes with perfusion, causing hypoxia and hypercapnia, which trigger increased blood flow. This increased volume at a time when injury impairs auto-regulation increases cerebral edema, which, in turn, increases intracranial pressure and results in a further decrease in perfusion with resultant ischemia. If pressure continues to rise, the brain may herniate. Concomitant hypotension may result in hypoventilation, further complicating treatment. During transport continuously monitor neurological status and vitals. Treatments include:

- Monitoring ICP and CCP
- Providing oxygen
- Elevating head of stretcher and maintaining body alignment
- Giving medications: Analgesics, anticonvulsants, and anesthetics
- Providing blood/fluids to stabilize hemodynamics
- Managing airway, providing mechanical ventilation if needed
- Providing osmotic agents, such as mannitol and hypertonic saline solution, to reduce cerebral edema.

ICP Monitoring

Intracranial pressure (ICP) is the pressure applied on the brain tissue, cerebrospinal fluid, and the blood circulating in the brain by the skull. In adult patients, signs of increased ICP can include vomiting; headaches; seizure activity; neurologic deficits such as an inability to speak, coordination difficulties, or changes in vision; behavioral changes; and/or a decrease in LOC. The intraventricular catheter may be used to monitor ICP and to drain excess CSF. CSF may be drained continuously or intermittently and must be monitored hourly for amount, color, and character. For ICP measurement, the patient's head must be elevated to 30–45° and the transducer leveled to the outer canthus of the eye. Normal ICP is 0-15 mmHg on transducer or 80-180 mm H_2O

on manometer. Transport nurses should be familiar with ICP monitoring devices before interfacility transport. Never flush a device used for ICP monitoring, never used heparinized solution in the pressure tubing (only sterile NaCl), keep system free of air with tight connections, and use care when positioning patient to avoid decannulation. Be prepared to follow other orders to manage increases in ICP during transport including giving Mannitol, dexamethasone, draining CSF, and vasopressors for keep bp with a defined range. All orders should be reviewed before transporting this patient.

Managing the Patient with a Ventriculostomy

A ventriculostomy involves placing a catheter in the ventricles of the brain. The catheter is attached to external tubing with a sampling port, a transducer (which must be leveled to the ear), a manometer, and drainage tub/bag in order to obtain the most accurate ICP measurements, allow for drainage of CSF (intermittently, not continuously) to control pressure, and to sample CSF. A ventriculostomy is required when there is obstruction in the brain, most often from bleeding or swelling that prevents adequate drainage of CSF, which is constantly produced at a rate of about 600–700 mL in 24 hours. The patient must be monitored continuously to ensure proper positioning, as sitting up during CSF drainage may result in rapid loss of CSF and damage to brain tissue. The drain must be clamped while the patient's position is changed. The transport nurse must monitor pressure, drain CSF if pressure increases above baseline per protocol, monitor neurological signs, and assess insertion site and character of CSF for signs of infection.

Intracranial Hematomas

<table>
<tr><th>Type</th><th>Characteristics</th><th>Prehospital</th></tr>
<tr><td>Epidural</td><td>Bleeding between the dura and the skull, pushing the brain downward and inward. The hemorrhage is usually caused by arterial tears, so bleeding is often rapid, leading to severe neurological deficits and respiratory arrest. The patient may be lucid and without symptoms for 2–6 hours after the injury.</td><td rowspan="2">Provide supportive care, keep the patient's head elevated to reduce intracranial pressure, note neurological status (movement, strength, mental status, pupils equal and reactive or unequal/fixed), and provide rapid transport. Provide an IV access line and fluids.</td></tr>
<tr><td>Subdural</td><td>Bleeding between the dura and the arachnoid mater, usually from tears in the cortical veins of the subdural space. It tends to develop more slowly than an epidural hemorrhage. If the bleeding is acute and develops within minutes or hours of injury, then the prognosis is poor. Subacute hematomas that develop more slowly cause varying degrees of injury.</td></tr>
<tr><td>Intracerebral</td><td>Bleeding into the substance of the brain from an artery. Sudden onset; it results in a hemorrhagic stroke with a lack of nutrients and oxygen to parts of the brain. May result from degenerative changes, hypertension, brain tumors, medications, or illicit drugs (crack, cocaine). Symptoms vary depending on the site, but they may include one-sided weakness, paralysis, difficulty speaking, severe headache, and altered mental status.</td><td rowspan="2">Provide supportive care, keep the patient's head elevated to reduce intracranial pressure, note neurological status (movement, strength, mental status, pupils equal and reactive or unequal/fixed), provide rapid transport, start an IV access line, and give fluids.</td></tr>
<tr><td>Subarachnoid</td><td>Bleeding in the space between the meninges and brain and into the cerebrospinal fluid, usually resulting from aneurysm, arteriovenous malformation (AVM), or trauma. This type of hemorrhage compresses the brain tissue. The first presenting symptoms are severe headache, nausea and vomiting, nuchal rigidity, palsy related to cranial nerve compression, retinal hemorrhages, and papilledema.</td></tr>
</table>

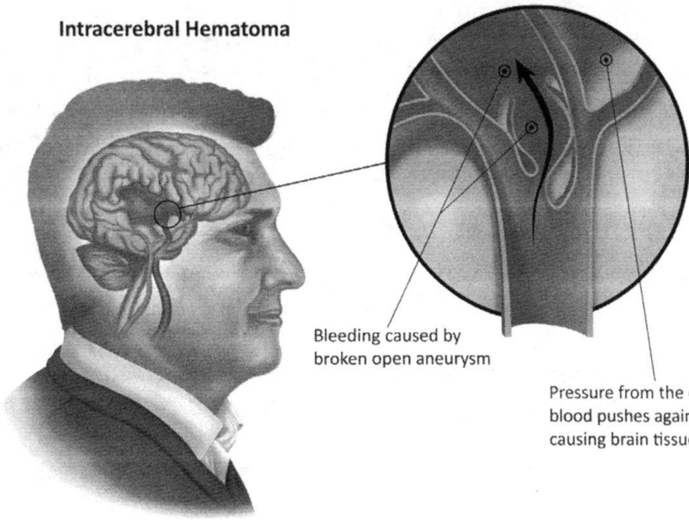

Hypoxic Encephalopathy

Cerebral hypoxia (hypoxic encephalopathy) occurs when the oxygen supply to the brain is decreased. If hypoxia is mild, the brain compensates by increasing cerebral blood flow, but it can only double in volume and cannot compensate for severe hypoxic conditions. Hypoxia may be the result of insufficient oxygen in the environment, inadequate exchange at the alveolar level of the lungs, or inadequate circulation to the brain. Brain cells may begin dying within 5 minutes if deprived of adequate oxygenation, so any condition or trauma that interferes with oxygenation can result in brain damage:

- Near-drowning
- Asphyxia
- Cardiac arrest
- High altitude sickness
- Carbon monoxide
- Diseases that interfere with respiration, such as myasthenia gravis and amyotrophic lateral sclerosis
- Anesthesia complications

Symptoms include increasing neurological deficits, depending upon the degree and area of damage, with changes in mentation that range from confusion to coma. Prompt identification of the cause and increase in perfusion to the brain is critical for survival.

Concerning Causes of Ear Drainage

Inflammation or infection of some kind is one of the most common causes of ear drainage. Otitis externa, also known as swimmer's ear, is an inflammation that occurs in the ear canal or in the outer ear. The condition generally causes ear pain, itching or irritation, and ear drainage. Otitis media is an infection of the middle ear that can cause ear pain, a feeling of overall illness, vomiting, diarrhea, and/or hearing loss in the infected ear. Both otitis externa and otitis media are infections that can cause ear drainage. Certain things such as traumatic head injury, sudden changes in pressure, and extremely loud noises can rupture a patient's eardrum, which can also lead to ear drainage. Conditions that cause skin inflammation, such as eczema, can result in bleeding from the ear as well.

After a traumatic head injury, ear drainage that is suspected to be CSF can be tested quickly using the halo test, by placing a drop of the drainage on a filter paper. If the fluid creates a rapidly advancing halo ring it is most likely CSF, however this test can't differentiate between CSF and saliva.

INDICATIONS FOR HYPERVENTILATION FOR TRAUMATIC BRAIN INJURY

While routine hyperventilation is not recommended as a first line of treatment in the majority of patients who have sustained traumatic brain injuries, there are instances with such patients in which hyperventilation may be indicated. Hyperventilation is indicated if the patient with a traumatic brain injury exhibits dilation in one or both pupils. Additionally, if the patient's pupils do not react in a balanced—or symmetric—manner, hyperventilation is likely indicated. It may also be indicated in patients who do not respond to pain and/or in patients who display other evidence of neurological deterioration.

SPINAL INJURIES AND SPINAL CORD INJURIES (SCIS)

Spinal injuries of the vertebrae include fractures, dislocations, open wounds, and flexion and extension injuries. Because the spinal cord lies within the vertebral column, injury to the vertebrae may cause spinal cord injuries (SCIs) and disrupt transmissions in nerves that connect the body and the brain. SCI may affect only a few nerves, or they may completely transect the spinal cord, resulting in permanent paralysis below the site of injury. SCIs should be suspected with head trauma, penetrating trauma, direct blunt trauma, falls, diving injuries, motor vehicle accidents, rapid deceleration accidents, and multisystem trauma. Assessment includes evaluating extremity movement, respiration control, sensation, reflexes, pain/tenderness, and vital signs.

Interventions: Logroll the patient to examine his or her back, immobilize the patient (seated or standing), apply a rigid cervical collar, lift and move him or her with care, and provide rapid transport. Elevate the torso of children 2–3 cm with padding so that the head is in a neutral position if using an adult immobilization device. Immobilize infants in their car seats, padding all the voids.

Spinal cord injuries (SCIs) may result from blunt trauma (such as automobile accidents), falls from a height, sports injuries, and penetrating trauma (such as a gunshot or knife wound). Damage results from mechanical injury and secondary responses resulting from hemorrhage, edema, and ischemia. The types of symptoms relate to the area and degree of injury, as below:

- **Anterior cord**: This results from pressure/damage to the anterior spinal cord. The posterior column functions remain, so there are sensations of touch, vibration, and position remaining below the injury but with complete paralysis and loss of the sensations of pain and temperature. The prognosis is poor.
- **Brown-Séquard**: The cord is hemisected from penetrating trauma, resulting in spastic paresis, loss of sense of position and vibration on the injured side, and loss of pain and temperature sensation on the other side. The prognosis is good.
- **Posterior cord**: Motor function is preserved but without sensation.
- **Conus medullaris**: Injury to the lower spine (lower lumbar and sacral nerves).
- **Central cord**: This results from hyperextension or hyperflexion and ischemia or stenosis of the cervical spine, causing spinal contusion and quadriparesis (more severe in the upper extremities) with some loss of sensations of pain and temperature. Prognosis is good, but fine motor skills are often impaired in the upper extremities with paresis being more acute distally than proximally in the arms.

CAUDA EQUINA

Cauda equina is caused by compression damage to the spinal cord that occurs below L-1 to lumbar and sacral nerve roots with variable loss of motor ability, reflexes, and sensation in the groin area and bowel, bladder, and sexual dysfunction. Injury is to peripheral nerves descending from the end of the spinal cord. These nerves can regenerate so prognosis is better than for other lesions of the spinal cord. Initial symptoms may be non-specific with complaints of severe lower back pain and frequently weakness and pain both legs (sciatica). Patients may complain of saddle anesthesia (impaired sensation in the perineal area. Sensation of the lower extremities may be impaired as well. Cauda equina should be suspected with patients who present with lower back pain because it can lead to paraplegia if improperly cared for. Causes may include traumatic spinal injury, malignancy, stenosis, fracture, or infection.

Interventions: Question the patient specifically about saddle anesthesia, lower extremity weakness, and difficulty urinating. Patient should be transported in a position of comfort to a facility with MRI and neurosurgeons available because of the need for surgical decompression. Monitor VS.

Neurogenic Shock

Neurogenic shock occurs with injury to the CNS above T6 (from trauma resulting in acute spinal cord injury and from blunt and penetrating injuries), neurological diseases, drugs, or anesthesia, and it impairs the ANS that controls the cardiovascular system. Symptoms include hypotension and warm, dry skin related to the lack of vascular tone that results in hypothermia from loss of cutaneous heat. Bradycardia is a common but not universal symptom. The severity of symptoms relates to the level of injury, with injuries above T1 capable of causing disruption of the entire somatic nervous system and with lower injuries causing various degrees of disruption. Even incomplete SCIs can cause neurogenic shock.

Interventions: Monitor the patient's airway/ventilation/oxygen supplementation, start an IV access line with fluid resuscitation with crystalloid to keep mean arterial pressure at 85-90 mmHg to maintain oxygen saturation >90%, perform spinal immobilization, administer norepinephrine or dopamine (per protocol) if hypotension persists and atropine for severe bradycardia, and provide rapid transport.

Nerve Injuries

Nerve root injury occurs when nerves have been damaged in the spine because of trauma or compression (such as from herniated disc, arthritis, bone spurs, and tumors). Pain may occur from damage to one or multiple nerve roots. Common nerve root injuries occur in the lumbar area, resulting in lower back and leg pain (more severe below the knee), and the brachial area, resulting in pain in the arm, which may radiate to the hand. Patients may complain of numbness and tingling, muscle weakness, impaired sensation, and pain.

Peripheral nerve injury may occur from trauma or medical disorders, such as diabetes mellitus, carpal tunnel syndrome, Guillain-Barré syndrome, arthritis, tumors, and lupus erythematosus. Symptoms vary widely and may include pain, numbness, tingling, muscle weakness and/or cramps, difficulty walking, balance disturbance, heat intolerance, GI upset, hyperhidrosis, and BP changes.

Interventions: Assess symptoms, obtain history. Monitor VS, oxygen saturation, and circulation, movement, pain, and sensation in affected limbs. Transport in position of comfort.

Thoracic

Chest Wounds

Chest wounds can be characterized as sucking wounds or impalements.

- **Sucking wounds**: This is an open pneumothorax in which air is sucked into the thoracic cavity, deflating the lung, usually through a penny-size or larger wound. Patients will exhibit respiratory distress, absent breath sounds on the affected side, wound gurgling on inspiration, and bubbling of blood around the wound. Interventions: Apply an occlusive dressing with an Asherman Chest Seal dressing or with Vaseline gauze covered with secured (taped on three sides) plastic wrap or aluminum foil and place the patient in a position of comfort.
- **Impalement**: This is a penetrating wound with an object impaled into the chest. Symptoms may be similar to those listed above, depending on the site of impalement and the depth. Impalement may cause hemothorax, tension pneumothorax, or pericardial tamponade. Interventions: Expose the wound area, and secure the object manually with a bulky dressing. Do not remove the object unless it is necessary for performing chest compressions (CPR). Control any bleeding.

Fractured Ribs and Flail Chest

Fractured ribs usually result from severe blunt trauma (motor vehicle accident, physical abuse). Underlying injuries should be expected according to the area of fractures as follows:

- Upper two ribs: Injuries to the trachea, bronchi, or great vessels
- Right-sided ≥ rib 8: Liver trauma
- Left-sided ≥ rib 8: Spleen trauma

Pain may be the primary symptom of rib fractures, resulting in shallow breathing.

Flail chest (more common in adults and adolescents than children) occurs when at least three adjacent ribs are fractured, anteriorly and posteriorly, so that they float free of the rib cage. Variations include the sternum floating with ribs fractured on both sides. With flail chest, the chest wall cannot support changes in intrathoracic pressure, so paradoxical respirations occur with the flail area contracting on inspiration and expanding on expiration. Ventilation decreases.

Interventions: Manage the patient's airway/ventilation/oxygen supplementation (PPV with BVM or intubation). Provide cardiac monitoring, an IV access line, and supportive care. Observe for signs of tension pneumothorax or hemothorax.

Tension Pneumothorax

If not treated promptly, a sucking chest wound (open pneumothorax) may progress to a tension pneumothorax, especially if mechanical ventilation is used. A tension pneumothorax occurs when pressure in the pleural space exceeds that of the atmosphere, causing a mediastinal shift (which is usually difficult to assess visually) with displacement of the trachea away from the affected site, putting pressure against the great vessels (decreasing cardiac output), and putting pressure against the heart (resulting in tachycardia). Patients are usually in severe respiratory distress with jugular vein distension, absent breath sounds on the affected side, narrow pulse pressure, pulsus paradoxus, and unequal chest rise.

Interventions: Place an airtight seal or Asherman Chest Seal over the open wound, manage the patient's airway/ventilation/oxygen supplementation to an oxygen saturation level of ≥94%, provide cardiac monitoring, start an IV access line, and provide rapid transport. Tension pneumothorax will require needle decompression or insertion of a chest tube (according to protocol).

Hemothorax

Hemothorax occurs with bleeding into the pleural space, usually from major vascular injury such as tears in the intercostal vessels, lacerations of the great vessels, or trauma to the lung tissue. Hemothorax is most common with penetrating wounds. A small bleed may be self-limiting and seal, but a tear in a large vessel can result in massive bleeding, followed quickly by hypovolemic shock from decreased circulating blood. The pressure from the blood may result in the inability of the lung to ventilate and a mediastinal shift. Clots in the chest area may trigger fibrinolysis, which breaks down clots and increases bleeding. Often a hemothorax occurs with a pneumothorax, especially in severe chest trauma. Further symptoms include severe respiratory distress, decreased breath sounds, unequal breath sounds, dullness on auscultation, jugular venous distension, and shock.

Interventions: Manage the patient's airway/ventilation/oxygen supplementation, provide an IV access line and fluid bolus for shock but avoid aggressive fluids because of the risk of hemodilution, provide the patient a position of comfort (the shock position if necessary), and provide rapid transport.

Cardiac Tamponade

Cardiac tamponade occurs when fluid, usually blood, accumulates in the pericardial sac. If the fluid accumulates rapidly, the walls of the pericardial sac do not have time to stretch to accommodate the fluid, so the patient may quickly develop pulseless electrical activity (PEA) with fluid accumulation of 50-250 mL. If fluid accumulates slowly, such as with pericardial effusions associated with cancer, patients may tolerate up to 2 L of fluid before symptoms become acute. Cardiac tamponade compresses the heart and limits the venous return to the heart and blood flow into the ventricles, thereby reducing cardiac output. Symptoms: Beck's triad includes decreased arterial BP, increased jugular venous distension, and muffled heart sounds. Patients may be anxious, dyspneic, dizzy, and have angina-like pain.

Interventions: Manage airway/high concentration oxygen, monitor the ECG, provide an IV access line and fluids as indicated, and provide rapid transport for pericardiocentesis.

Blunt Cardiac Trauma

Blunt cardiac trauma most often occurs as the result of motor vehicle accidents, falls, or other blows to the chest, which can result in respiratory distress as well as hypovolemia from rupture of the great vessels of the heart and/or cardiac failure from cardiac tamponade or increasing intrathoracic pressure. The heart is particularly vulnerable to chest trauma, with the right atrium and right ventricle being the most commonly injured because they are anterior to the rest of the heart. **Commotio cordis,** an often-lethal dysrhythmia from a blow to the pericardial area, may occur (most common in young males with sports injuries). Cardiac trauma may be difficult to identify because of other injuries, but if it is suspected, an ECG should be done and any abnormalities (dysrhythmias, ST changes, sinus tachycardia, or heart block) should be noted. Decreased cardiac output and cerebral oxygenation may result in severe agitation with combative behavior.

Interventions: Provide CPR and defibrillation if indicated; manage the patient's airway/ventilation/oxygen supplementation; provide an IV access line with severe injury; and monitor changes in the patient's level of consciousness.

Myocardial and Pulmonary Contusion

A myocardial contusion occurs when the heart muscle is bruised. Patients often sustain myocardial contusion from motor vehicle accidents, aggressive chest compressions during cardiopulmonary resuscitation (CPR) efforts, and/or blunt chest trauma resulting from a fall. Symptoms of the condition are typically mild. Many patients with myocardial contusion feel as though their heart is racing, and they also frequently experience pain in their breastbone.

A pulmonary contusion occurs when the lung becomes bruised. High-velocity motor vehicle accidents are a common cause of pulmonary contusion. Symptoms of the condition may include the presence of rales during inhalation, an increased rate of respiration, and/or breathing difficulties.

Traumatic Asphyxia

Traumatic asphyxia occurs when severe crushing pressure on the chest pushes against the heart, forcing blood from the right side of the heart back into the venous system (superior vena cava), including the neck and head veins, resulting in inadequate oxygenation to the upper extremities, face, and brain. Symptoms include altered mental status, seizures, swollen tongue, subconjunctival hemorrhages in the eyes, and cyanosis of the arms.

Interventions: Manage the patient's airway/ventilation/oxygen supplementation, provide supportive care, provide cardiac monitoring, and start an IV access line with fluid bolus for shock.

Traumatic Aortic Disruption

Traumatic aortic disruption occurs when the aorta is torn or ruptures as the result of trauma, usually blunt injury, such as in a motor vehicle accident. Massive bleeding may occur and the trauma is often fatal unless the tear is partial-thickness and the blood is contained in a pseudo aneurysm (sac). Patients may complain of chest, back, or abdominal pain and may exhibit signs of shock (dyspnea, pallor, hypotension, tachycardia, cool/clammy skin). A harsh systolic murmur may be evident, and circulation to the lower extremities may be impaired, with faint or absent palpable pulses and decreased blood pressure.

Interventions: Continually assess vital signs, oxygen saturation, and ECG. Assess level of pain (1-10 numeric scale), provide 100% oxygen with non-rebreather mask, administer analgesia per protocol and antiemetic if nauseated to prevent vomiting, insert large bore IV and provide NS infusion and transfusions if indicated and available. Rapid transit to ED is essential.

Diaphragmatic Rupture

A ruptured diaphragm is usually caused by blunt trauma, often associated with rib fractures and/or a ruptured spleen. Injuries to the left diaphragm are more common because the liver provides some underlying protection on the right. Symptoms may be overlooked initially, so a careful abdominal examination should be done. Symptoms include respiratory and circulatory impairment and herniation of abdominal organs into the chest cavity that is often associated with nausea, vomiting, and abdominal pain, sometimes radiating to the left shoulder from pressure on the phrenic nerve.

Interventions: Manage the patient's airway/ventilation/oxygen supplementation and provide supportive care.

Tracheobronchial Disruption

Tracheobronchial disruption occurs with trauma (blunt or penetrating, such as gunshot wound) to the trachea and/or bronchial tree. Penetrating injuries are often associated with injury to adjacent structures, such as the esophagus, heart, and spinal cord as well. Severe injury often results in death from asphyxia or tension pneumothorax. Injuries include:

- **Cervical trachea**: Patients cyanotic even with oxygen and may exhibit subcutaneous emphysema, cough, pain, and hemoptysis.
- **Thoracic trachea/Bronchial**: Intrapleural lacerations result in severe dyspnea, air leaks, and large pneumothorax that does not respond to chest tube. Extrapleural rupture into the mediastinum results in air leaks (pneumomediastinum, subcutaneous emphysema). Patient may exhibit little dyspnea initially.

Interventions: Assess airway, breathing, and circulation. Intubation with administration of 100% oxygen is indicated in most cases but positive pressure may worsen air leaks. Monitor VS, oxygen saturation, and ECG. Insert large bore IV and administer NS bolus if hypotensive. Use suction (not more than 10 seconds at a time) as necessary to clear airway of blood.

Tube Thoracostomy

Indications

A tube thoracostomy is the procedure by which a tube is inserted in a patient's chest. The purpose of the chest tube is to remove fluid or air that has entered the pleural space—located between the inner and outer linings of the lung—as it can cause the patient's lung to collapse. If the fluid and/or air can be removed through the chest tube, the lungs will be able to expand completely, and the risk of collapse will be minimized. Pneumothorax (air accumulation in the pleural space) and pleural effusion (fluid accumulation in the pleural space) are two primary conditions for which a tube thoracostomy is indicated. The procedure is generally indicated for any condition or situation that could lead to a collapsed lung such as hemothorax, which is characterized by bleeding into the chest; empyema, an accumulation of pus in the pleural space; chest trauma; or chest surgery.

Procedure

A tube thoracostomy is the procedure whereby a tube is inserted into a patient's chest in an attempt to remove fluid or air. Prior to the procedure, if the patient can tolerate it, provide pain control and local anesthesia as well as supplemental oxygen. Once the area has been anesthetized, prep skin with chlorhexidine and perform procedure using sterile procedure and full barrier precautions. Make a small incision parallel to the intercostal space. Then use a Kelly clamp to dissect and make a little tunnel through which the tube will be inserted.

Clamp the chest tube with the Kelly clamp and then insert the chest tube into the tunnel that was created. After placing, remove the clamp and look for condensation in the tube on respiration or any drainage, making sure all drainage holes are within the thoracic space. To prevent the tube from falling out, it is sutured to or taped to the patient's skin. Obtain x-rays when able. Monitor lung expansion, breath sounds, oxygenation status and vitals.

Assessment

After the chest tube and drainage system have been inserted, the patient's level of comfort should be evaluated and, if possible, adjustments should be made to achieve an optimal comfort level. While the tube is in place, breath sounds and breathing rate should be monitored for abnormalities or changes that occur. Additionally, the patient's heart rate, blood pressure, and core body temperature should be monitored continuously. Oxygen saturation levels should be obtained to ensure that they are within normal range. The amount, color, and consistency of any drainage should be documented periodically while the drainage system is in place and assess and document bubbling in the water seal or whether the chest tube is to suction and if so how much suction. Subcutaneous emphysema, a condition whereby the skin covering the chest wall allows air to penetrate the patient's tissues, can occur at the site where the chest tube was inserted; consequently, the transport team member should assess for the condition by palpating the chest wall and listening for a crackling sensation. Tubing should be kept from kinking.

Abdominal

Abdominal and Genitourinary Organs

The **peritoneum** lines the abdominal cavity. The anterior (front) area is the **intraperitoneal space**, which contains the stomach, the first part of the duodenum, the small intestines, and part of the large intestines and rectum as well as the liver, bile ducts, spleen, ovaries, part of the pancreas and ureters, and bladder. The posterior (back) **retroperitoneal space** contains part of the duodenum, the ascending and descending colon, and part of the rectum as well as part of the pancreas and ureters, the kidneys, the adrenal glands, the uterus, and the fallopian tubes. The ovaries, uterus, and fallopian tubes comprise the female reproductive system. **Solid organs** include the liver, spleen, ovaries, uterus, pancreas, kidneys, and adrenals. **Hollow organs** include the bile ducts, stomach, large and small intestines, fallopian tubes, ureters, and bladder.

Abdominal Compartment Syndrome

Abdominal compartment syndrome (ACS) occurs when intraabdominal pressure (IAP) is sustained at >20 mmHg (normal 0-5 mmHg), resulting in multi-organ failure and death. ACS may be primary, caused by abdominal trauma, ruptured aortic aneurysm, or retroperitoneal hemorrhage associated with pelvic fractures. ACS may also be secondary, such as from traumatic injuries to the extremities, septic shock, and severe burns. Risk factors include hypothermia, acidosis, and fluid resuscitation of greater than 5 L/24 hours. Symptoms include abdominal pain, dyspnea, dizziness, and weakness. Patient may exhibit distended abdomen, oliguria, hemodynamic instability, and respiratory distress. The most common measurement is intravesicular pressure in which a Foley catheter is inserted into the bladder and connected to an IV bag of NS with a pressure transducer in the line. The patient is placed in supine position and transducer leveled to the mid-axillary line. The bladder is filled with 1 mL/kg (to maximum of 25 mL) NS, then the tubing clamped. After 60 seconds, the mean pressure is obtained at the end of expiration.

Eviscerations and Impaled Objects

Eviscerations occur with open abdominal wounds, such as opening incisions or traumatic injuries, which allow the internal organs (often the intestines) to protrude externally. Surgical repair is required to reinsert the organs into the abdomen. The patient may go into shock, especially if the evisceration is part of other major injuries (common in trauma cases).

Interventions: Provide supportive care; cover the eviscerated organs with thick, sterile gauze dressings moistened with NS, but do not attempt to reinsert them, manage the patient's airway/ventilation/oxygen supplementation as needed, and provide rapid transport.

Impalements occur when an object penetrates the abdomen and remains in place and may be associated with multiple internal injuries and bleeding.

Interventions: Do not remove the object, but do expose the abdomen and manually secure the object with bulky dressings and control any bleeding. Provide supportive care, manage the patient's airway/ventilation/oxygen supplementation as needed, and provide rapid transport.

Blunt Abdominal Wounds

Abdominal trauma may result in **blunt wounds**, which may occur as the result of motor vehicle accidents, motorcycle accidents, pedestrian injuries, sports injuries, falls, blast injuries, and assaults. Blunt injuries comprise crush (compression), shear (tearing), and burst (sudden increased pressure) injuries. Motor vehicle accidents often result in liver injury in the passenger with impact on that side of the vehicle and spleen injury in the driver with impact on the driver's side. Other injuries from blunt trauma include damage to the diaphragm, retroperitoneal hematomas, and intestinal injuries, including perforation. Symptoms of internal injuries include pain, guarding, abdominal distension, discoloration, tenderness on movement, and evidence of lower rib fractures. Some patients may exhibit rectal bleeding and/or vomiting of blood.

Interventions: Provide airway/ventilation/oxygen supplementation as needed, place in a position of comfort, treat for shock if indicated (especially with suspected internal bleeding), and provide rapid transport for patients in an unstable condition.

Penetrating Abdominal Wounds

Abdominal trauma may result in **penetrating wounds**, which are almost always related to gunshot wounds (high energy), shotgun wounds (medium energy), or knife wounds (low energy). Gunshot and shotgun wounds tend to cause more extensive damage than stab wounds, especially to the colon, liver, spleen, and diaphragm, and they may have an exit wound. Interior injuries may be extensive because the bullet damages tissues and may ricochet off of bone. Hemorrhage and peritonitis (especially with perforation of the intestines) are common complications. Pain is often more acute with injury to hollow organs than to solid organs, although blood loss may be severe with injury to the liver, spleen, or kidneys, and blood collecting in the retroperitoneal space may not be evident on inspection, palpation, or auscultation.

Interventions: Control external bleeding, manage the patient's airway/ventilation/oxygen supplementation, mobilize the spine if indicated, and apply a pneumatic antishock garment (PASG) if indicated for shock or pelvic fracture (contraindicated with difficulty breathing, pregnancy [second and third trimesters], evisceration, an impaled object, and open fractures).

Hepatic (Liver) Injury

Hepatic (liver) injury is the most common cause of death (mortality rates of 8–25%) from abdominal trauma and is often associated with multiple organ damage, so symptoms may be nonspecific. **Liver injuries** are classified according to the degree of injury, as follows:

I. Tears in the capsule with hematoma
II. Laceration(s) of the parenchyma (<3 cm)
III. Laceration(s) of the parenchyma (>3 cm)
IV. Destruction of 25–75% of a lobe from burst injury
V. Destruction of >75% of a lobe from burst injury
VI. Avulsion (tearing away)

Hemorrhage is a common complication of hepatic injury. Treatment often includes intravenous fluids for fluid volume deficit as well as blood products (plasma, platelets) for coagulopathies.

Interventions: Manage the patient's airway/ventilation/oxygen supplementation, control external bleeding, treat signs of shock, start an IV access line with fluid bolus if indicated (but beware of hemodilution), provide rapid transport for an unstable patient.

Splenic Injury

The spleen is the most frequently injured solid organ in blunt trauma because it's not well protected by the rib cage and it is very vascular. Symptoms may be very nonspecific. Kehr's sign (radiating pain in the left shoulder) indicates intra-abdominal bleeding, and Cullen's sign (ecchymosis around the umbilicus) indicates hemorrhage from a ruptured spleen. Some may have right upper abdominal pain, although diffuse abdominal pain often occurs with blood loss, associated with hypotension. **Splenic injuries** are classified according to the degree of injury, as follows:

- Tear in splenic capsules or hematoma
- Laceration of parenchyma (<3 cm)
- Laceration of parenchyma (>3cm)
- Multiple lacerations of parenchyma or burst-type injury

Treatment may be supportive if the injury is not severe; otherwise, suturing or removal of the spleen may be needed.

Interventions: Control external bleeding, manage the patient's airway/ventilation/oxygen supplementation, treat signs of shock, start an IV access line with fluid bolus if indicated (but beware of hemodilution), and provide rapid transport for an unstable patient.

Abdominal Vascular Injuries

Vascular injuries usually result from penetrating injuries, which may partially or completely transect a vessel, or blunt injuries, which may damage the wall or dissect the vessels. Acceleration/deceleration may result in shearing injuries. Indications of **vascular injuries** include pulsatile bleeding, enlarging hematoma, and ischemia distal to the vascular injury, as noted by the six P's (pain, pallor, pulseless, paresthesia, poikilothermia [unstable core body temperature], and paralysis) as well as audible bruit or palpable thrill and signs of increasing shock or compartment syndrome. Abdominal vessel injuries are most common in the aorta and inferior vena cava (45% mortality), but additional injuries, such as to the hepatic veins and portal vein, increase mortality rates (90%). Internal venous hemorrhage may be more severe than arterial.

Interventions: Control external bleeding, manage the patient's airway/ventilation/oxygen supplementation, start an IV access line with fluid bolus if needed for shock (but beware of hemodilution with bleeding), and provide rapid transport (surgical repair within 1 hour is critical).

Musculoskeletal

Musculoskeletal System

The musculoskeletal system includes 206 bones including long bones (e.g., the femur in the thigh), short bones (e.g., the carpal bones in the fingers), and flat bones (e.g., the sternum). The outer hard shell of the bone is the cortex, and the inner porous area is the trabecular bone. The vertebrae lack the cortex layer. Long bones have three parts: The middle section is the diaphysis, followed by the metaphyses, and then the epiphyses (the bone ends). In growing children, an epiphyseal plate of cartilage separates the metaphyses and epiphyses, allowing bone growth. This closes in adults, but damage to this area in a child may impair bone growth. The middle part of the short bones contains yellow bone marrow (fatty tissue). Red bone marrow, which produces blood cells, is found in the middle of the flat bones (pelvis, sternum, ribs, and scapula) and at the ends (epiphyses) of long bones. The skeletal system is connected by cartilage and tendons, and it is protected, supported, and allowed movement by about 700 soft-tissue muscles.

Review Video: Muscular System
Visit mometrix.com/academy and enter code: 967216

Review Video: Skeletal System
Visit mometrix.com/academy and enter code: 256447

Assessment of Musculoskeletal Injuries

Assessment of musculoskeletal injuries should include the following:

- Palpation/inspection for tissue damage, swelling, deformity, and tenderness
- Comparison with the opposite side if a limb is involved
- Assessment of neurovascular status (pulse, color, sensation, and function) distal to (below) the fracture
- Assessment of the six P's:
    - **Pain** (site of pain, degree, character)
    - **Pallor** (below the fracture or generalized)
    - **Paresthesia** (impaired sensation below fracture)
    - Distal **pulses** (intact, weak, absent)
    - **Paralysis** (with or without impaired sensation)
    - **Pressure** (often associated with swelling and pain)
- Assessment of age and general condition (geriatric patients are more likely to have fractures from relatively minor injuries because of osteoporosis)

If a fracture or dislocation is suspected, then the area should be splinted or immobilized for transport. Types of splints include rigid (should be padded), nonrigid (moldable), traction, air (pneumatic devices), pillow/blanket, short spine board, and long spine board. Splinting procedures are similar for adults, pediatric patients, and geriatric patients.

Fractures

Fractures usually result from trauma (falls, auto accidents), but **pathologic (nontraumatic) fractures** can result from minor force to diseased bones (osteoporosis or cancerous lesions). **Stress fractures** are caused by repetitive trauma (forced marching). **Salter-Harris fractures** involve the cartilaginous epiphyseal plate near the ends of long bones in children who are growing, and this can impair bone growth. Fractures can be classified as open or closed:

- **Open fractures** have soft-tissue injury and a break in the skin overlying the fracture, including puncture wounds from external forces or bone fragments; these can result in osteomyelitis (bone infection).
- **Closed fractures** involve a broken bone but no break in the skin.

Symptoms include pain, deformity or angulation, swelling, bruising, inability to move the joint or bear weight, grating on movement, and impaired function or circulation. Isolated fractures are usually not life threatening, but pelvic and femur fractures may involve severe blood loss.

Interventions: Cover open wounds with sterile dressings, manually stabilize and immobilize the fracture area, but do not replace protruding bones, apply a cold pack, and place the patient in a position of comfort.

Nontraumatic Fractures

Nontraumatic fractures occur when the bone weakens and can no longer support the body, such as may occur with a cancerous tumor of the bone or osteoporosis. Common fractures associated with osteoporosis include fractures of the vertebrae and hip. Osteoporotic fractures are most common in older adults, but they may also occur in adolescents with eating disorders. Infants and young children with multiple nontraumatic, non-abusive fractures may have a genetic disorder, such as osteogenesis imperfecta. Assessment of suspected fractures includes evaluating pain/tenderness, swelling around the fracture site, loss of sensation or movement, circulatory impairment (note the color of the skin, pallor or cyanosis), and deformity (especially noticeable in limb fractures).

Interventions: Splint extremity fractures; manage the patient's airway/ventilation/oxygen supplementation as needed; and provide transport for treatment.

Types of Fractures

Fractures can be classified by the location and style of the break.

Spiral: Common in toddlers who fall on an extended leg, breaking the tibia, but it may also occur with abuse in small children as a result of jerking on or twisting an extremity (usually the arm).

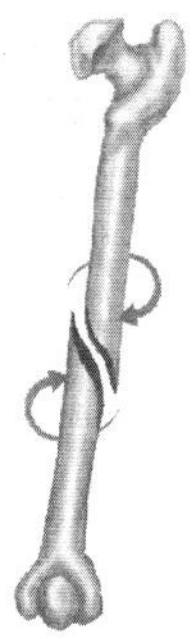

SPIRAL

Greenstick: Most common in children whose bones are less hard. It is usually quite painful but without deformity.

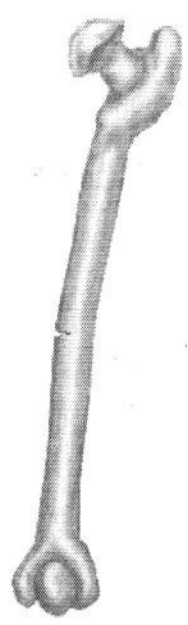

GREENSTICK

Displaced: Poses a risk of damage to surrounding tissues, including nerves and blood vessels and may lead to an open fracture if not properly splinted. The deformity is usually evident.

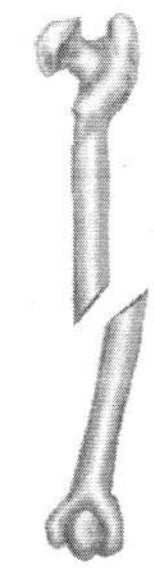

DISPLACED

Transverse: Usually occurs in long bones and is at risk of displacement unless it is splinted to prevent movement. Most often occurs from direct impact, such as sports injuries. May suggest abuse if occurring in small children.

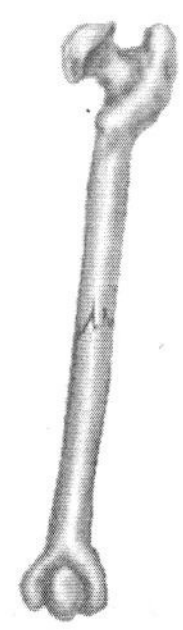

TRANSVERSE

Comminuted: Usually result from high-impact trauma, such as with motor vehicle accidents, and it is more common in older adults or those with weakened bones. This fracture is very painful and is often accompanied by swelling and muscle spasms.

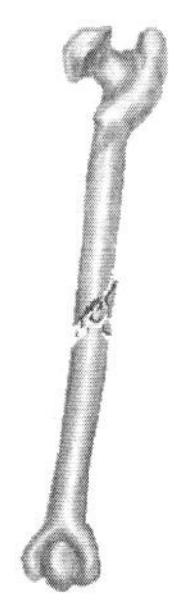

COMMINUTED

The femur is the long bone in the thigh. Although any part of the femur may fracture, fractures in the upper femur are common and are generally referred to as hip fractures. **Femur fractures** in young patients usually result from high-impact trauma, such as motor vehicle or pedestrian/motor vehicle accidents, whereas femur fractures in geriatric patients are most often from falls and are associated with osteoporosis. Patients may have many comorbidities and may present with dehydration and blood loss. Mortality rates for **hip fractures** are high, with 10% during the initial treatment and 25% over the next year. Symptoms of femur fractures include pain and deformity at the fracture site and an inability to walk or bear weight. A hematoma may be present.

Interventions: Splint the leg in the position it was found in with a traction splint (Hare Traction Splint/Sager Emergency Traction Splint), flush open fractures with NS to remove debris, and apply an NS-moistened sterile gauze dressing, monitor vital signs and neurovascular status, and assess soft tissue for damage. Provide an IV access and fluids if indicated.

Prehospital Management of Fractures

Prehospital management of fractures depends on the location and severity of the fracture:

- **Tibia/Fibula (lower leg)**: Manually immobilize during splinting. Splint the joint above and below the fracture(s) (upper thigh to ankle) with a padded rigid long-leg splint or a pneumatic splint, and then secure it to the other leg for additional support.
- **Shoulder**: Apply a sling to the affected side and secure the patient's arm against the body with a swathe to limit movement.
- **Knee**: If the pulse below the fracture is adequate and there is no deformity, splint with the knee straight. If there is deformity, splint the leg in the position it was found. If there is no pulse below the fracture, consult with medical assistance immediately. Never use a traction splint.
- **Clavicle (upper chest)**: Apply a sling to the affected side. (Common in young children who fall with an arm outstretched.)
- **Humerus (upper arm)**: Apply a sling to the affected side and swathe the arm to the body to limit movement.
- **Radius/Ulna (forearm)**: Splint from the elbow to the wrist and secure above and below the fracture. Elevate the arm.
- **Elbow**: Apply a sling to the affected side (often results from a fall).

Amputations

Amputations may be partial or complete and result from crush, guillotine (cutting), or avulsion (twisting) injuries. A **simple amputation** requires no extrication and other injuries or shock are absent, but a **complex amputation** may involve multiple injuries, shock, and delayed treatment because of extrication. The amputated limb should be treated initially as though it could be reattached, although single digits (except the thumb) and lower limbs are not usually reattached. The part should be irrigated with normal saline (NS) to remove debris; wrapped in NS-moistened gauze; and placed in a sealed plastic bag, which should be immersed in ice water. The body part should not freeze and should not be placed directly on ice.

Interventions: Manage the patient's airway/ventilation/oxygen supplementation; control bleeding by direct pressure or, if there is severe hemorrhage, by applying a BP cuff proximal to (above) the injury 70 mmHg greater than the systolic BP for <30 minutes. Irrigate the stump with NS if it is dirty, cover the open area with NS-moistened gauze, and elevate the stump.

Pelvic Fractures

Pelvic fractures represent about 3% of total fractures, but they pose a greater risk than most other types of fractures. **Pelvic fractures** most often result from a motor vehicle accident (50-60%) in adults and a pedestrian/motor vehicle impact (60-80%) in children. Pelvic fractures may be accompanied by major injuries to soft tissue and internal organs, especially the bladder, urethra (especially in children and women), and colon. A fracture on one side often results in a fracture on the other side as well. The primary cause of death after a pelvic fracture is hemorrhage with 50-70% of patients with unstable fractures requiring multiple transfusions. Geriatric patients have higher mortality rates than do younger patients. Symptoms include pain and tenderness, bloody urine, rectal bleeding, vaginal bleeding, retroperitoneal bleeding, hematoma over the fracture site, pain on hip motion, and signs of shock (with blood loss).

Interventions: Monitor vital signs for indications of shock, position supine, apply PASG or a pelvic wrap device (per protocol) to stabilize and prevent excessive movement, and monitor the patient's airway, ventilation, and oxygen supplementation. Provide an IV access (large bore) and fluid as indicated.

PNEUMATIC ANTISHOCK GARMENT (PASG)

The pneumatic antishock garment (PASG) is indicated for hypovolemic shock and hypotension associated with and stabilization of pelvic and bilateral femur fractures. PASG is contraindicated with respiratory distress, pulmonary edema, pregnancy (second and third trimesters), heart failure, myocardial infarction, stroke, evisceration, abdominal or leg impalement, head injuries, and uncontrolled bleeding above the garment.

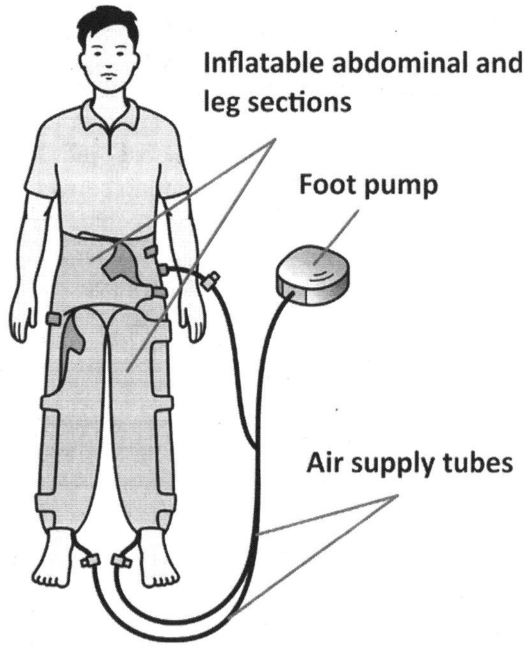

The **procedure** for PASG use is as follows:

1. Place the garment flat on the patient-transport device/stretcher and transfer the patient onto the garment.
2. If the patient is already on the stretcher, place the garment under his or her legs first and then lift the patient's buttocks and slide the garment upward until the upper garment edge is 1 inch below the bottom ribs.
3. Secure the legs first and then the abdominal section with the Velcro straps. Attach the pump hoses to each leg and the abdominal section at the valves and close the stopcocks.
4. Open the stopcock for each leg and abdominal section one at a time, and inflate them one at a time.

After inflating each section, close the stopcock and check the vital signs. Stop inflating if the systolic BP ≥90 mmHg. If the systolic BP is still <90 mmHg, then proceed to filling the next section or sections until all three are filled.

FAT EMBOLISM

Fat embolism, a life-threatening complication of fractures, can occur when fat enters the venous circulatory system, typically lodging in the pulmonary microvasculature, causing increased pulmonary vascular resistance. Patients most at risk are the young with multiple injuries, the elderly, and those with preexisting disease (pulmonary hypertension, right ventricular disorder, or metastatic cancer). Preventive methods include stabilizing fractures of long bones or the pelvis within 24 hours of injury. Signs of fat embolism include abrupt bradycardia, hypertension, jugular venous distension, hypoxemia, decreased $ETCO_2$ concentration, chest and upper extremity petechiae, fat globules in the retina, and various cardiac irregularities such as dysrhythmias. As the pulmonary artery pressure increases, cardiac output decreases.

Interventions: Immediate treatment includes 100% oxygen with mechanical ventilation per endotracheal tube with adequate IV fluids. Epinephrine or related drugs may be used for hemodynamic support per protocol.

Joint Dislocations

Subluxation (partial dislocation of a joint) and **luxation** (complete dislocation of a joint) can cause neurovascular compromise, which can be permanent if reduction is delayed. This is especially a problem with **hip dislocations**, which most commonly occur in automobile accidents when the person's knees impact the dashboard. **Elbow dislocations** often result from athletic injuries and may cause nerve damage. **Shoulder dislocations** are the most common type and also often result from athletic injuries. They may become chronic. **Knee dislocations** may result in severe injury to the popliteal artery, and this can lead to amputation, so rapid transport and emergent surgical repair are indicated. Differentiating between fractures and dislocations can be difficult because the symptoms and appearance are often similar. A deformity may not be evident or may be obscured by edema, or edema may give the appearance of a deformity. Extensive bruising may occur with all types of injuries, and pain may occur even with minor soft-tissue injuries.

Interventions: Splint and immobilize the area, and place the patient in a position of comfort.

Shoulder Injuries

A **sternoclavicular sprain** results from tearing of the ligaments that connect the sternum to the clavicle, usually resulting from a direct blow or twisting of an arm extended backward. Symptoms include pain near the top of the chest (below the neck). The pain increases on activity (such as lifting) and when lying on the affected side.

The **rotator cuff** comprises the muscle and ligaments of the shoulder joint. The bones in the joint include the scapula and humerus. Muscles (subscapularis, supraspinatus, infraspinatus, spines minor) and tendons anchor to the head of the humerus so that the arm can move in all directions, and ligaments connect the bones. Part of the rotator cuff is under the scapula. The most common injury to the rotator cuff is a tear in the supraspinatus tendon, so that the tendon is separated from its attachment, resulting from a violent pull on the arm, an abnormal rotation, or fall on an outstretched hand.

Interventions: Provide a protective sling.

Strains and Sprains

A **strain** is an overstretching of a part of the musculature ("pulled muscle") that causes microscopic tears in the muscle, usually resulting from excess stress or overuse of the muscle. The onset of pain is usually sudden with local tenderness on use of the muscle. A **sprain** is damage to a joint, with a partial rupture of the supporting ligaments and/or tendons, usually caused by wrenching or twisting that may occur with a fall. The rupture can damage blood vessels, resulting in edema, tenderness at the joint, and pain on movement with pain increasing over 2–3 hours after the injury. An avulsion fracture (the bone fragment is pulled away by a ligament) may occur with strain.

Interventions: Immobilize the area for transport, use rest, ice, compression, and elevation (the RICE protocol), and monitor the patient's neurovascular status (especially for sprains) by checking the pulse, capillary refill, color, and sensation distal to (below) the injury.

Splinting and Spinal Motion Restriction

Long Spinal Board and Splinting by Traction

Various methods of splinting and spinal motion restriction should be considered by the emergency medical responder, based on the patient's method of injury and symptoms:

- **Long spinal board**: If spinal injury is suspected, place a cervical collar on the patient before placing the patient on the long board. With one person stabilizing the head and neck, the patient is logrolled onto one side and the board is positioned against the patient so that the patient can be logrolled back onto the board. Once the patient is positioned on the board, padding such as rolled towels should be placed about the head, neck, and shoulders to provide further support and to ensure the head remains in a neutral position. The patient is secured by straps.
- **Splinting by traction**: Assess patient for signs/symptoms of mid-shaft femur fracture without lower leg or hip injury. Ask partner to apply the ankle hitch and apply manual traction and then to elevate the leg. Slide the long-leg device under the leg and secure with the ischial strap by the hip. Fasten the ankle hitch to the device and apply traction according to manufacturer's guidelines until the patient feels some relief of discomfort. Secure the rest of the leg with straps. Reassess circulation, sensation, and motor function. Place patient on a long spinal board and secure the patient and the device to the long board.

Seated Spinal Motion Restriction Using the Kendrick Extrication Device

Seated spinal motion restriction (SMR) using the Kendrick Extrication Device (KED) is indicated for a seated patient who is unable to self-extricate, is conscious and stable, and complains of head, neck, or back pain. Ask another person to continually stabilize the patient's head from behind and then check the patient's hands and feet for sensation and movement:

1. Apply cervical collar. Support the chest and lean the patient forward ≤45 degrees and place the KED in position behind the patient.
2. Move the patient back to upright position and fasten the straps (usually color coded) across the abdomen first and then the chest. Before fastening the chest strap, ask the patient to take a deep breath to ensure the strap doesn't restrict breathing.
3. Then fasten leg straps by bringing each strap under the buttocks and up between the legs and then to the side to fasten. Male patients may need to adjust their genitals.
4. Last make sure the head contacts the padding of the device, bring the flaps about the sides of the face, and then apply the chin strap and the forehead strap.
5. Check sensations and movement in the hands and feet again and then move the patient onto a long board and then onto a stretcher.
6. Remove KED but leave the cervical collar in place.

Compartment Syndrome

Compartment syndrome occurs when muscle perfusion is inadequate because of constriction caused by a cast or tight dressing or because of an increase in the contents of the enclosed compartment of a muscle sheath resulting from edema or hemorrhage. This increases pressure and compression, often related to fractures, crush injuries, burns, rhabdomyolysis, and snakebites. **Compartment syndrome** most often affects the forearm and leg muscles. Symptoms include severe throbbing pain unrelieved by opiates, numbness and tingling as pressure on the nerves increases, cyanosis and decreased or absent pulse distal to injury, limb paralysis, and edema (with tissue often being rigid). Necrosis and permanent damage may occur within 4 hours if treatment is inadequate or delayed.

Interventions: Remove the constriction (cast, splint, or dressing), elevate the limb, apply an ice compress, provide pain management, and provide rapid transport because the patient may need surgical fasciotomy to relieve the pressure.

Rhabdomyolysis

Rhabdomyolysis occurs when damage of the cells of the skeletal muscles causes the release of toxins from injured cells into the bloodstream. Rhabdomyolysis may be caused by trauma, tissue ischemia, infection, certain medications (statins, selective serotonin reuptake inhibitors, lithium, and antihistamines), sepsis, immobilization, extraordinary physical exertion, myopathies and cocaine or alcohol abuse. Additionally, rhabdomyolysis may occur with exposure to certain toxins such as snake/insect venoms or mushroom poisoning. In rare circumstances, the identifiable cause cannot be determined. The most serious complication of rhabdomyolysis is renal failure. Rhabdomyolysis may be life threatening. Early recognition and treatment are critical to avoid serious complications and for patients to make a full recovery.

Interventions: The treatment of rhabdomyolysis includes fluid administration to eliminate toxins and prevent renal failure. Bicarbonate may be administered to correct metabolic acidosis. Mannitol or dopamine may be administered to increase renal perfusion. Electrolyte replacement may also be indicated. In severe cases, emergency dialysis may be necessary.

Achilles Tendon Rupture

Tendons are fibrous tissues that connect muscles to bones. The **Achilles tendon** (the largest in the body) attaches the muscles of the lower leg to the heel and is strong but inflexible, so it can easily become inflamed from chronic irritation, such as from sports (hill running, jumping), resulting in tendinitis. If tendinitis is untreated, it can result in a tear in the tendon and eventual rupture. Rupture can also result from sudden blunt trauma.

Pain and stiffness in the back of the heel is common with tendinitis; but with tear or rupture, the area may become bruised and swollen, and walking may be difficult (although it is not usually impossible) and very painful. The patient is able to place the foot into plantar flexion (foot pointing downward) if the tendon is completely or partially intact but cannot do so if it is ruptured (a positive sign for rupture). Severe tendinitis, tear, or rupture may require surgical repair.

Interventions: Provide RICE therapy.

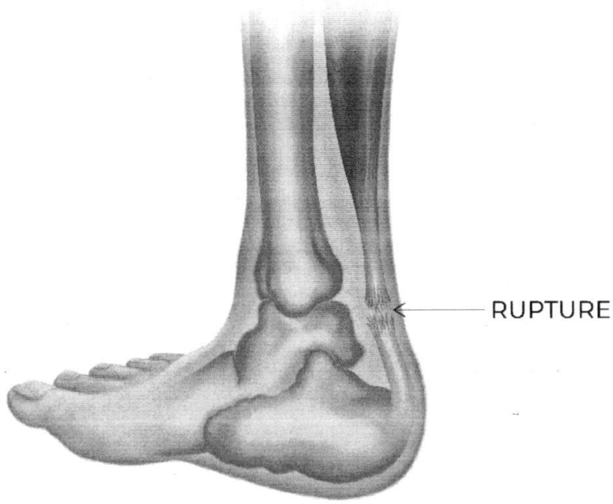

KNEE/PATELLA INJURY

The **patella** is anterior to the knee joint and embedded within the quadriceps tendon. The patella protects the underlying bones of the joint and facilitates knee extension. Ligaments (patellar, medial tibial, and lateral fibular) form a fibrous capsule to surround and support the joint. The anterior and posterior cruciate ligaments lie within the joint in a crisscross fashion from femur to tibia to maintain the position of the tibia in the joint. The lateral collateral ligament connects the femur to the fibula and stabilizes the knee. The medial collateral ligament connects the femur to the tibia and prevents excessive extension, stabilizes the knee, and allows rotation. Injury may occur with twisting (common in sports), torsion, and hyperextension.

- **Compression syndrome**: Results from weak quadriceps muscles or knee injury (as from a direct blow to knee). Knee pain without swelling, worsens after long sitting, when standing, and walking up or down hills/stairs. The knee may catch or give way.
  Interventions: Provide RICE therapy.
- **Anterior cruciate ligament (ACL) injury**: Usually rupture results from violent impact/trauma and may cause severe pain and hemarthrosis, swelling, and a slightly flexed position. May require knee aspiration.
  Interventions: Provide RICE therapy.
- **Posterior cruciate ligament (PCL) injury**: Injury usually occurs from a direct blow to the knee when the knee is flexed. Symptoms are similar to ACL injury.
  Interventions: Provide RICE therapy.
- **Lateral collateral ligament injury**: Injury usually results from forceful bending of the knee toward the midline, most often tearing the attachment to the fibula. Tenderness is present, and there is sometimes joint crepitus. Injury may occur to the peroneal nerve, impairing the ability to move the anterior and lateral leg muscles.
  Interventions: Provide RICE therapy.
- **Medial collateral ligament injury**: Injury usually results from forceful bending of the knee away from the midline, most often tearing the attachment to the femur. With a tear, pain is often severe but function remains. With a rupture, lateral movement is lacking and pain and swelling are evident.

Interventions: Provide RICE therapy.

OPEN SOFT-TISSUE INJURIES

Injury	Characteristics	Interventions
Abrasion	Painful superficial scraping of the outermost layer of skin. There is little or no bleeding.	Irrigate with water or NS to remove debris and cover with nonadherent dressing.
Laceration	A cut or break in the skin from impact with a sharp object. Bleeding may vary from mild to severe.	Apply pressure to control the bleeding, irrigate to remove debris if necessary, and cover with a dry sterile gauze dressing.
Puncture	Wound from impact with a sharp pointed object (knife, bullet); it may exhibit little external bleeding but major internal bleeding and soft-tissue damage. An exit wound may be present.	Apply pressure to control any bleeding, manage the patient's airway/ventilation/oxygen supplementation, and provide rapid transport if the patient's condition is unstable.
Impaled object	Penetrating object remains in wound.	Leave the object in place and pad with bulky dressings.

Injury	Characteristics	Interventions
Foreign body in eye(s)	Patient has pain, tearing, redness, and blurred or impaired vision from dirt, dust, chemicals, or other materials in the eye(s).	Cover both eyes loosely (avoiding pressure) to prevent movement. If it is chemical contamination, flush the eye(s) with copious amounts of NS or water.
Avulsions	The skin and underlying soft tissue are torn away, such as with a degloving injury, from any part of the body, although lower extremity injury is the most common. Bleeding may be severe, especially if vessels are torn or exposed.	Flush with sterile water or NS to remove debris if necessary, apply pressure and dressings to control bleeding and protect tissue, apply an ice pack, seal the avulsed skin and tissue in a plastic bag, and place in ice water for possible reimplantation or skin grafts. Return loose flaps to their anatomic positions.
Blast injury	Involves varying degrees of soft-tissue injury and sometimes amputations, fractures, impalements, traumatic brain injuries, ruptured eardrum, pulmonary injury, perforated bowel, and burns.	Manage the patient's airway/ventilation/oxygen supplementation, control bleeding and shock, provide CPR if necessary, supportive care, and rapid transport.

Closed Soft Tissue Injuries

Injury	Characteristics	Interventions
Contusion	Results from blunt or compressive pressure to a muscle and is a common sports injury. These may include other injuries, such as sprains, strains, fractures, and damage to internal organs. Symptoms include tenderness, pain on movement, and bruising. If bruising is in the shape of an instrument, it usually indicates abuse.	Provide RICE therapy and supportive care.
Hematoma	Collection of blood within the tissue because of damaged blood vessels from injury, underlying fracture, or medications (such as warfarin). These may be small or very large, and patients may lose ≥1 L of blood. Symptoms may include pain and swelling.	Provide supportive care for small contusions (which often resolve spontaneously), RICE therapy, and monitor for signs of continued bleeding.
Crush injury	External pressure may cause severe internal injuries, such as fractures and organ rupture.	Manage the patient's airway, ventilation, oxygen supplementation, and shock as needed, control bleeding, and provide supportive care.

Burns

Classification of Burns and Rule of Nines

Burn injuries may be chemical, electrical, or thermal and are assessed by the area affected, percentage of the body burned, and the depth of the burn, as follows:

- **First-degree burns** are superficial and affect the epidermis, causing erythema and pain.
- **Second-degree burns** extend through the dermis (partial thickness), resulting in blistering and sloughing of the epidermis and severe pain.

- **Third-degree burns** affect the underlying tissue, including the vasculature, muscles, and nerves (full thickness). Depending on the extent of the nerve damage, third-degree burns may present with less pain.

Burns are **classified** according to the American Burn Association's criteria as follows:

- **Minor**: <10% body surface area (BSA) or 2% BSA with third-degree burns without serious risk to the face, hands, feet, or perineum
- **Moderate**: 10–20% BSA combined second-degree and third-degree burns in adults; age <10 years or ≤10% third-degree without serious risk to the face, hands, feet, or perineum
- **Major**: ≥20% BSA; ≥10% third-degree burns; all burns are to the face, hands, feet, or perineum and will result in functional/cosmetic defect; or burns with inhalation or other major trauma

The **rule of nines** estimates the BSA burned:

- **Adults**: Head 9%, trunk (front) 18%, trunk (back) 18%, arm 9%, leg 18%, perineum 1%
- **Infants/Children**: Head 18%, trunk (front) 18%, trunk (back) 18%, arm 9%, leg 13.5%, perineum 1%

Review Video: Rule of Nines
Visit mometrix.com/academy and enter code: 846800

Electrical Burns

Low-voltage **electrical contact** most often causes a localized burn (first to third degree) to the hand or mouth (toddlers) with various degrees of tissue damage, although mouth contact may also result in cardiac or respiratory arrest. High-voltage electrical contact results in an entry and an exit wound with internal damage occurring between these wounds. Electrical current takes the shortest route to leave the body (flowing along blood vessels and nerves), so if the current passes from hand to hand, damage is usually more severe than if it passes from a hand to a foot. Severe injury may result in damage to bones, compartment syndrome, organ failure, and cardiac arrest from asystole or ventricular fibrillation. Vessels may be mildly or severely damaged. Abdominal organs may be damaged. Neurological damage with unconsciousness is common, especially if the current passes through the head. Peripheral nerve damage is also common, and damage to the spinal cord may occur.

Interventions: Manage the patient's airway, ventilation, and oxygen supplementation, provide CPR/defibrillation as needed, provide rapid transport (with the head elevated if it was involved), start an IV access line, and give fluid resuscitation if needed.

Lightning Burns and Injuries

Lightning injuries may occur with a direct strike (≤5%), side splash from a strike nearby, contact voltage when touching an item that has been struck, ground current (from a more distant strike), and blunt trauma from being too close to a strike (which often results in the patient being thrown). Symptoms may vary, but they can include external burns (Lichtenberg figures) in a fernlike pattern, acute pain, fixed and dilated pupils (temporary), eye injuries, confusion, headache, hearing loss, perforated eardrum, hypotension, paralysis/paresis, spinal cord injury, altered mental status, brain injury, fractures, and cardiac arrest. Patients may be responsive initially but lapse into unconsciousness as cerebral edema increases, resulting in secondary respiratory and/or cardiac arrest. Burns are usually mild because of the brief contact.

Interventions: Manage the patient's airway, ventilation, and oxygen supplementation, provide CPR/defibrillation as needed, provide rapid transport (with the head elevated), start an IV access line, and give fluid resuscitation.

General Management of Chemical and Electrical Burns

Patients with severe burns may develop shock and impairment of all major body systems. If the burning process is ongoing, room-temperature water or NS should be applied to stop the burning and any smoldering clothes or jewelry should be removed, although if the clothing is adhered to the skin, it should be left in place. With facial or airway burns, the airway must be monitored constantly with interventions as necessary, and an IV access line should be provided for fluid replacement, based on the patient's weight and the extent of the burn (Parkland formula: 4 mL/kg/wt × BSA per 24 hours). The burned area should be covered with nonadherent dry clean dressings, and the patient should be kept warm for transport. Children experience greater fluid and heat loss because of their greater body surface relative to their size, and the EMS provider should be alert to the possibility of child abuse. With **chemical burns**, any dry powder should be brushed off, and wet chemicals should be flushed with copious amounts of water (by a provider wearing gloves and eye protection). With **electrical burns**, internal burns may be more severe than external burns, and the patient is at risk of cardiac arrest.

Dressings and Bandages

Dressings and bandages may be appropriate when handling specific wounds or burns. Each type of dressing has specific characteristics meant to be used for specific purposes.

- **Sterile gauze**: 4×4 (sponge) or roller/wrapping gauze (Kerlix) used to protect skin or pack wounds to control bleeding. Roller gauze may be used to secure other dressings.
- **Nonadherent dressings**: Designed not to stick to open wounds because of their special coating (Teflon, foam, petrolatum, hydrogel). Used on abrasions, burns, and lightly draining wounds.
- **Occlusive dressings**: These have a waxy coating to make an air- and water-tight seal, but they are not as absorbent as gauze. Used for sucking chest wounds, abdominal eviscerations, and lacerations of the external jugular vein or carotid.
- **Trauma dressings**: Dressings that often include a nonadherent pad, a clotting agent embedded in the dressing, and an elastic wrap in one piece so that they can be rapidly applied (e.g., an ACE bandage), include QuikClot Combat Gauze and Celox Rapid hemostatic gauze. Especially useful to control bleeding and to apply pressure to a wound.
- **Adhesive, roller bandages**: May be elastic or nonelastic, and they are used to secure other dressings and/or apply compression.

Escharotomy

Escharotomy is a procedure commonly used with burn patients. The purpose of performing such a procedure is to relieve pressure placed on the patient's tissue and to restore adequate circulation to the tissue. Eschar is the dead tissue that forms over a burn wound like a scab; oftentimes this scab interferes with a patient's circulation in his/her limbs, which can lead to limb loss. Without an escharotomy, respiratory complications can also develop. Escharotomy should be performed by making incisions using sterile instruments in the eschar to allow the tissue to break open, thereby releasing the pressure that was being placed on the tissue by the scabbing.

Fluid Resuscitation for Burn Injuries

The primary purposes of fluid resuscitation in patients with burn injuries is to allow blood to flow to the tissues, to restore and/or maintain functioning to the vital organs, and to preserve tissue that has been damaged from the burn injury but remains viable. The patient's size and the severity of the burn injury are taken into account when calculating fluid resuscitation needs. The two most common formulas for calculating fluid resuscitation needs, the Parkland formula and the Modified Brooke formula, have been combined into the Consensus formula. This formula stipulates 2–4 mL/kg/%BSA where BSA represents body surface area. The first half of the fluids required should be delivered during the first eight hours following the injury, and the second half of the fluids should be administered within the 16 hours after those initial eight.

Inhalation Injuries

There are three mechanisms by which inhalation injuries can occur. First, irritants can be inhaled and cause damage to cells as well as damage to the pulmonary parenchyma, the tissue of the lungs. Asphyxiants that deprive the body of oxygen can lead to hypoxemia, which is a second mechanism of inhalation injuries. Hypoxemia is a condition characterized by the blood not having an adequate supply of oxygen; its most common symptom is shortness of breath. The third mechanism by which inhalation injuries can occur is via absorption of a toxic substance into the bloodstream through the respiratory tract, which can lead to organ damage and/or organ failure, depending on the inhaled substance.

Maxillofacial and Neck

Skull Bones and Sutures

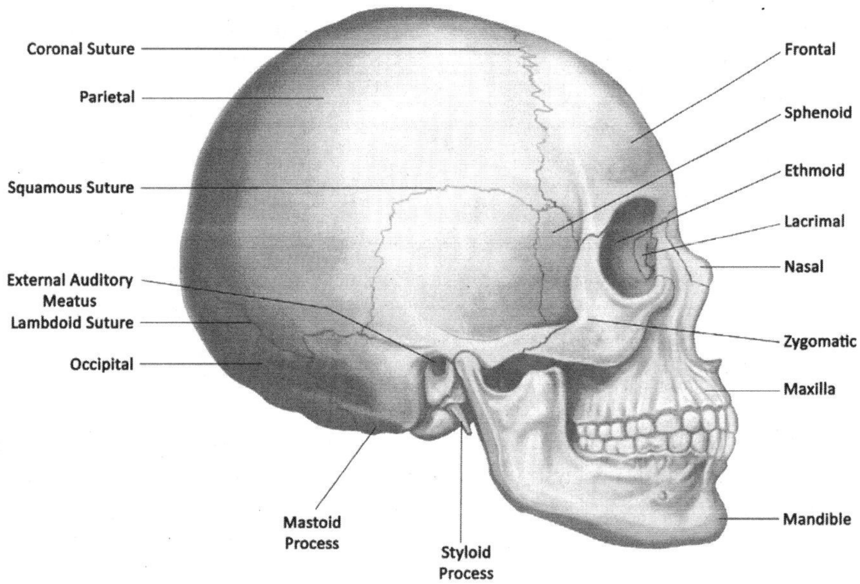

Assessing Maxillofacial Trauma

Maxillofacial trauma is often accompanied by pain, swelling, bleeding, and bruising; the presence of one or more of these symptoms may indicate such trauma. Examine the teeth of the patient to determine if any have been knocked loose or knocked out. Examine the patient's jaw to uncover signs of dislocation. Assess upper respiratory functioning and look for signs of bruising around the eyes to help diagnose a fractured nose. Conduct an ocular examination to look for injuries to the eyes and the eye sockets. Blurred or double vision, limited eye mobility, and numbness in the ocular area may also be indicators of maxillofacial trauma of the eyes.

Head, Scalp, and Facial Injuries

Injury	Characteristics	Prehospital
Head	Open: Bleeding. Closed: Swelling and bruising, may have depression of the skull and underlying injury. Battle's sign (bruising over the mastoid process) and/or raccoon eyes (bruising about eyes) may indicate a basal skull fracture.	Apply direct pressure to control the bleeding; apply dry, sterile dressings. Monitor the patient's mental status. Be alert for signs of skull fracture.
Scalp	Copious bleeding may occur. May cause shock in infants and young children. Injuries above the ears increase the risk of brain injury.	As above. Manage the patient's airway, ventilation, and oxygen supplementation if needed. Rapid transport is required with shock. Avoid closing the patient's mouth with bandages.
Facial	May include soft-tissue damage, facial bone fractures (nasal, orbital), eye injuries, and oral/dental injuries (tooth avulsions, mandibular/ maxillary fractures). May have severe swelling, airway compromise, impaired vision, and bloody nose.	Maintain a patent airway, but avoid nasopharyngeal airways; suction as needed; take broken teeth to the hospital; examine the eyes; and control bleeding. Patch both eyes if one or both eyes are injured. Stabilize impaled objects in the eye(s), but remove impaled objects from the cheeks if any bleeding obstructs the patient's airway.

Non-Spinal Neck Injuries and Nasal Fractures

Non-spinal neck injuries may result from blunt trauma or penetrating trauma, and they must be carefully assessed for underlying spinal cord injury. Open wounds may bleed profusely, especially if the carotid artery is breached, resulting in rapid exsanguination and death. The airway may be compromised. Difficulty swallowing indicates esophageal injury, whereas voice changes indicate laryngeal injury. Crackling on palpation indicates air in the tissues.

Interventions: Apply single-digit (gloved) pressure to control bleeding of the carotid artery or jugular veins; apply an occlusive dressing for an injury to the large vessels after the bleeding is controlled to prevent air from entering the bloodstream, which is life-threatening; and manage the patient's airway/ventilation/oxygen supplementation (advanced life support may be needed). Rapid or air medical transport may be needed.

Nasal fractures (40% of facial fractures) may cause persistent bleeding and should be assessed for drainage of the cerebrospinal fluid and injury of the surrounding structures, including brain injury, skull fracture, and neck and cervical spine injury.

Interventions: Control any bleeding, elevate the patient's head, and manage the airway, but do not use a nasopharyngeal airway.

Mandibular Fractures, Laryngotracheal Injuries, and Non-CNS-Associated Spinal Trauma

Additional non-CNS fractures of the face, neck and spine include:

- **Mandibular fractures** are most common in males 21 to 30 and result from a blow to the jaw from an assault, motor vehicle accident, or gunshot wound and are often associated with other injuries, such as head injury or midface fractures. Symptoms include malocclusion of teeth, pain, point tenderness, and ecchymosis of the floor of the mouth.
  Interventions: Manage the patient's airway/ventilation/oxygen supplementation (avoid the nasal airway), use an ice pack to reduce edema, elevate the patient's head, and monitor him or her closely.
- **Laryngotracheal injuries** result from direct trauma and may result in swelling and hemorrhage. Symptoms include swelling, changes in voice, hemoptysis, subcutaneous emphysema (from open wounds), and structural irregularities. The patient must be assessed for associated injuries.
  Interventions: Manage the patient's airway/ventilation/oxygen supplementation because airway obstruction is common, elevate the patient's head, and provide supportive care. May require a surgical airway.
- With **non-CNS-associated spinal trauma**, patients complain of pain and point tenderness, but neurological findings are intact.
  Interventions: Provide sitting or standing spinal mobilization and supportive care and manage the patient's airway, ventilation, and oxygen supplementation as needed.

Dental Injuries

Dental fractures, most commonly of the maxillary teeth, may occur in association with other oral and facial injuries and may be overlooked unless a careful dental examination is carried out. Fractures may range from chipping of the enamel to fracture of the tooth root.

Dental avulsions are complete displacement of a tooth from its socket. The tooth may be reimplanted if done within 1-2 hours after displacement, although only permanent teeth are reimplanted, not primary teeth, so question the parents of children to determine if an avulsed tooth is permanent.

Interventions: Manage the patient's airway, ventilation, and oxygen supplementation as needed, elevate the patient's head, and place the avulsed tooth in NS for transport.

Unstable Facial Fractures

Unstable facial fractures are those of the midface, usually from blunt facial trauma and are often associated with other trauma because of the degree of force involved. Categories include:

- **Le Fort I** (low downward force): The hard palate and lower maxilla are separated from the rest of skull.
- **Le Fort II** (low or mid-maxilla force): The nasal bones and lower maxilla are separated from the facial skull and other cranial bones.
- **Le Fort III** (force to the bridge of the nose or the upper maxilla): The entire midface is separated from the cranium.

Symptoms may include malocclusion, open bite, apparent lengthening of the face, clear nasal discharge (cerebrospinal fluid), periorbital ecchymosis, pain, swelling, and epistaxis (nosebleed), vision disturbances, airway compromise.

Interventions: Suction if necessary, manage the patient's airway/ventilation/oxygen supplementation (usually with intubation, avoid a nasopharyngeal airway), control any bleeding, elevate the patient's head. Cricothyroidotomy may be necessary if the airway is obstructed. Patch both eyes if one or both are injured.

Stabilize an impaled object in the eye, but remove an impaled object in the cheek; apply dry sterile dressings, but do not cover the mouth; provide rapid transport.

Orbital Fractures and Ruptured Tympanic Membrane

Orbital fractures most often occur with blunt force against the globe causing a rupture through the floor of the orbital bone or a direct blow to the orbital rim, often related to an assault or sports injury. Injuries are most common in adolescents and young adults. Patients may be essentially asymptomatic, or they may exhibit ecchymosis and edema of the eyelid, infraorbital anesthesia from pressure or damage to the infraorbital nerve, decreased sensation of the cheek and upper gum on the injured side, diplopia (double vision), and enophthalmos (a sunken globe).

Interventions: Patch both eyes to prevent movement, provide supportive care, and use an ice compress to reduce edema.

A **ruptured tympanic membrane** may result from pressure (diving, waterskiing), a direct blow to the ear, explosions, and a foreign object in the ear. Symptoms may include pain, hemorrhagic otorrhea (bloody drainage), and hearing impairment.

Interventions: Provide supportive care.

Penetrating Neck Injury

Patients with a penetrating neck injury (such as a gunshot or knife wound) should be carefully screened to determine if they have cervical disc and/or spinal cord injuries. The airway should be immediately assessed, as the patient may require intubation and ventilation. Orotracheal intubation is most common. If the injury creates a tracheostomy site, this site can be intubated. Suctioning may be needed if blood is in the airway. Bleeding must be controlled with direct pressure and an occlusive dressing applied to venous injuries to prevent air emboli. General circulation must be assessed, as injury to great vessels may occur. If the wound is contaminated with debris, it should be irrigated with normal saline. If the patient is fully conscious and has no indications of spinal cord injury, spinal immobilization is not indicated. A rigid cervical color is usually not necessary unless there is neurological impairment.

Medical Emergencies

Neurologic

Clonus

Clonus can be described as a series of rapid muscle contractions that occur involuntarily when a muscle is stretched. Clonus can indicate the presence of certain neurological abnormalities and is often associated with spinal cord injuries, stroke, and multiple sclerosis. The ankles are one of the most common areas for clonus to be present; as such, an ankle clonus test is often performed to assess for clonus. The test is performed by gently bending the patient's foot backwards, dorsiflexing the foot towards him/her. Rapid muscle contractions will persist while the patient's foot is in a dorsiflexed position if clonus is present.

Strokes

Strokes result from interruption of blood flow to an area of the brain.

- **Ischemic strokes** (80%) are caused by blockage of an artery supplying the brain, usually from a thrombus (blood clot) or embolus (traveling clot).
- **Hemorrhagic strokes** (20%) result from a ruptured cerebral artery, causing not only a lack of oxygen and nutrients but also edema (swelling) that causes widespread pressure and damage. With both types, patients may experience weakness, paralysis, and loss of sensation in one or more extremities; difficulty speaking or loss of speech; vision impairment; difficulty swallowing; headache; an altered state of consciousness (confusion, disorientation); or coma.
- **Transient ischemic attacks** (TIAs) from small clots cause similar but short-lived (minutes to hours) symptoms. Emergent treatment includes placing the patient in the semi-Fowlers or Fowler's position and administering oxygen. The patient may require oral suctioning if the secretions pool. The patient's airway, breathing, and circulation should be assessed. Patients should be transported immediately to the receiving facility because thrombolytic therapy to dissolve blood clots should be administered within 1-3 hours.

Review Video: Overview of Strokes
Visit mometrix.com/academy and enter code: 310572

Cincinnati Prehospital Stroke Scale

The Cincinnati Prehospital Stroke Scale should be administered to any patient who is suspected of having a stroke. The patient may be experiencing a stroke if he tests positive for any of the three signs and should be transported to the receiving facility as soon as possible.

Signs	Directions to patient	Abnormal results
Facial drooping	Smile. Show your teeth.	One side of the face is weak or paralyzed and doesn't move as well as the other.
Arm drifting	Close your eyes and hold your arms out straight and hold them there for 10 seconds.	One arm doesn't move at all or drifts downward.
Speaking abnormality	Repeat after me: "Don't count your chickens before they are hatched."	Patient slurs words, uses inappropriate words, or is unable to respond.

Los Angeles Prehospital Stroke Screen

The Los Angeles Prehospital Stroke Screen is used to assess patients in a prehospital setting who have symptoms that suggest a stroke (such as altered state of consciousness, difficulty speaking, one-sided weakness, or paralysis). The results are positive for stroke if all criteria are met or are unable to be measured and the physical exam shows an unequal response. Note: A patient may still be having a stroke even if all the criteria are not met.

General criteria	Yes	No	Unknown
Age >45			
No history of epilepsy or seizures			
Onset of symptoms <24 hours			
Patient was able to walk before the onset of symptoms			
Blood glucose between 60 and 400 mg/dL			

Physical criteria	Equal	Right	Left
Facial smile	Normal	Droop	Droop
Grip strength	Normal	Weak or no grip	Weak or no grip
Arm strength	Normal	Drifts or falls down	Drifts or falls down

SEIZURES

GRAND MAL SEIZURES

Seizures are sudden, involuntary, abnormal electrical disturbances in the brain that can manifest as alterations of consciousness, spastic tonic and clonic movements, convulsions, and loss of consciousness.

- **Tonic-clonic (grand mal)**: Occurs without warning.
  - *Tonic period* (10–30 seconds): The eyes roll upward with loss of consciousness, the arms flex, and the body stiffens in symmetric contractions with cyanosis and salivating.
  - *Clonic period* (usually 30 seconds or longer): Violent rhythmic jerking with contraction and relaxation and sometimes incontinence of urine and feces.

During the seizure, the patient's head and body should be protected from injury but no attempt should be made to insert anything into the mouth or restrain the patient. If possible, the patient should be screened from spectators and turned onto his or her side (the recovery position) to prevent aspiration. Following seizures, there may be confusion, disorientation, and impairment of motor activity and speech and vision for several hours. Headache, nausea, and vomiting may occur.

Review Video: Seizures
Visit mometrix.com/academy and enter code: 977061

Interventions: Monitor the airway, breathing, and circulation and suction. Administer oxygen as needed. Insert a nasopharyngeal airway for assisted ventilation if the patient is cyanotic.

PARTIAL SEIZURES

Partial seizures are caused by an electrical discharge to a localized area of the cerebral cortex, such as the frontal, temporal, or parietal lobes with seizure characteristics related to the area of involvement. They may begin in a focal area and become generalized, often preceded by an aura.

- **Simple partial**: Unilateral motor symptoms including somatosensory, psychic, and autonomic.
  - *Aversive*: Eyes and head are turned away from the focal side.
  - *Sylvan* (usually during sleep): Tonic-clonic movements of the face, salivation, and arrested speech.
- **Special sensory**: Various sensations (numbness, tingling, prickling, or pain) spreading from one area. May include visual sensations, posturing, or hypertonia. These are rare in patients <8 years old.

- **Complex (psychomotor)**: There is no loss of consciousness, but there may be altered levels of consciousness, and patients may be nonresponsive with amnesia. May involve complex sensorium with bad tastes, auditory or visual hallucinations, and a feeling of déjà vu or strong fear. Patients may carry out repetitive activities, such as walking, running, smacking lips, chewing, or drawling. Patients are rarely aggressive. The seizure is usually followed by prolonged drowsiness and confusion. Occurs from age 3 through adolescence.

Status Epilepticus

Status epilepticus (SE) is usually generalized tonic-clonic seizures that are characterized by a series of seizures with intervening time too short for regaining of consciousness. The constant assault and periods of apnea can lead to exhaustion, respiratory failure with hypoxemia and hypercapnia, cardiac failure, and death.

Causes	Treatment
• Uncontrolled epilepsy or non-compliance with anticonvulsants. • Infections, such as encephalitis. • Encephalopathy or stroke. • Drug toxicity (isoniazid). • Brain trauma. • Neoplasms. • Metabolic disorders.	• Seizure precautions to keep patient safe. • IV access for benzos and RSI meds if needed. • Secure airway and provided associated supportive care. • Anticonvulsants beginning with fast-acting benzodiazepines, usually lorazepam 0.1 mg/kg IV at a rate of 2 mg/min. Allow 1-2 minutes after dose has been given to assess if seizures continue. If they continue, subsequent doses of Ativan can be given, monitoring sedative effects and bp. • Diazepam can be given instead of lorazepam: 0.2 mg/kg IV.

Neuromuscular Disorders

Guillain-Barré Syndrome (GBS)

Guillain-Barré syndrome (GBS) is an autoimmune disorder of the motor peripheral nervous system, resulting in demyelination of protective myelin sheaths, often triggered by a viral gastroenteritis or *Campylobacter jejuni* infection. As the myelin sheath becomes inflamed and demyelination occurs, the conduction of nerve impulses is blocked. In most cases, the axon remains intact and recovery occurs with remyelination; however, in severe cases, the axon is permanently damaged, and recovery is incomplete or death occurs. Symptoms include numbness and tingling with increasing lower extremity weakness that may ascend and become generalized, affecting the legs and then the arms, sometimes resulting in complete paralysis and an inability to breathe without ventilatory support. Deep tendon reflexes are typically absent, and some people experience facial weakness and ophthalmoplegia (paralysis of muscles controlling the movement of the eyes).

Interventions: Provide supportive care and oxygen as needed, and start an IV access line. If the patient is in respiratory failure, intubation and ventilation may be necessary.

Review Video: Guillain-Barre Syndrome
Visit mometrix.com/academy and enter code: 742900

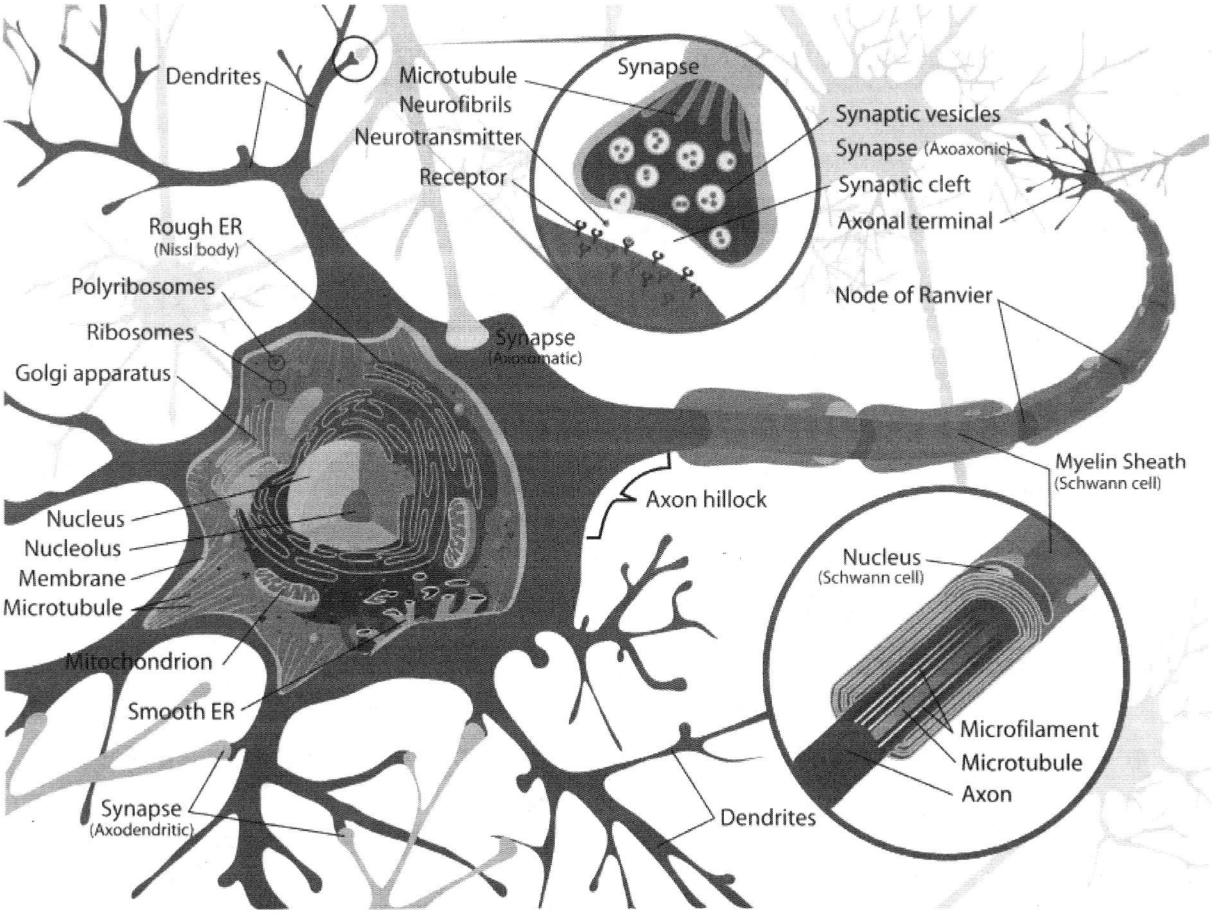

Myasthenia Gravis (MG)

Myasthenia gravis (MG) is an autoimmune disorder of the neuromuscular system in which acetylcholine receptors are damaged at neural synapses, preventing transmission of impulses to contract muscles. This results in the weakness of voluntary muscles, increasing with activity because the need for acetylcholine is not met. Muscles that are initially affected include those of the eyes, neck, and face. Additionally, the thymus gland develops abnormalities, such as hypertrophy or thymoma, in about 90% of those with MG. Onset may be abrupt or gradual, and it occurs most commonly in women between ages 20 and 30 and men between ages 70 and 80. There are five classes of MG, depending on severity. Typical symptoms (which tend to worsen through the day) include drooping eyelids; double vision; difficulty speaking, chewing, and swallowing; weakened muscles of respiration; and weakened extremity muscles. Symptoms may exacerbate (worsen) with menstruation, infection, stress, or some medications. Treatment includes angiotensin converting enzyme (ACE) inhibitors, immunomodulating agents, IV immune globulin, plasmapheresis, and removal of the thymus. With myasthenic crisis, respiratory failure may occur.

Review Video: Myasthenia Gravis
Visit mometrix.com/academy and enter code: 162510

Interventions: Provide the patient with supportive care, place in the recovery position, intubate, and ventilate if he or she is in respiratory distress.

Multiple Sclerosis (MS)

Multiple sclerosis (MS) is a central nervous system (CNS), immune-mediated, inflammatory, demyelinating disease believed to be triggered by an unidentified environmental source, such as a virus. The myelin sheath, primarily composed of lipids (fats), is white in appearance, creating the "white matter" of the brain. Impulses travel along the sheath, jumping from one node to another. With MS, an immune reaction causes killer T cells to attack the sheaths, which begin to demyelinate, leaving scarred areas along the axons, slowing nerve transmissions. Initially, symptoms come and go, and the sheaths undergo repair. Over time, however, cells cannot remyelinate and new cells don't develop adequately, so symptoms worsen. Symptoms vary widely, often beginning with muscle tingling and weakness, poor balance, and blurred/double vision. Patients may develop muscle spasticity, bladder and bowel problems, emotional changes, depression, and cognitive impairment. Advanced symptoms include difficulty speaking, breathing problems, tremor, seizures, and hearing loss.

Interventions: Provide IV hydration if the patient is dehydrated, assisted ventilation if he or she is in respiratory distress, and careful positioning to prevent injury, especially with spasticity.

Review Video: Multiple Sclerosis (MS)
Visit mometrix.com/academy and enter code: 417355

Parkinson's Disease (PD)

Parkinson's disease (PD) is an extrapyramidal movement motor system disorder caused by loss of brain cells that produce dopamine, resulting in decreased levels of dopamine. Symptoms appear when 60–80% of neuronal cells are impaired and dopamine levels drop by 20–50%. As dopamine levels fall, other areas of the brain function abnormally as well, further impairing motor function. Typical symptoms include tremor of the face and extremities, rigidity, bradykinesia (slow movement), akinesia (absence of movement), stooped posture, and lack of balance and coordination, causing increasing problems with mobility, talking, and swallowing. Some patients may suffer depression, mood changes, and dementia. Tremors usually present unilaterally in an upper extremity. Treatment includes symptomatic support, dopaminergic therapy (levodopa, amantadine, and carbidopa), and anticholinergics (trihexyphenidyl, benztropine). Patients may experience resistance to medications over time.

Interventions: Provide supportive care. Be aware of the risk of choking, especially with advanced Parkinson's disease, and look for signs. Place the patient in the recovery position to prevent aspiration.

Cerebral Palsy (CP)

Cerebral palsy (CP) is a nonprogressive motor dysfunction related to CNS damage associated with congenital, hypoxic, or traumatic injury before birth, during birth, or ≤2 years after birth. CP may include visual defects, speech impairment, seizures, and intellectual disabilities. Characteristics may vary widely, depending upon the degree of CNS injury.

Types of motor dysfunction	Characteristics of CP
Spastic: Constant hypertonia and rigidity lead to contractures and curvature of the spine **Dyskinetic**: Tremors and twisting with exaggerated posturing and impairment of voluntary muscle control **Ataxic**: Atonic muscles in infancy with lack of balance, instability of muscles, and poor gait **Mixed**: Combinations of all three types with multiple areas of damage	• Hypotonia or hypertonia with rigidity and spasticity • Athetosis (constant writhing motions) • Ataxia • Hemiplegia (one-sided involvement, more severe in the upper extremities) • Diplegia (all extremities are involved, but it is more severe in the lower extremities) • Quadriplegia (all extremities are involved with the arms flexed and legs extended)

Interventions: Provide routine supportive care and position the patient to prevent injury.

Nuchal Rigidity and Meningitis

Nuchal rigidity is a condition whereby a patient is not able to flex his/her head as a result of the neck muscles being rigid, or stiff. The condition can be an indicator of a problem with or irritation to the meninges, which are the membranes that surround the patient's central nervous system. Nuchal rigidity is associated with bacterial meningitis but is not exclusive to that process.

Patients with bacterial meningitis may exhibit signs to help support the diagnosis. While the following are not universally present, they are specific to meningitis and are rarely positive with other disorders:

- Kernig's sign: Flex each hip and then try to straighten the knee while the hip is flexed. Spasm of the hamstrings makes this painful and difficult with meningitis.
- Brudzinski sign: With the patient lying supine, flex the neck by pulling head toward chest. The neck stiffness causes the hips and knees to pull up into a flexed position with meningitis.
- Jolt accentuation maneuver: (Used if nuchal rigidity is not present.) Ask patient to rapidly move his/her head from side to side horizontally. Increase in headache is positive for meningitis.

Interventions: Obtain a history of the symptoms and use contact/droplet isolation (masks). Provide supportive care and oxygen if the saturation level falls below 95%. Provide an IV access line. Keep the lights dim.

Hydrocephalus

The brain's ventricular system produces and circulates cerebrospinal fluid (CSF). **Hydrocephalus** occurs with an imbalance between the production and absorption of cerebrospinal fluid in the ventricles, resulting from impaired absorption (communicating) or obstruction (noncommunicating). In early infancy before closure of the cranial sutures, head enlargement is the most common presentation, but in older children and adults with less elasticity in the skull, neurological symptoms usually relate to increasing pressure on structures of the brain. Symptoms in children may include headache relieved by vomiting, papilledema, strabismus, ataxia, irritability, lethargy, confusion, and difficulty communicating. Adults may have similar symptoms and may be misdiagnosed as having Alzheimer's. Treatment is a ventriculoperitoneal shunt, which is a catheter with a one-way valve to prevent backflow extending from the ventricles to the peritoneal cavity or the right atrium to drain excess fluid. Complications include infection characterized by a rapid rise in temperature, confusion, and neurological impairment and obstruction characterized by increasing signs of intracranial pressure.

Interventions: Provide supportive care. Elevate the patient's head for transport for surgical repair.

Brain Tumors

Any type of brain tumor can occur in adults. Brain tumors may be primary, arising within the brain, or secondary as a result of metastasis:

- **Astrocytoma**: This arises from astrocytes, which are glial cells. It is the most common type of tumor, occurring throughout the brain. There are many types of astrocytomas, and most are slow growing. Some are operable while others are not. Radiation may be given after removal. Astrocytomas include glioblastomas, aggressively malignant tumors occurring most often in adults 45-70.
- **Glioblastoma**: This is the most common and most malignant adult brain tumor/astrocytoma. Treatment includes surgery, radiation, and chemotherapy, but survival rates are very low.
- **Brain stem glioma**: This may be fast or slow growing but is generally not operable because of location, although it may be treated with radiation or chemotherapy.
- **Craniopharyngioma**: This is a congenital, slow-growing, recurrent (especially if >5 cm) and benign cystic tumor that is difficult to resect and is treated with surgery and radiation.

- **Meningioma**: Slow growing recurrent tumors are usually benign and most often occur in women, ages 40-70; however, they can cause severe impairment/death, depending on size and location. Meningiomas are surgically removed if causing symptoms.
- **Ganglioglioma**: This can occur anywhere in the brain and is usually slow growing and benign.
- **Medulloblastoma**: There are many types of medulloblastoma, most arising in the cerebellum, malignant, and fast growing. Surgical excision is often followed by radiation and chemotherapy although recent studies show using just chemotherapy controls recurrence with less neurological damage.
- **Oligodendroglioma**: This tumor most often occurs in the cerebrum, primarily the frontal or temporal lobes, involving the myelin sheath of the neurons. It is slow growing and most common in those age 40-60.
- **Optical nerve glioma**: This slow growing tumor of the optic nerve is usually a form of astrocytoma. Optic nerve glioma is often associated with neurofibromatosis type I (NF1), occurring in 15-40% of patients with NF1. Despite surgical, chemotherapy, or radiotherapy treatment, it is usually fatal.

Cardiovascular

Circulatory System

The circulatory system controls blood flow throughout the body and to the tissues, controls gas exchange (carbon dioxide and oxygen), serves as a reservoir for blood, maintains blood pH through a buffer system, responds to infections, and facilitates coagulation (blood clotting). The circulatory system includes the cardiovascular system (heart and blood vessels) and the blood.

- **Heart**: The heart has four chambers, upper (right atrium and left atrium) and lower (right ventricle and left ventricle). The heart muscle receives blood from two major coronary arteries and their branches. The myocardium (heart muscle) receives blood from two major coronary arteries and their branches. The inner lining of the heart is the endocardium, and the lining that surrounds the heart is the pericardium, which has an inner double-layered serous membrane (visceral pericardium) and a fibrous outer layer (parietal pericardium).
- **Vessels**: The venous system includes veins, venules, and venous capillaries and brings blood back to the heart via the inferior and superior vena cava. The arterial system, including the coronary arteries, branches from the aorta after it leaves the heart and includes arteries, arterioles, and arterial capillaries.
- **Blood**: Blood consists of red blood cells (erythrocytes); white blood cells (leukocytes including monocytes, lymphocytes, basophils, neutrophils, and eosinophils); platelets (thrombocytes); and plasma, the liquid portion of the blood (which contains clotting factors).

Review Video: Functions of the Circulatory System
Visit mometrix.com/academy and enter code: 376581

Conduction System of the Heart

Normal conduction of the heart has the following four stages:

1. **Generation of an impulse at the sinoatrial (SA) node** (primary pacemaker) located at the junction of the right atrium and superior vena cava: The electrical impulse travels the cells of the atria along internodal pathways, causing electrical stimulation and contraction of the atria, including Bachmann's bundle, which stimulates the left atrium.
2. **Atrioventricular node conduction of impulse**: This occurs when the impulses from the SA node reach the AV node in the right atrial wall near the tricuspid valve. There is a slight delay (about one-tenth of a second), allowing the atria to empty.

3. **Atrioventricular bundle (bundle of His) conduction**: The AV node relays the impulse to the ventricles through the atrioventricular bundle—specialized conduction cells in the ventricular septum that branch to the right and left ventricles, carrying the electrical impulse.
4. **Purkinje fiber conduction**: Impulses are conducted down the AV bundles to the base of the heart where they divide into the Purkinje fibers, which stimulate the myocardial cells to contract the ventricles.

Cardiac Cycle and Blood Flow Through the Heart

The cardiac cycle involves one complete heartbeat with systole (ventricular contraction) and diastole (relaxation) phases. **Stroke volume** is the volume of blood ejected from the left ventricle in one cardiac cycle (about 60–70 mL), and **cardiac output** is the heart rate times the stroke volume.

The **blood flows** as follows:

- Deoxygenated venous blood returns to the heart per the inferior vena cava, superior vena cava, and coronary sinus (bringing blood from the coronary arteries) into the right atrium, and then it flows through the tricuspid valve into the right ventricle.
- From the right ventricle, blood flows through the pulmonic (semilunar) valve into the pulmonary artery and to the lungs to exchange carbon dioxide for oxygen.
- Oxygenated blood flows from the lungs through the pulmonary veins into the left atrium and through the mitral (bicuspid) valve into the left ventricle.
- From the left ventricle, blood flows through the aortic valve and into the aorta, the coronary arteries, and the general circulation through the thoracic and abdominal aorta.
- After blood flows through the valves, they close to prevent backflow. Both atria and both ventricles contract simultaneously.

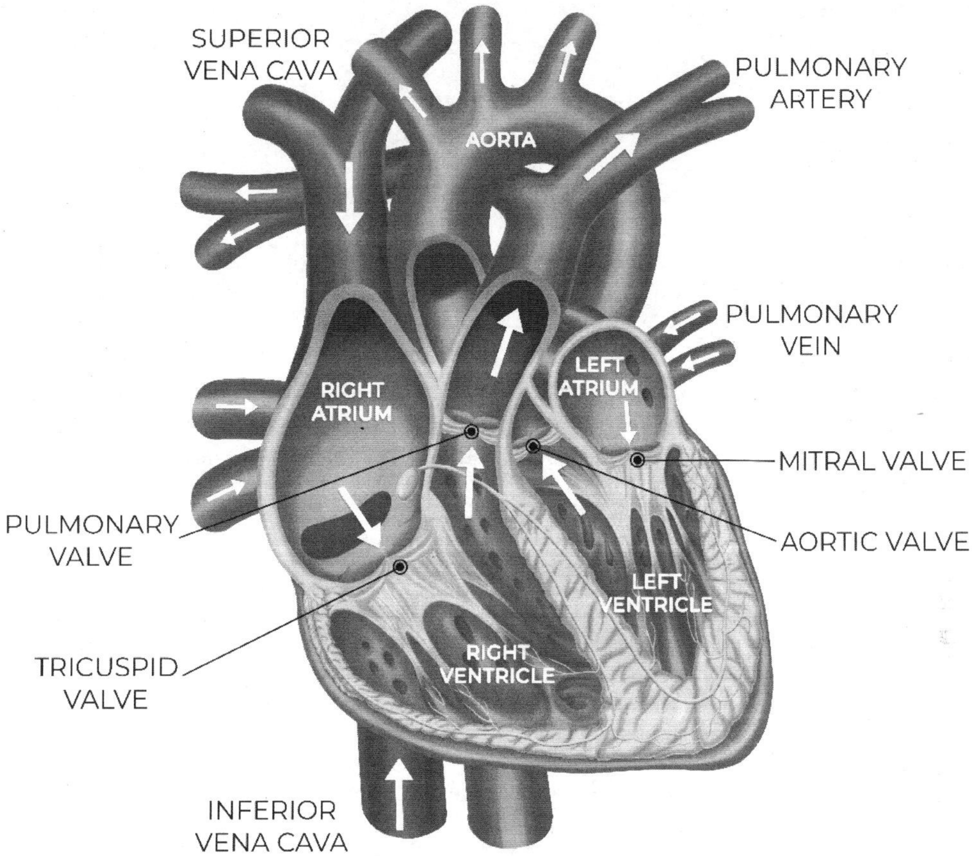

Review Video: Heart Blood Flow
Visit mometrix.com/academy and enter code: 783139

Review Video: Diastolic vs Systolic
Visit mometrix.com/academy and enter code: 898934

Perfusion, Oxygenation of Tissues, and Cardiac Compromise

Perfusion depends on an adequate supply of red blood cells, which carry oxygen. Perfusion may be impaired if the heart does not pump adequately, if the rate of heart contractions is too low or too rapid to be effective, and if the volume of blood and/or red blood cells pumped is not adequate to provide oxygenation to the tissues. With adequate perfusion, **oxygenation of tissues** occurs when blood flows throughout the body, and gas exchange of carbon dioxide and waste products for oxygen occurs at the capillaries. **Cardiac compromise** results in inadequate circulation and/or perfusion of vital organs. Cardiac compromise may result from atherosclerosis (plaques/fatty deposits) in the arterial lumens, resulting in obstructed blood flow and inadequate dilation and constriction of arteries. Ischemia (low oxygenation) occurs with decreased blood flow and can damage tissues, but occlusion (obstruction) can result in the death of tissue. Cardiac compromise may result from heart damage causing an inadequate heart rate and/or pumping. Cardiac compromise may also result from an inadequate volume of circulating blood.

Cardiovascular Assessment

Electrocardiogram (ECG)

The electrocardiogram (ECG) records and shows a graphic display of the electrical activity of the heart through a number of different waveforms, complexes, and intervals as follows:

- **P wave**: Start of the electrical impulse in the sinus node and spreading through the atria, muscle depolarization
- **QRS complex**: Ventricular muscle depolarization and atrial repolarization
- **T wave**: Ventricular muscle repolarization (resting state) as cells regain a negative charge
- **U wave**: Repolarization of the Purkinje fibers

A modified lead II ECG is often used to monitor basic heart rhythms and dysrhythmias. Typical placement of leads for a two-lead ECG is 3 to 5 cm inferior to the right clavicle and left lower rib cage. Typical placement for a three-lead ECG is the right arm (RA) near the shoulder, the V_5 position over the fifth intercostal space (LA), and the left upper leg (LL) near the groin.

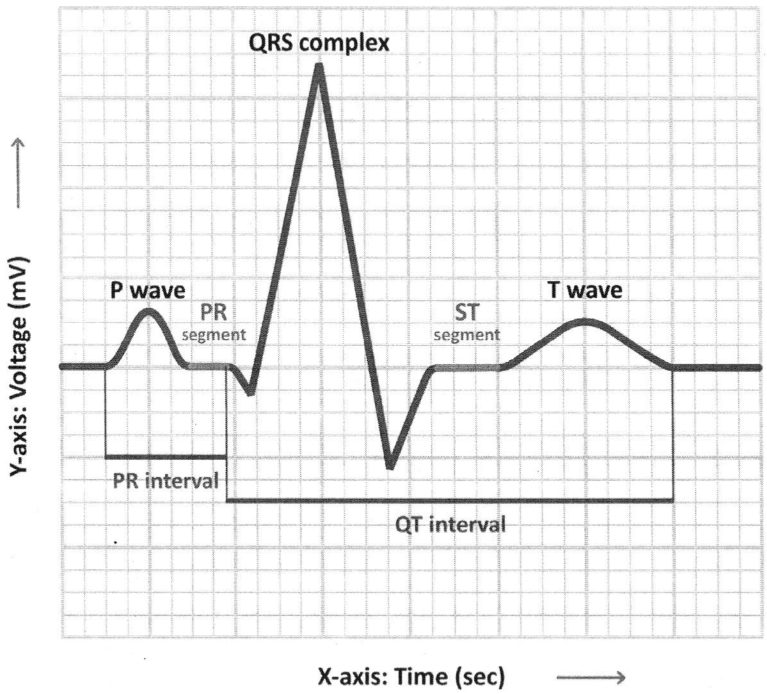

12-Lead Electrocardiography

The most common electrocardiography setup is the **12-lead ECG**, which assesses 12 different views of the heart. The 12-lead ECG actually comprises 10 electrodes and 12 sources of measurement as follows:

- Four limb electrodes: right and left arm and right and left leg (RA, LA, RL, LL). Put in place, avoiding heavily muscled areas.
- Six precordial (in front of the heart/pericardium) electrodes:
  - V1—Right sternum, fourth intercostal space
  - V2—Left sternum, fourth intercostal space
  - V3—Halfway between V2 and V4
  - V4—Midclavicular line, fifth intercostal space
  - V5—In line with V4 at the anterior axillary line
  - V6—In line with V4 and V5 at the midaxillary line

The patient should be placed in the flat supine position for the ECG, although he or she can sit in the semi-Fowler's position if unable to tolerate a flat position. The skin should be dry and the hair clipped or shaved to improve the electrode contact, and conductive gel is applied to the electrode. The skin can be wiped with an alcohol pad to remove oils or other residue before applying the electrodes. Electrodes should not be placed directly over a bone.

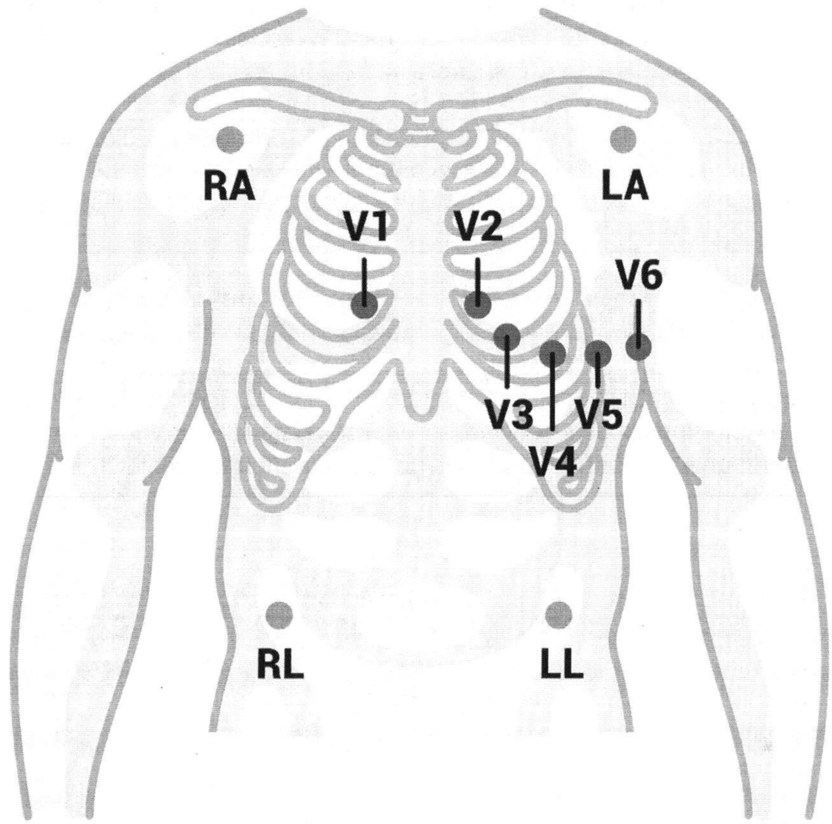

Review Video: Cardiovascular Assessment
Visit mometrix.com/academy and enter code: 323076

Heart Sounds

Normal and abnormal heart sounds include the following:

- **First and second sounds**: The first heart sound (S1—"lub") is closure of the mitral and tricuspid valves (heard at the apex/left ventricular area of the heart). The second heart sound (S2—"dub") is closure of the aortic and pulmonic valves (heard at the base of the heart). There may be a slight splitting of the S2.
- Gallop rhythms:
  - S3 occurs after S2 in children and young adults, but it may indicate heart failure or left ventricular failure in older adults (heard with the patient lying on the left side).
  - S4 occurs before S1 and occurs with ventricular hypertrophy, such as from coronary artery disease, hypertension, or aortic valve stenosis.
- **Opening snap**: Unusual, high-pitched sound occurring after S2 with stenosis of mitral valve from rheumatic heart disease
- **Ejection click**: Brief, high-pitched sound occurring immediately after S1 with stenosis of the aortic valve

- **Friction rub**: Harsh, grating sound heard in systole and diastole with pericarditis
- **Murmur**: Sound caused by turbulent blood flow from stenotic or malfunctioning valves, congenital defects, or increased blood flow

Capillary Refill Test

A capillary nail refill test is a measure of how much blood is flowing to a patient's tissues, which is known as tissue perfusion. The test can quickly identify whether a patient's vascular flow is normal. The skin and nail beds are a good indicator of systemic vascular resistance and shunting. The test is performed by applying direct pressure to a patient's nail bed until the nail bed turns from pink to white in color. The individual applying the pressure to the patient's nail bed will monitor how long it takes for the nail bed to return to pink, which indicates that blood has returned to the tissue. A patient whose capillary nail refill test is longer than two seconds may be suffering from hypothermia, shock, dehydration, and/or peripheral vascular disease.

Jugular Venous Pressure

Jugular venous pressure should be measured with the head of the patient's bed at a 45-degree angle. The patient's head should be turned to the right for accurate measurement. With the patient's head in the proper position, the examiner should identify the patient's jugular venous pulsations. Additionally, the examiner needs to locate the sternal angle, which can be found at the superior edge of the sternum. In centimeters, the examiner should then measure the distance between the identified pulsations and the patient's sternum. If this distance measures greater than four centimeters, neck vein distention is present; the distance is considered normal if it is four centimeters or less.

Angina

Chest pain may indicate angina (pain from temporary constriction/blockage of blood flow in the coronary arteries) or a heart attack (pain caused by blockage of blood flow to the heart muscle because of a blood clot (most common) or hemorrhage, resulting in the death of heart tissue). Heart problems in children are often associated with congenital heart disease. Geriatric and female patients may not have chest pain with a heart attack. Make note of the following:

- Character, location, and severity of the pain.
- Radiation of pain to the neck, jaw, arms, back, jaw, and/or stomach.
- Shortness of breath at rest, with exertion, or worsening when lying flat.
- Cold, clammy skin is common with a heart attack.
- Note BP, pulse (rapid, irregular, slow), and respirations.
- Note nausea and/or vomiting and dizziness/lightheadedness.

Angina Pectoris (Stable)

Impairment of blood flow through the coronary arteries leads to ischemia of the cardiac muscle and angina pectoris—pain that may occur in the sternum, chest, neck, arms (especially the left arm), or back. The pain frequently occurs with crushing pain substernally, radiating down the left arm or both arms, although this type of pain is more common in males than females, whose symptoms may appear less acute and may include nausea, shortness of breath, and fatigue. Elderly or diabetic patients may also have pain in their arms, no pain at all (silent ischemia), or weakness and numbness in both arms.

Stable angina episodes usually last for <5 minutes and are fairly predictable, exercise-induced episodes caused by atherosclerotic lesions blocking >75% of the lumen of the affected coronary artery. Precipitating events include exercise, a decrease in the environmental temperature, heavy eating, strong emotions (such as fright or anger), or exertion, including coitus. Stable angina episodes usually resolve in less than 5 minutes by decreasing the activity level and administering sublingual nitroglycerin. Provide supportive care, oxygen, and assist the patient to take nitroglycerin if available.

Angina Pectoris (Unstable, Variant/Prinzmetal's)

Unstable angina (also known as preinfarction or crescendo angina) is a progression of coronary artery disease, and it occurs when there is a change in the pattern of stable angina. The pain may increase, may not respond to a single nitroglycerin dose, and may persist for >5 minutes. Usually pain is more frequent, lasts longer, and may occur at rest when sitting or lying down. Unstable angina may indicate a rupture of an atherosclerotic plaque and the beginning of thrombus formation, so it should always be treated as a medical emergency with rapid transport because it may indicate a myocardial infarction.

Variant angina (also known as **Prinzmetal's angina**) results from spasms of the coronary arteries. It can be associated with or without atherosclerotic plaques and is often related to smoking, alcohol, or illicit stimulants. Variant angina frequently occurs cyclically at the same time each day and often while the person is at rest. Nitroglycerin or calcium channel blockers are used for treatment.

Management of a Patient with Angina

Management of a patient with angina begins with a thorough assessment, primary and secondary survey, and use of the OPQRST and SAMPLE methods of history taking. Patients are often very frightened, so the transport nurse should provide clear feedback and reassurance. The patient should be placed in the semi-Fowler's position, especially if he or she is experiencing shortness of breath, and the oxygen saturation should be monitored. Respiratory compromise may require supplemental oxygen, bag-mask ventilation (BVM) assistance, PEEP, CPAP/BiPAP, manually triggered ventilators (MTVs), or automatic transport ventilators (ATVs).

Pharmacological interventions (assist the patient with medication administration, or administer the medication according to protocol) may include the following:

- **Aspirin** (for suspected heart attack; Bayer, Heartline, ZORprin, Empirin): Provide 162 to 325 mg chewable (preferred). Contraindicated with GI bleeding, stroke.
- **Nitroglycerin** (for suspected angina; Nitro-Dur, Nitrolingual, NitroMist): Provide 0.4 mg sublingually repeated every 3–5 minutes up to three doses. Contraindicated if the patient has recently taken Viagra, had a stroke, or has excessive bleeding.
- **Oral glucose** (for suspected hypoglycemia/insulin reaction): Glucose tablets, solution.

All patients with chest pain should be transported because even mild chest discomfort may indicate that the patient is having a heart attack, especially in older patients and female patients, who often have atypical symptoms.

Myocardial Infarction

Myocardial infarction (also referred to as an MI or heart attack) may occur after an episode of unstable angina caused by a rupture of an atherosclerotic plaque and thrombosis associated with coronary artery spasm, but it may also result from vasoconstriction, acute blood loss, decreased oxygen, and ingestion of cocaine. Symptoms may vary considerably, with males having the more "classic" symptom of a sudden onset of crushing chest pain. Elderly and diabetic patients may complain primarily of weakness. Symptoms include the following:

- Angina with pain in the chest that may radiate to the neck or arms, crushing pain, tightness (often more than 30 minutes and unrelieved by rest or nitroglycerin).
- Hypertension or hypotension.
- Palpitations, tachycardia, bradycardia, and dysrhythmias.
- Dyspnea.
- ECG changes (ST segment and T-wave changes), tachycardia, bradycardia, and dysrhythmias.
- Pulmonary edema, peripheral edema, weak/absent peripheral pulses.
- Nausea and vomiting.

- Pallor, cold and clammy skin, diaphoresis.
- Neurological/psychological disturbances: Anxiety, light-headedness, headache, visual abnormalities, slurred speech, and fear.

Interventions: Manage the patient's airway/ventilation/oxygen supplementation, provide supportive care, perform CPR/defibrillation if needed, and provide rapid transport.

Review Video: Myocardial Infarction
Visit mometrix.com/academy and enter code: 148923

ECG Analysis of Myocardial Infarction

Myocardial ischemia results in ST-segment depression and T-wave inversion. **Myocardial injury** results in ST-segment elevation and T-wave inversion. **Myocardial infarction** results in hyperacute T waves (initial stage), ST-segment elevation, T-wave inversion, and pathologic Q waves. Arrhythmias common to MI include sinus tachycardia (rapid heart rate), sinus bradycardia (slow heart rate), heart blocks, ventricular fibrillation, pulseless electrical activity (PEA), and asystole. Rapid transport is indicated for patients having no relief from medication, hypotension, hypoperfusion, and/or significant ECG changes/abnormalities. No transport is indicated only for patient refusal.

Q wave MI:

- Characterized by a series of abnormal Q waves (wider and deeper) on ECG, especially in the early morning (related to adrenergic activity)
- Infarction is usually prolonged and results in necrosis (This may indicate extensive transient ischemia)
- Usually transmural

Non-Q wave MI:

- Characterized by changes in the ST-T wave with ST depression (usually reversible within a few days)
- Usually reperfusion occurs spontaneously, so the infarct size is smaller; contraction necrosis related to reperfusion is common
- Usually nontransmural

Heart Failure

Heart failure (HF, aka congestive HF) includes disorders of contractions (systolic "left-sided" dysfunction) or filling (diastolic dysfunction) or both, which result in hypertrophy (thickening, enlarging, and stiffening) of the myocardium (heart muscle). The most common causes are coronary artery disease, myocardial infarction, systemic or pulmonary hypertension, cardiomyopathy, and valvular disorders. The incidence of HF correlates with age. Left-sided HF may cause pulmonary edema that impairs ventilation, leading to hypoxia, especially when the patient is lying in a supine position, and right-sided HF may cause abdominal and peripheral edema of the feet and legs. The circulatory time with HF decreases overall, so changes in oximetry to show hypoxia may be delayed. The autonomic nervous system's regulation of breathing to control oxygen levels may be impaired, resulting in periodic breathing patterns, Cheyne-Stokes breathing, or central sleep apnea. Medications used to treat HF include ACE inhibitors (captopril, lisinopril), angiotensin receptor blockers (ARBs) (losartan, valsartan), beta-blockers (metoprolol, carvedilol), aldosterone agonists (spironolactone), and diuretics (hydrochlorothiazide, furosemide).

Chronic vs Acute Heart Failure

Chronic heart failure develops insidiously over time as the heart muscles weaken and enlarge, so initially patients may only note fatigue, weight gain, and swelling in their feet and ankles. **Acute heart failure** is characterized by impairment of gas exchange and decreased cardiac output because of changes in preload, contractibility, and heart rhythm; symptoms are more acute and may include irregular heartbeat, chest pain, cough, and rapid breathing, wheezing, and cyanosis from lack of adequate oxygen. Patients may also suffer from anxiety, decreased activity tolerance, and disturbances in sleep patterns. Medical management is aimed at increasing cardiac function, providing support, and monitoring treatment. Patients often are acutely short of breath and sitting upright, with rales evident in their lungs. Assessment includes conducting primary and secondary surveys, taking a complete medical history including medication use and home oxygen use, and assessing the patient's level of consciousness, airway status (cough, sputum, labored breathing, tripod position), heart rate/rhythm, peripheral pulses, edema (pitting/nonpitting, ascites, sacral), and complications.

Interventions: Manage the patient's airway/ventilation/oxygen supplementation with a nonrebreather mask or BVM with high-flow oxygen. Position the mask for comfort and suction if necessary.

Dysrhythmias

Sinus Bradycardia

Sinus bradycardia is characterized by a regular pulse <60 bpm with P waves in front of QRS, which are usually normal in shape and duration. The PR interval is 0.12–0.20 seconds, the QRS interval is 0.04–0.11 seconds, and there is a P:QRS ratio of 1:1.

Prehospital: Monitor, provide an IV access line, perform a 12-lead ECG, administer atropine (per protocol), and/or perform transcutaneous pacing if the patient is hypotensive or hypoperfusing. Administer epinephrine or dopamine if necessary.

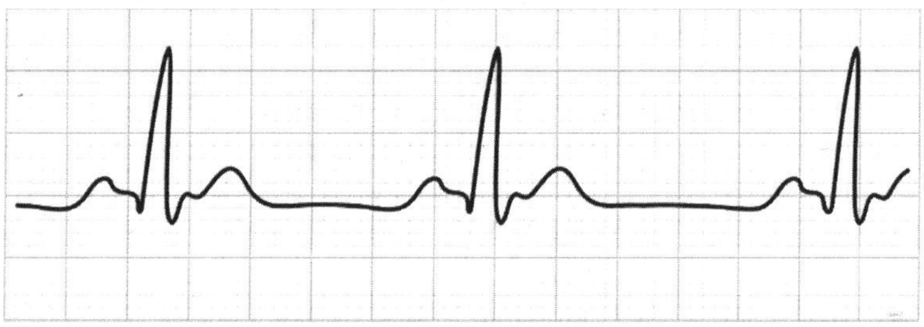

Sinus Tachycardia (ST)

With sinus tachycardia, the sinus node impulse increases in frequency. ST is characterized by a regular pulse >100 bpm with P waves before QRS, but sometimes they are a part of the preceding T wave. The QRS is usually of normal shape and duration (0.04–0.11 seconds), but it may have consistent irregularity. The PR interval is 0.12–0.20 seconds, and there is a P:QRS ratio of 1:1. The rapid pulse decreases the diastolic filling time and causes reduced cardiac output with resultant hypotension.

Prehospital: Stable—Monitor, provide supportive care, vagal maneuvers, an IV access line, and 12-lead ECG. Narrow—administer adenosine (per protocol). Wide—consult a cardiac expert. Unstable—perform cardioversion.

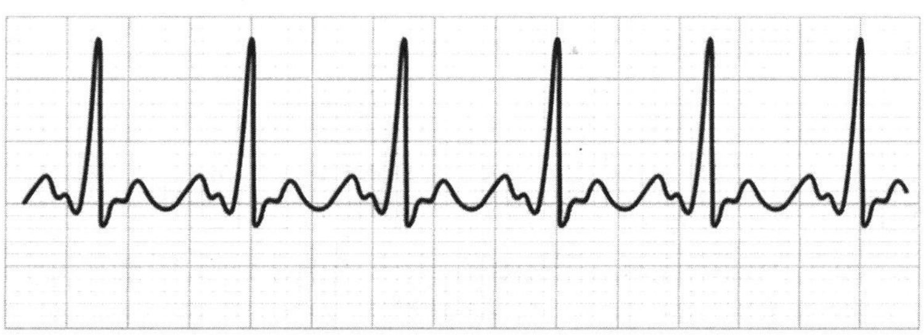

Sinus Arrhythmia

In sinus arrhythmia, irregular impulses from the sinus node, often paradoxical (increasing with inspiration and decreasing with expiration) because of stimulation of the vagal nerve during inspiration; it rarely causes a negative hemodynamic effect (common in both children and young adults and often lessens with age, but it may persist in some adults).

Prehospital: No treatment unless associated with severe bradycardia.

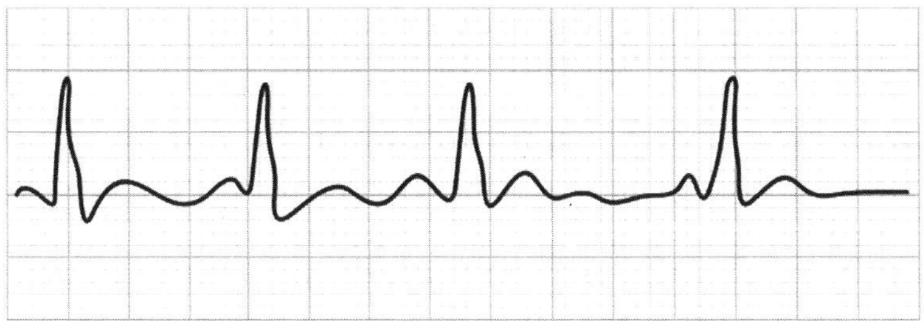

Supraventricular Tachycardia (SVT)

Supraventricular tachycardia may have a sudden onset and result in congestive heart failure. The heart rate is >100 bpm and may increase to 200–300 bpm. SVT originates in the atria rather than the ventricles, but it is controlled by the tissue in the area of the AV node rather than the SA node. The rhythm is usually rapid but regular.

Prehospital: Monitor, oxygen supplementation, adenosine (per protocol) if unstable.

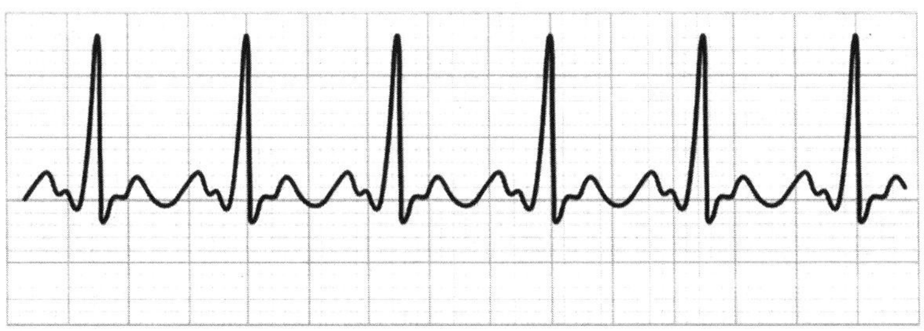

Atrial Fibrillation

With atrial fibrillation, the atrial rate is faster, usually 250–400 bpm, than the AV node conduction rate, so not all of the beats are conducted into the ventricles, effectively blocked at the AV node, preventing ventricular fibrillation, although some extra ventricular impulses may go through. Ventricular rate is usually irregular.

Prehospital: Monitor and administer an antiarrhythmic (amiodarone) if necessary.

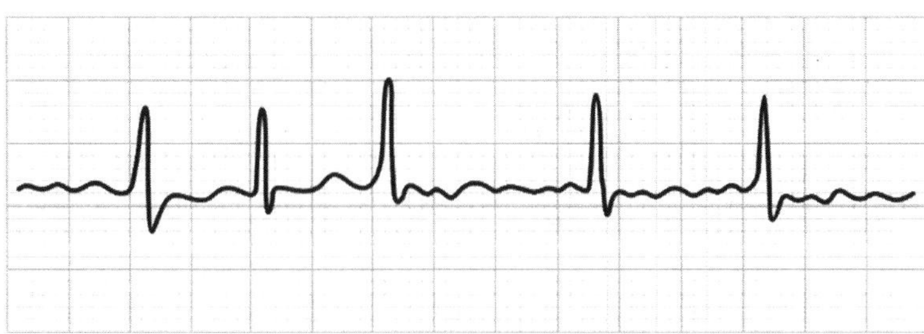

Atrial Flutter (AF)

Conditions that cause atrial flutter are coronary artery disease, valvular disease, pulmonary disease, heavy alcohol ingestion, and cardiac surgery. AF is characterized by atrial rates of 250–400 with ventricular rates of

75–150, with the ventricular rate usually being regular. P waves are saw-toothed (referred to as F waves), the QRS shape and duration (0.4–0.11 seconds) are usually normal, PR interval may be hard to calculate because of F waves, and the P:QRS ratio is 2–4:1.

Prehospital: Monitor and administer antiarrhythmics (amiodarone) if necessary to convert the unstable AF to a sinus rhythm (per protocol).

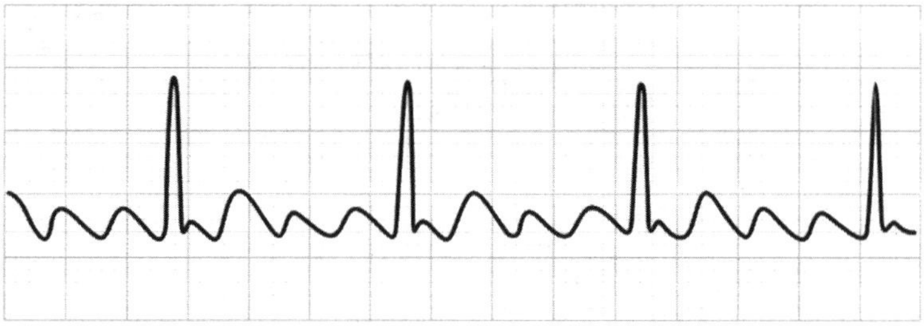

Ventricular Tachycardia

Ventricular tachycardia is ≥3 premature ventricular contractions (PVCs) in a row with a ventricular rate of 100–200 beats per minute. A detectable rate is usually regular, and the QRS complex is ≥0.12 seconds and is usually abnormally shaped. The P wave may be undetectable with an irregular PR interval if a P wave is present. The P:QRS ratio is often difficult to ascertain because of the absence of P waves.

Prehospital: Monitor, provide defibrillation if pulse is not palpable and patient is unresponsive, start an IV access line, and administer epinephrine. If there is failure to convert, administer amiodarone (per protocol).

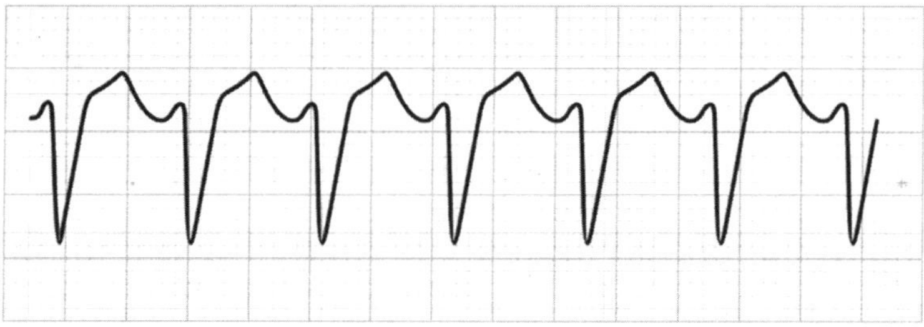

Ventricular Fibrillation

Ventricular fibrillation consists of a rapid, very irregular ventricular rate >300 bpm with no atrial activity observable on the ECG, caused by disorganized electrical activity in the ventricles. The QRS complex is not recognizable because the ECG shows irregular undulation.

Prehospital: Monitor, provide defibrillation, start an IV access line, and administer epinephrine. If there is failure to convert, administer amiodarone (per protocol).

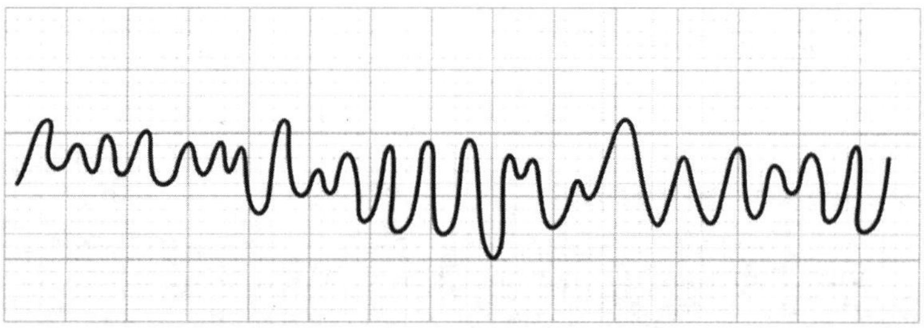

First-Degree AV Block

In first-degree AV block, atrial impulses are conducted through the AV node to the ventricles at a slower rate than normal. The P and QRS are usually normal, but the PR interval is >0.20 seconds, and the P:QRS ratio is 1:1.

Prehospital: Monitor. It usually requires no specific treatment.

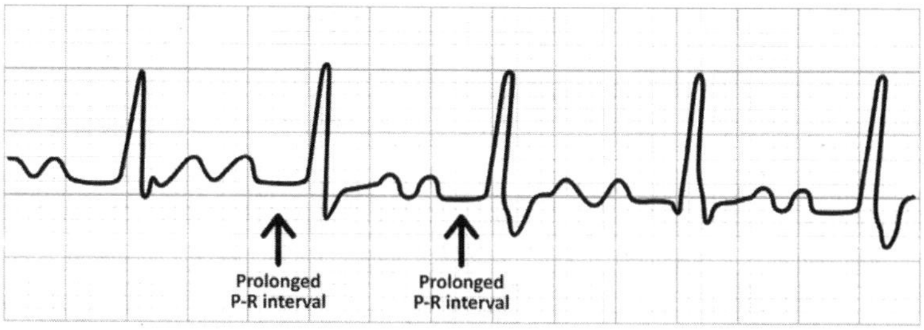

Second-Degree AV Block

Type I (Wenckebach)

In type I second-degree AV block, each atrial impulse in a group of beats is conducted at a lengthened interval until one fails to conduct (the PR interval progressively increases), so there are more P waves than QRS, but the QRS complex is usually of normal shape and duration.

Prehospital: Monitor. Usually does not cause significant problems unless it is associated with a myocardial infarction.

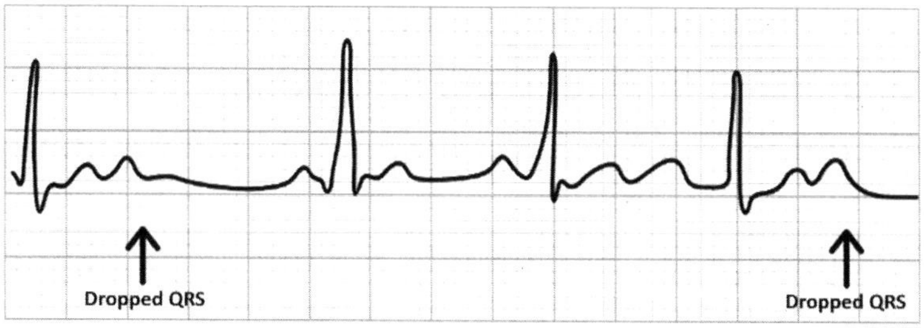

Type II (Mobitz)

In type II, only some of the atrial impulses are conducted unpredictably through the AV node to the ventricles. The PR intervals are the same if impulses are conducted, and the QRS complex is usually widened. The P:QRS ratio varies 2:1, 3:1, and 4:1.

Prehospital: Monitor. May progress to complete heart block, requiring transcutaneous pacing.

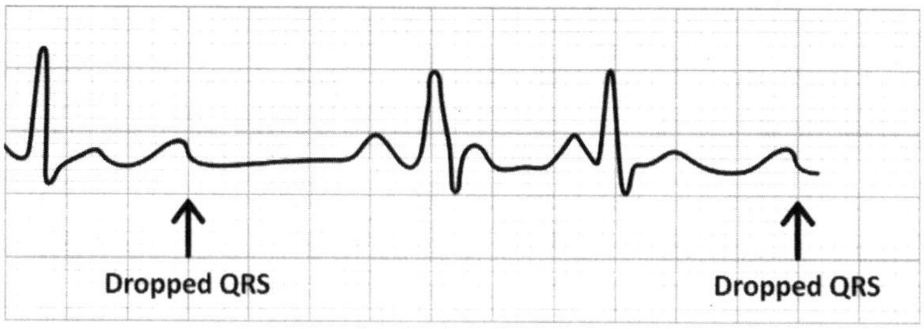

Third-Degree AV Block

With third-degree AV block, there are more P waves than QRS with no clear relationship between them and an atrial rate 2–3 times the pulse rate, so the PR interval is irregular. With SA node malfunction, the AV node fires at a lower rate. With AV node malfunction, the pacemaker site in the ventricles takes over at a bradycardic rate; thus, with complete AV block, the heart still contracts, but often ineffectually.

Prehospital: Monitor. May progress to complete heart block, requiring transcutaneous pacing.

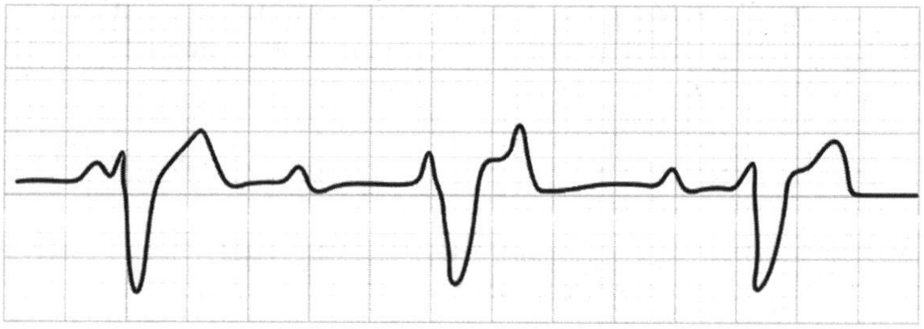

Pulseless Electrical Activity and Asystole

Pulseless electrical activity (PEA) is any rhythm without a palpable pulse (this is common after defibrillation). Identifying and correcting the underlying cause is critical for treatment. Common causes include the following:

Five H's:

- Hypokalemia/Hyperkalemia
- Hypoxia
- Hypothermia
- Hypovolemia
- Hydrogen ion (acidosis)

Five T's:

- Toxins
- Tamponade (cardiac)
- Tension pneumothorax
- Thrombosis (lungs)
- Thrombosis (heart)

Interventions: Begin CPR, start an IV access line, administer epinephrine (per protocol) every 3-5 minutes, provide intubation and ventilation, and give oxygen as indicated. Provide rapid transport.

Asystole ("flatlined") is the absence of an audible heartbeat, palpable pulse, and respirations. The ECG may show some P waves initially. The QRS complex is absent, although there may be an occasional QRS "escape beat." Prehospital: Check leads, begin CPR, start an IV access line, administer epinephrine (per protocol) every 3-5 minutes, provide intubation and ventilation, and give oxygen as indicated. Provide rapid transport.

Note: Defibrillation is not indicated in PEA or asystole.

Transcutaneous Pacing

Transcutaneous pacing is used temporarily to treat bradyarrhythmia that doesn't respond to medications (atropine) and results in hemodynamic instability. Generally, an arterial line is placed and the patient is provided oxygen before the pacing. The placement of pacing pads (large self-adhesive pads) and ECG leads varies somewhat according to the type of equipment, but usually one pacing pad (negative) is placed on the left chest, inferior to the clavicle, and the other (positive) is placed on the left back, inferior to the scapula. The heart is sandwiched between the two pads such that the myocardium is depolarized through the chest wall. Lead wires attach the pads to the monitor. The rate of pacing is usually set between 60 and 70 bpm. Current is increased slowly until capture occurs—a spiking followed by a QRS sequence—then the current is readjusted downward if possible, just to maintain capture. Demand and fixed modes are available, but the demand mode is preferred. Patients may require analgesia, especially if a higher current setting is needed.

Transvenous Pacing

Transvenous pacemakers, comprised of a catheter with a lead at the end, may be used prophylactically or therapeutically on a temporary basis to treat a cardiac abnormality, especially bradycardia. The catheter is inserted through a vein at the femoral or neck area and attached to an external pulse generator. Clinical uses include:

- To treat persistent dysrhythmias not responsive to medications.
- To increase cardiac output with bradydysrhythmia by increasing rate.
- To decrease ventricular or supraventricular tachycardia by "overdrive" stimulation of contractions.
- To treat secondary heart block caused by myocardial infarction, ischemia, and drug toxicity.
- To improve cardiac output after cardiac surgery.
- To provide diagnostic information through electrophysiology studies, which induce dysrhythmias for purposes of evaluation.
- To provide pacing when a permanent pacemaker malfunctions.

Complications are similar to implanted pacemakers and include increased risk of pacemaker syndrome.

Aortic Abnormalities

Abdominal Aortic Aneurysm

An aneurysm occurs when a blood vessel expands beyond its normal size in a confined space. Aneurysms can lead to instant death, but patients with aneurysms can also be saved if the aneurysm is caught and treated in its early stages. A true aneurysm is one in which all three layers of the arterial wall are involved. These three layers are the adventia, the intima, and the media. Congenital malformations, high blood pressure, or infections can all lead to the development of true aneurysms. For many patients, they are not aware of an aortic aneurysm until there is a major problem, however, some patients have known aneurysms that are being monitored. The risk of rupture of the aneurysm increases with aneurysm diameter, and risk of rupture must be weighed with risk of surgery. Because of this, many CV surgeons don't choose to do aneurysm repair until the AAA is bigger than 5cm. 50% of patients with a rupture aneurysm will present with hypotension, severe pain, and a pulsating abdominal mass. Treating a patient with an AAA rupture, management is focused on maintaining hemodynamic status. If presenting with shock give IVF. For patients with blood pressures that are adequate, pain medications and prophylactic antiemetics are given. Note home meds, especially anticoagulants. Transfer to facility with CV surgery. For patients being transported between facilities for definitive care of a confirmed AAA, aggressive BP control is usually used with target SBPs often in the 100-120s, often with Esmolol.

Aortic Dissection

An aortic dissection is life threatening with a mortality rate of 27%. Aortic dissections often arise in a preexisting aneurysm with 65% in the ascending, 10% in the arch, and 20% in the descending aorta. Symptoms include abrupt, acute chest pain, although patients with a congenital defect (Marfan's disease) may lack pain. Symptoms may mimic a myocardial infarction, but ECG indications of an MI are missing. Patients may exhibit JVD, pulsus paradoxus, and muffled cardiac sounds if the dissection results in cardiac tamponade. BP may be increased or decreased, depending on the type of dissection. One indication of aortic dissection is blood pressure difference between right and left arms of greater than 20 mmHg. Patients may exhibit both neurologic and respiratory impairments. Interventions include ECG and cardiac monitoring, intubation/ventilation if unstable, insertion of two large-bore IV lines, and administration of morphine for pain. If BP is elevated, propranolol or another beta-blocker may be given to decrease BP and pulse rate. If BP remains high, nitroprusside sodium may be administered.

Cardiac Arrest

Sudden cardiac arrest is the termination of cardiac movement and electrical activity, usually brought on by v-fib and v-tach. Without intervention it usually progresses to sudden cardiac death. Sudden cardiac arrest (SCA) may be preceded by warning signs but those signs may also be minimized and ignored by patients. A little more than 50% of patients had warning signs in the four weeks prior to arrest, with 80% having symptoms the hour before cardiac arrest. Chest pain and dyspnea are the two most commonly reported symptoms prior to SCA. Many patients with chest discomfort experience the sensation in the center of their chest; oftentimes, the pain or discomfort comes and goes, lasting several minutes each time. The discomfort is generally characterized as a tightening feeling, a feeling of squeezing in the chest, or pressure along the chest. Pain and discomfort in other areas of the body, including the back, the neck, either arm, the jaw, or the stomach, can also be signs, particularly when they are accompanied by chest pain. Shortness of breath and nausea or vomiting are additional signs of impending cardiac arrest. Once SCA happens the patient will be unresponsive, pulseless, with abnormal or absent breathing.

Pericardial Tamponade

Pericardial tamponade occurs when fluid builds up in the membranes surrounding the heart, known as the pericardium. Upon physical examination, a patient with pericardial tamponade might exhibit signs of shock. Signs of shock can include loss of pigment in the skin, abnormally low blood pressure, excessive sweating, abnormal values for peripheral pulses, diminished capillary refill capacity, and/or shortness of breath. Another indicator of pericardial tamponade is the presence of Beck's triad, which is a medical condition comprised of three symptoms: 1) decrease in systolic pressure, 2) obscured heart sounds, and 3) enlargement of the jugular vein, a vein in the neck that transports blood from the head region to the heart.

Pericardiocentesis

Blind (without ultrasound) pericardiocentesis is indicated with patient deterioration suspected to be from cardiac tamponade. All steps involved in an emergency pericardiocentesis must be exercised with extreme caution, as the environment make the procedure quite difficult. Patient should have IV, IVF running, ECG monitoring, airway and respiratory support. Position the patient at 30–45 degrees to bring the heart closest to chest wall, as this increases pooling in the heart. Use aseptic technique, prep skin with chlorhexidine solution to the chest, drape area, wear PPE gear if at all possible. Anesthetize the insertion site and needle track in alert patient. Insert the pericardiocentesis needle, and advance it towards the pericardial sac, with continuous aspiration of the attached syringe. Upon reaching the pericardial sac with the needle, there is usually increased resistance and then a "pop", then fluid should be easily aspirated. If catheter-needle assembly is used, send a guide wire through the insertion site down towards the needle. Remove the needle, and replace it with a pericardial catheter, to drain the fluid from the sac. Hemodynamic improvement usually is the best indicator that pericardiocentesis was successful, as fluids draining can be from other sites or due to cardiac puncture.

The site for a blind pericardiocentesis has typically been subxiphoid, however current studies show that the left parasternal and apical approaches yield superior results.

Hypertensive Crisis

Hypertensive crisis (aka malignant hypertension) is a marked elevation in BP that can cause severe organ damage if left untreated. Causes include encephalopathy, intracranial hemorrhage, aortic dissection, eclampsia, and heart failure. Classifications are as follows:

- **Hypertensive emergency**: Acute hypertension, usually >120 mmHg diastolic, must be treated immediately to lower the BP in order to prevent damage to vital organs, such as the heart, brain, or kidneys.
- **Hypertensive urgency**: Acute hypertension must be treated within a few hours, but the vital organs are not in immediate danger. The blood pressure is lowered more slowly to avoid hypotension, ischemia of vital organs, or failure of autoregulation with a one-third reduction in 6 hours.

Symptoms include headache, dizziness, dyspnea, weakness, visual disturbances, anxiety, chest pain (atypical), heart failure, acute coronary syndrome, and stroke.

Interventions: Asymptomatic hypertension requires referral to a physician, whereas severe symptoms require rapid transport. Interventions include airway support/ventilation with oxygen supplementation and advanced life support as needed. Patients with severe dyspnea and pulmonary edema may need CPAP.

Arterial Line Management

Arterial lines are used for continuous BP monitoring, frequent blood sampling, and ABGs. Arterial lines are inserted into the radial (preferred) or femoral artery. Before radial insertion, the CRFN should conduct the Allen test to ensure adequate circulation to the hand. Contraindications include coagulopathy, inadequate circulation, Raynaud's syndrome and Buerger disease. The most common catheter is the 7 Fr 15 or 20 cm triple lumen. For insertion, the patient should be placed in supine position with wrist in a supported, dorsiflexed (30-45°) position with palm up. Lidocaine 1% should be injected for conscious patients. A catheter-over-needle or catheter-over-wire technique may be utilized with the needle inserted at a 30° to 45° angle. (If utilizing the catheter-over-wire technique, a small nick with a scalpel at the insertion site is needed to allow passage of the catheter.) Once the catheter is in place, the catheter must be secured with a suture or tape, site monitored carefully, and circulation in the hand assessed frequently.

Central Line Management

Central lines are central venous access devices (CVD) inserted for long-term IV therapy. Types include peripherally inserted central catheters (PICC), non-tunneled percutaneous central venous catheters, tunneled central venous catheters, and implanted subcutaneous ports. The PICC line is inserted into a lower arm vein while the others are inserted into veins in the right upper chest or neck with the tips of all types in the superior vena cava. The most common complication is infection. Before transport, the nurse should assess the type of CVAD, manufacturer's directions (if available), schedules for treatments (IVs, blood products, medications) or testing, patient skin turgor, and condition of skin about insertion site for signs of infiltration, extravasation, and/or infection. The CRFN should determine if any lumen needs flushing, check all connection points, and assess length of catheter. During transfer and transport, the transport nurse should protect the CVAD to prevent dislodgement or catheter damage by using a catheter stabilization device or looping and taping securely.

Monitoring Central Venous Pressure

Central venous pressure (CVP) is monitored through a central venous catheter with a pressure monitoring device attached to the distal port and threaded into one of the major vessels with the tip resting in the superior vena cava. The transducer should be placed at the midaxillary line, fourth intercostal space. CVP is the pressure in the superior vena cava or right atrium related to either volume or compliance. The normal CVP ranges from 2–6 mmHg. If the CVP increases to greater than 6 mmHg, this may indicate hypervolemia (such as may occur with renal failure), right-sided heart failure (decreased cardiac output and stroke volume), pulmonary artery stenosis, or positive pressure breathing (Valsalva maneuver). If the pressure falls below 2 mmHg, it most often represents hypovolemia, which may result from dehydration, blood loss, diarrhea, vomiting, and excessive diuresis. CVP may also decrease with negative pressure breathing.

Swan-Ganz Catheter Management

Swan-Ganz catheterization is a procedure whereby a catheter is passed into the right side of a patient's heart to monitor heart functioning and to examine blood flow. Normal diastolic pressure of the pulmonary artery ranges from zero to eight millimeters of mercury (mmHg); normal pulmonary artery systolic pressure is 15–30 mmHg. The mean pulmonary artery pressure is 12 mmHg. Pulmonary capillary wedge pressure normally ranges from 5–15 mmHg, and the normal range for right atrial pressure is 0–8 mmHg. If the monitor calculates cardiac output, normal ranges are 4-8 L/min and normal cardiac index is 2.5–4.2 L/min/m^2. However, before interfacility transfer, note that numbers that have been normal for that patient this admission to compare with any changes during transport, as these patients may not have normal numbers.

After transferring the patient to the vehicle, connect transducers to monitor (if transport monitor isn't compatible). Rezero the transducers. Make sure to release any extra air in the fluid bag of the pressure bag to avoid expansion during transport. Frequently monitor pressure of bag when flying (maintain 300 mmHg).

Managing a Patient with a VAD

A ventricular assist device (VAD) is a small pump implanted into the patient's chest or abdomen. The left ventricular assist device, or LVAD (the most common type of VAD), takes blood from the left ventricle through an inflow tube to the pump, which pumps it though an outflow tube to the aorta where it circulates. A driveline (cable) connects the implanted device to a computerized control unit outside of the body. The control unit is attached by additional cables to a power module or to 2 lithium battery packs and carried in a patient pack or special vest. LVADs are non-pulsatile, so a peripheral pulse is not palpable. Batteries must be changed one at a time (the pair last 10-12 hours). LVADs have alarm systems with symbols or messages to describe problems, such as disconnected cables or hypovolemia. INR target varies according to manufacturer, and is usually 2-3. Complications include right HF, arrhythmias, thrombus, stroke, bleeding, infection, hypovolemia, and device malfunction. Patients may not have obvious signs initially of arrhythmias (such as VFib), but they must be treated promptly to prevent organ failure.

Managing a Patient with an Intraaortic Balloon Pump

Intraaortic Balloon Counterpulsation (IABC, also known as IABPs) is a cardiac assist device used to treat patients with cardiogenic shock or severe perfusion issues. The primary purpose of an IABP is to increase the myocardial oxygen supply while decreasing the myocardial oxygen demand. The balloon needs to be inflated and deflated according to the patient's cardiac cycle; if the inflation and deflation are not timed correctly, the issue of myocardial oxygen supply vs demand will not be resolved. In addition to improper balloon placement, other complications can occur. Limb ischemia, a condition in which the arteries become obstructed and subsequently decrease the flow of blood to the patient's extremities, is one of the most common complications. Other complications can include infection, hemorrhage, circulatory problems, and aortic rupture. The transport nurse should assess the IABP insertion site and distal limb prior to transporting a patient with an IABP and note adequate perfusion. The site of insertion should be noted for hematoma, bleeding or s/s of infection. If hematoma is present, area should be outlined and assessed frequently for growth. New sharp back or groin pain, hypotension, tachycardia, bruises to abdomen and flank could indicate retroperitoneal bleeding, a very severe complication. If a patient with an IABP has cardiac arrest, most pump manufacturers recommend switching from ECG trigger to AP trigger, due to loss of ECG rhythm. The pump doesn't have to be disconnected during defibrillation.

Transport Considerations

Before transporting patient, the transport nurse should know the reason the patient has the IABP, the type/brand of pump (and have more than one set wires for that pump), have supplies to deal with any bleeding issues easily accessible, and consider ways to keep the femoral area immobile. Make sure IABP battery is fully charged and a backup battery is available. IABP should be placed in auto mode to compensate for altitude changes. The pressure bag for the system should be inflated and the transducer at the level of the phlebostatic axis. Settings, including timing, trigger, and balloon inflation should be known and checked frequently. Since most IABPs are triggered from ECG, assessing and replacing ECG electrode pads prior to transport is essential. Prior to transport, the transport nurse should assess the level of helium in the helium tank. The transport nurse should be familiar with the device, understand troubleshooting, and should trace all tubing and wiring, especially from console to patient, to check for blood or issue. Assessment should be done prior to transport to the vehicle, after patient is set up on the vehicle, with any major changes in patient status, and when alarms sound, at minimum. Transport nurses should be familiar with alarms and be able to visualize alarms when noise prevents alarms from being heard. Low pressure or helium leak alarms may indicate the IABP console should be put on hold until issue is resolved. Most IABP manufacturers state the pump can be immobile <20 mins due to risk for embolus, balloon entrapment, and vascular damage.

MANAGING A PATIENT UNDER INDUCED HYPOTHERMIA

Induced hypothermia (usually for 12–24 hours) maintains body temperature at a level lower than normal in order to provide neuroprotection following a period in which circulation to the brain was inadequate, such as after cardiac arrest. Induced hypothermia may also be used with some surgical procedures. Mild hypothermia is cooling the body to 32° to 35° C.; moderate hypothermia is 28° to 32° C; and deep hypothermia is <28° C. (Some studies suggest that cooling below 32° C has no advantage.) Management includes careful temperature monitoring and recording of temperature every hour. Vasopressors may be needed if systolic BP falls below 90 mmHg or MAP above 75 mmHg. Urinary output should be monitored and the physician should be alerted if output falls above 200 mL or below 30 mL for 2 consecutive hours. An NMBA (such as vecuronium) is used to prevent shivering in conjunction with sedation (such as midazolam). Pupillary reactions should be checked at least every hour.

Pulmonary

RESPIRATORY ASSESSMENT

ASSESSING FOR UPPER RESPIRATORY DISTRESS

A patient who is taking more breaths per minute than normal may be having difficulty breathing and/or may now have an adequate supply of oxygen. Additionally, patients who are not getting enough oxygen may display a bluish tint to their lips either around the mouth or on the inside of the lips. Skin that looks pale or gray in tone may also indicate a lack of oxygen. Oftentimes, patients produce a grunting noise when they are having trouble breathing. This grunting noise is apparent when the patient exhales. The noise is caused by the body attempting to keep the lungs filled with air. When a patient's nostrils flare when he/she breathes, it may indicate that the patient is exerting more effort than usual to breathe, which may in turn signify upper respiratory distress. Sweating, particularly along the forehead, and wheezing are also indicators of upper respiratory problems.

QUESTIONS TO ASK REGARDING BREATHING DIFFICULTIES

- How long have you been having trouble breathing?
- Did your breathing difficulties come on suddenly?
- Do you have additional symptoms or other medical conditions?
- In what position are your breathing difficulties at their worst?
- Does physical activity make it even more difficult for you to breathe?
- Are you able to breathe easier when you are not exerting yourself?
- Do you feel like you are short of breath?
- Do you have episodes of breathing difficulty or is the difficulty continuous?
- If you have episodes of breathing difficulty, how long does each episode last?
- Have you been exposed to anything or ingested anything to which you are allergic?
- Can you hear any abnormal sounds each time you breathe?
- Do your breathing difficulties prevent you from sleeping?
- Do your breathing difficulties awaken you when you are asleep?

INSPECTION AND PALPATION OF THE CHEST

Inspection of the chest is performed, in part, to determine a patient's respiratory rate. The rate can be determined by counting the number of breaths the patient takes in a minute through observing his/her chest rise and fall. A rate of 12 breaths per minute is considered normal respiration for adults. Inspection of the chest can provide additional information about irregular or abnormal patterns of breathing as well as breathing difficulties. The examiner should also observe the patient's chest for asymmetry and/or deformity during the inspection process. During palpation of the chest, the examiner should assess any areas of tenderness. Similar to the inspection process, palpation of the chest should include an assessment of deformities uncovered during the process. A diminished vibration level in the chest when a patient speaks may indicate a potentially serious lung condition or other medical complication.

Breath Sounds

Normal and abnormal breath sounds are as follows:

Vesicular	Normal low-pitched sound over lung bases and most lung fields.
Broncho-vesicular	Medium-pitched sound heard over main bronchi. Duration the same in expiration and inspiration.
Bronchial	Normal high-pitched loud sound heard over trachea. Expiratory sound is as long or longer than inspiratory. Abnormal if heard over lung bases.
Rales (crackles)	High-pitched crackles usually heard at end of expiration in lung bases indicating fluid in the alveoli. May be fine or coarse.
Rhonchi	Deep rumbling sound may be high-pitched and sibilant (whistling) or low-pitched and sonorous (snoring) caused by constricted airways or large amounts of secretions in airways. More pronounced on expiration.
Wheezes	High or low-pitched whistling or musical sounds most pronounced on expiration. Often indicate asthma or foreign body obstruction.
Stridor	Crowing sound caused by inflammation and swelling or larynx and trachea. Common finding in croup (associated with cough).
Grunts	Indicates respiratory distress in newborn.
Friction rub	Grating sound heard over area of lungs where pleura are inflamed.

Review Video: Different Types of Lung Sounds
Visit mometrix.com/academy and enter code: 765616

Chest Percussion

To percuss a patient's chest, the examiner should place one of his/her middle fingers upon the chest so that the distal interphalangeal joint lies firmly against the chest. Using the tip of his/her opposite middle finger, the examiner should use a flicking motion to strike the finger that is placed against the patient's chest. The resulting sound(s) should be documented; the sound(s) should be recorded as normal, dull, or hyperresonant. Dull sounds resulting from chest percussion may indicate pleural effusion (fluid accumulation in the pleural space) or lung consolidation (hardening or swelling of lung tissue). Exaggerated resonance can indicate conditions such as pneumothorax (air accumulation in the pleural space) or pulmonary diseases such as emphysema.

Assessing for Pulsus Paradoxus

During respiration, variation in a patient's pulse occurs as a normal process. Typically, a patient's pulse is weaker during inhalation and stronger when the patient exhales. Pulsus paradoxus (PP) is characterized by an abnormal pulse variation during respiration. Such variation can be a sign of a more serious medical condition such as chronic obstructive pulmonary disease (COPD) or asthma. A blood pressure cuff and stethoscope are generally used to measure PP. By examining the patient's systolic blood pressure variation with respiration, PP can either be indicated or ruled out. PP is indicated when a reduction in systolic pressure upon inspiration is greater than 10 millimeters of mercury (mmHg), as normal systolic blood pressure variation with respiration is 10 mmHg.

Restrictive Airway Disease

Asthma

Asthma is the result of an immune response that causes constriction of bronchi and inflammation and increased secretions in the lower airways. Symptoms include cough, wheezing, diminished breath sounds, dyspnea, and difficulty speaking. Children's symptoms are often intermittent, whereas adults' symptoms tend to be persistent. Death from asthma is most common in those older than 65. Geriatric patients are most at risk from influenza, pneumonia, and pneumococcal pneumonia.

Interventions: Administer albuterol (nebulized/metered dose) per protocol and oxygen (6-8 L per minute), and provide airway management and ventilation. Provide CPAP for moderate/severe cases. If severe, provide rapid transport.

Chronic Pulmonary Obstructive Disease (COPD)

COPD is a disease with limitations of airflow, narrowing airways, exertional dyspnea, chronic cough, right-sided heart failure (cor pulmonale), damaged and distended alveoli, barrel chest, and clubbed fingers. Symptoms include severe dyspnea, cough, sputum, cyanosis, and the tripod position. Specific types of COPD include:

- Chronic Bronchitis: Chronic inflammation of bronchial passages with cough and sputum production, resulting in narrowed airway passages and dyspnea. Symptoms usually persist for more than 3 months per year.
- Emphysema: Chronic inflammation of the alveoli of the lungs results in ruptures and large, distended air sacs that trap air. Symptoms include dyspnea, cyanosis, difficulty exhaling, barrel chest, altered mental status, and pursed-lip breathing.

Interventions: Manage the patient's airway and ventilation and provide oxygen per nasal cannula or Venturi mask to maintain oxygen saturation >90%, provide the patient with a position of comfort or capnography near 35-45 mmHg, peak flow, and consider CPAP. Administer a beta-agonist bronchodilator (albuterol) according to protocol. Severe: Provide rapid transport.

Obstructive Airway Disease

Pneumonia

Pneumonia is inflammation of the lung, filling the alveoli with exudate and interfering with ventilation. It is common throughout childhood and adulthood. **Pneumonia** may be a primary disease, or it may occur secondary to another infection or disease, such as lung cancer. Pneumonia may be caused by bacteria, viruses, parasites, fungi, or toxins. Pneumonia is characterized by location (lobar, bronchial/lobular, interstitial). Symptoms include fever, chills, cough, purulent sputum, and difficulty breathing, chest pain on cough or deep inhalation, and headache. Bacterial pneumonia is treated with antibiotics, and viral pneumonia is treated with antivirals. Geriatric patients may exhibit confusion. Pediatric patients with undeveloped or poor immune systems, or chronic illnesses such as cystic fibrosis and asthma, have an increased risk.

Interventions: Use standard and droplet precautions, including wearing a protective face mask. Place the patient in a position of comfort (usually with his or her head elevated), manage the airway and ventilation, provide supplemental oxygen, and provide IV access line if indicated.

Review Video: Pneumonia
Visit mometrix.com/academy and enter code: 628264

Epiglottitis

Acute epiglottitis (supraglottitis) occurs in children (primarily 1-8 years old) and in young adults. Acute epiglottitis requires immediate medical attention because it can rapidly become obstructive. The onset is usually very sudden and often occurs during the night. The patient may awaken suddenly with a fever, but he or she usually does not have a cough.

Symptoms include the following:

- **Tripod position**: Sits upright, leaning forward with the chin out, mouth open, and tongue protruding.
- **Agitation**: Appears restless, tense, and agitated.
- **Drooling**: Excess secretions combined with pain or dysphagia and a mouth-open position cause drooling.
- **Voice**: No hoarseness, but the voice sounds thick and "froglike."
- **Cyanosis**: Color is usually pale and sallow initially but may progress to frank cyanosis.
- **Throat**: On examination, the epiglottis appears bright red and swollen. Note: The patient's throat should not be examined with a tongue blade unless intubation and tracheostomy equipment are immediately available because the examination can trigger an obstruction.

Interventions: Provide rapid transport, administer high-flow oxygen with a blow-by mask, or provide slow ventilation with a BVM.

Acute Lung Injury and Acute Respiratory Distress Syndrome

Acute lung injury (ALI) comprises a syndrome of respiratory distress culminating in acute respiratory distress syndrome (ARDS). ARDS is a dangerous, potentially fatal respiratory condition, always caused by an illness or injury to the lungs. Lung injury causes fluid to leak into the spaces between the alveoli and capillaries, increasing pressure on the alveoli, causing them to collapse. With increased fluid accumulation in the lungs, the ability of the lungs to move oxygen into the blood is decreased, resulting in hypoxemia. Lung injury also causes a release of cytokines, a type of inflammatory protein, which then brings neutrophils to the lung. These proteins and cells leak into nearby blood vessels and cause inflammation throughout the body. This immune response, in combination with low levels of blood oxygen, can lead to organ failure. Symptoms are characterized by respiratory distress within 72 hours of surgery or a serious injury to a person with otherwise normal lungs and no cardiac disorder. Untreated, the condition results in respiratory failure, MODS, and a mortality rate of 5-30%.

Symptoms include:

- Refractory hypoxemia (hypoxemia not responding to increasing levels of oxygen)
- Crackling rales/wheezing in lungs
- Decrease in pulmonary compliance which results in increased tachypnea with expiratory grunting
- Cyanosis/skin mottling
- Hypotension and tachycardia
- Symptoms associated with volume overload are missing (3rd heart sound or JVD)
- Respiratory alkalosis initially but, as the disease progresses, replaced with hypercarbia and respiratory acidosis
- Normal x-ray initially but then diffuse infiltrates in both lungs, while the heart and vessels appear normal

Management

The management of acute respiratory distress syndrome (ARDS) involves providing adequate gas exchange and preventing further damage to the lung from forced ventilation.

Treatment includes:

- Mechanical ventilation to maintain oxygenation and ventilation
- Corticosteroids (may increase mortality rates in some patient populations, though this is the most commonly given treatment), nitrous oxide, inhaled surfactant, and anti-inflammatory medications

- Treatment of the underlying condition is the only proven treatment, especially identifying and treating an infection with appropriate antibiotics, as sepsis is most common etiology for ARDS, but prophylactic antibiotics are not indicated.
- Conservative fluid management is indicated to reduce days on the ventilator, but does not reduce overall mortality.

VENTILATION MANAGEMENT

Ventilation management in ARDS consists of the following:

- O_2 therapy by nasal prongs, cannula, or mask may be sufficient in very mild cases to maintain oxygen saturation above 90%. Oxygen should be administered at 100% because of the mismatch between ventilation (V) and perfusion (Q), which can result in hypoxia on position change.
- ARDS oxygenation goal is PaO_2 55-80 mmHg or SpO_2 88-95%.
- Endotracheal intubation may be needed if SpO_2 falls or CO_2 levels rise.
- The ARDS Network recommends low tidal volumes (6 mL/kg) and higher PEEP (12 cmH_2O or more).
- The low tidal volume ventilation described above is referred to as lung protective ventilation, and it has been shown to reduce mortality in patients with ARDS.
- Placing patients with severe ARDS in prone position for 18-24 hours per day with chest and pelvis supported and abdomen unsupported allows the diaphragm to move posteriorly, increasing functional residual capacity (FRC) in many patients.

SPONTANEOUS PNEUMOTHORAX

Spontaneous pneumothorax is air in the pleural space that causes the lung to collapse but without an obvious cause. Symptoms include an abrupt onset of sharp chest pain on the affected side, dyspnea, difficulty breathing, and decreased or absent respirations on the affected side.

- **Primary** (no underlying lung disease): It is most common in tall, thin adolescents and young adults and is associated with cigarette smoking. It often resolves without treatment and rarely progresses to tension pneumothorax.
- **Secondary** (underlying lung disease): It is most common in those with chronic obstructive pulmonary disease (COPD), cystic fibrosis, and severe asthma, and it poses a risk of death because of respiratory compromise. Patients may develop hypoxemia, altered mental status, coma, and tension pneumothorax.

Interventions: Manage the patient's airway, ventilation, and oxygen supplementation. Place the patient in a position of comfort and transport. A large spontaneous pneumothorax will require catheter aspiration of air or insertion of a chest tube.

NEEDLE DECOMPRESSION

Needle decompression, also referred to as needle thoracostomy, and is indicated for hemodynamically unstable patients with a suspected tension pneumothorax. A needle decompression is performed by inserting a large needle into intercostal space along the patient's midclavicular plane. The purpose of the needle insertion is to release the pressure that has built up in the patient's chest as a result of the trapped air. Most emergency vehicles have readily available kits with 14-or 16-gauge angiocatheters in them. The angiocatheter is placed on the affected side, third intercostal space, and midclavicular. This allows for immediate decompression. The needle is withdrawn and the cath remains in place, open to air. Usually there is rush of air on placement that indicates there is in fact a tension pneumo, as well as improvement in vital signs post placement. The small catheters are prone to kinks and small so they may not be able to completely remove the pneumo, so when stabilized and able, place a standard chest tube.

Pulmonary Edema

Pulmonary edema occurs when the alveoli in the lungs fill with fluid.

- **Cardiogenic**: The left ventricle weakens, so the heart cannot pump adequate amounts of blood, resulting in back pressure in the left atrium and the vessels in the lungs, forcing fluid into the alveoli. Left ventricular damage can result from coronary artery disease, cardiomyopathy, myocardial infarction, defective heart valves, and uncontrolled hypertension.
- **Non-cardiogenic**: Damage to the capillaries in the lungs causes them to leak fluid into the alveoli. Conditions causing noncardiogenic pulmonary edema include acute respiratory distress syndrome (ARDS), adverse drug reactions, pulmonary embolism, lung injury, viral infections, nervous system conditions, toxin exposure, smoke inhalation, near drowning, and high-altitude pulmonary edema (HAPE).

Symptoms include severe dyspnea, orthopnea, tachycardia, cough, and chest pain.

Interventions: Manage airway, ventilation, and supplemental oxygen/CPAP or intubation with PEEP, and start an IV access line. Medications may include dopamine, dobutamine, nitroglycerin, and furosemide (per protocol). Severe cases require rapid transport. For HAPE, immediately descend to a lower altitude (500-1000 m), provide supplemental oxygen and a portable hyperbaric chamber, and administer acetazolamide or dexamethasone (per protocol).

Acute Pulmonary Embolism

Acute pulmonary embolism occurs when a pulmonary artery or arteriole is blocked by a blood clot originating in the venous system or the right heart. While most **pulmonary emboli** are from thrombus formation, other causes may be air, fat, or septic embolus. Common originating sites for thrombus formation are the deep veins in the legs, the pelvic veins, and the right atrium. Causes include atrial fibrillation and stasis related to damage to the endothelial wall and changes in blood coagulation factors. Symptoms include dyspnea, tachypnea, tachycardia, anxiety, restlessness, chest pain, fever, rales, cough (sometimes with hemoptysis), and hemodynamic instability.

Interventions: Assess vital signs, oxygen saturation, lung sounds, signs of jugular vein distention, signs of DVT, and signs of shock. Provide the patient with high-flow oxygen per nasal cannula (C-PAP or BIPAP if hypoxia persists), insert a large bore IV line in the antecubital fossa (to facilitate CT scan with dye), administer NS if the patient is hypotensive but limit to 500-1000 mL to avoid pulmonary edema. Monitor ECG, typical pattern is S1Q3T3—elevated S wave (lead 1) and Q wave and inverted T wave (lead III). Provide analgesia per protocol (avoid morphine). Administer norepinephrine for persistent hypotension. Provide immediate anticoagulation, such as IV heparin, if available.

Pulmonary Hypertension and Pulmonary Arterial Hypertension

Pulmonary arterial hypertension (PAH) is a progressive disease of the pulmonary arteries that can severely compromise cardiovascular patients. It may involve multiple processes. Usually, the pulmonary vasculature adjusts easily to accommodate blood volume from the right ventricle. If there is increased blood flow, the low resistance causes vasodilation and vice versa. However, sometimes the pulmonary vascular bed is damaged or obstructed, and this can impair the ability to handle changing volumes of blood. In that case, an increase in flow will increase the pulmonary arterial pressure, increasing pulmonary vascular resistance (PVR). This in turn, increases pressure on the right ventricle (RV) with increased RV workload and eventually causes RV hypertrophy with displacement of the intraventricular septum and tricuspid regurgitation (cor pulmonale). Over time, this leads to right heart failure and death. Pulmonary hypertension is usually diagnosed by right-sided heart catheterization and is indicated by systolic pulmonary artery pressure >30 mmHg and mean pulmonary artery pressure >25 mmHg. Non-invasive testing may include echocardiogram to look for cardiac changes.

Types

Pulmonary hypertension or pulmonary arterial hypertension (PAH) may be classified as primary (idiopathic) or secondary.

- **Primary (idiopathic) PAH** may result from changes in immune responses, pulmonary emboli, sickle cell disease, collagen diseases, Raynaud's, and the use of contraceptives. The cause may be unknown or genetic.
- **Secondary PAH** may result from pulmonary vasoconstriction brought on by hypoxemia related to COPD, sleep-disordered breathing, kyphoscoliosis, obesity, smoke inhalation, altitude sickness, interstitial pneumonia, and neuromuscular disorders. It may also be caused by a decrease in pulmonary vascular bed of 50-75%, which may result from pulmonary emboli, vasculitis, tumor emboli, and interstitial lung disease, such as sarcoidosis. Primary cardiac disease, such as congenital defects in infants, and acquired disorders, such as rheumatic valve disease, mitral stenosis, and left ventricular failure may also contribute to PAH.

Treatment Options for PAH

Medical treatment for pulmonary arterial hypertension (PAH) aims to identify and treat any underlying cardiac or pulmonary disease, control symptoms, and prevent complications:

- **Oxygen therapy** may be needed, especially supplemental oxygen during exercise.
- **Calcium channel blockers** may provide vasodilation for some patients.
- **Pulmonary vascular dilators**, such as IV epoprostenol (Flolan) and subcutaneous treprostinil sodium (Remodulin) and oral bosentan (Tracleer) help to control symptoms and prolong life.
- **Anticoagulants**, such as warfarin (Coumadin) are an important part of therapy because of recurrent pulmonary emboli. Studies have shown that anticoagulation increases survival rates.
- **Diuretics**, such as furosemide (Lasix) may be needed to relieve edema and restrict fluids, especially with right ventricular hypertrophy.

In some patients who cannot be managed adequately through medical treatment, a heart-lung transplant may be considered as the only effective treatment for long-term survival.

Abdominal

GASTROINTESTINAL (GI) TRACT

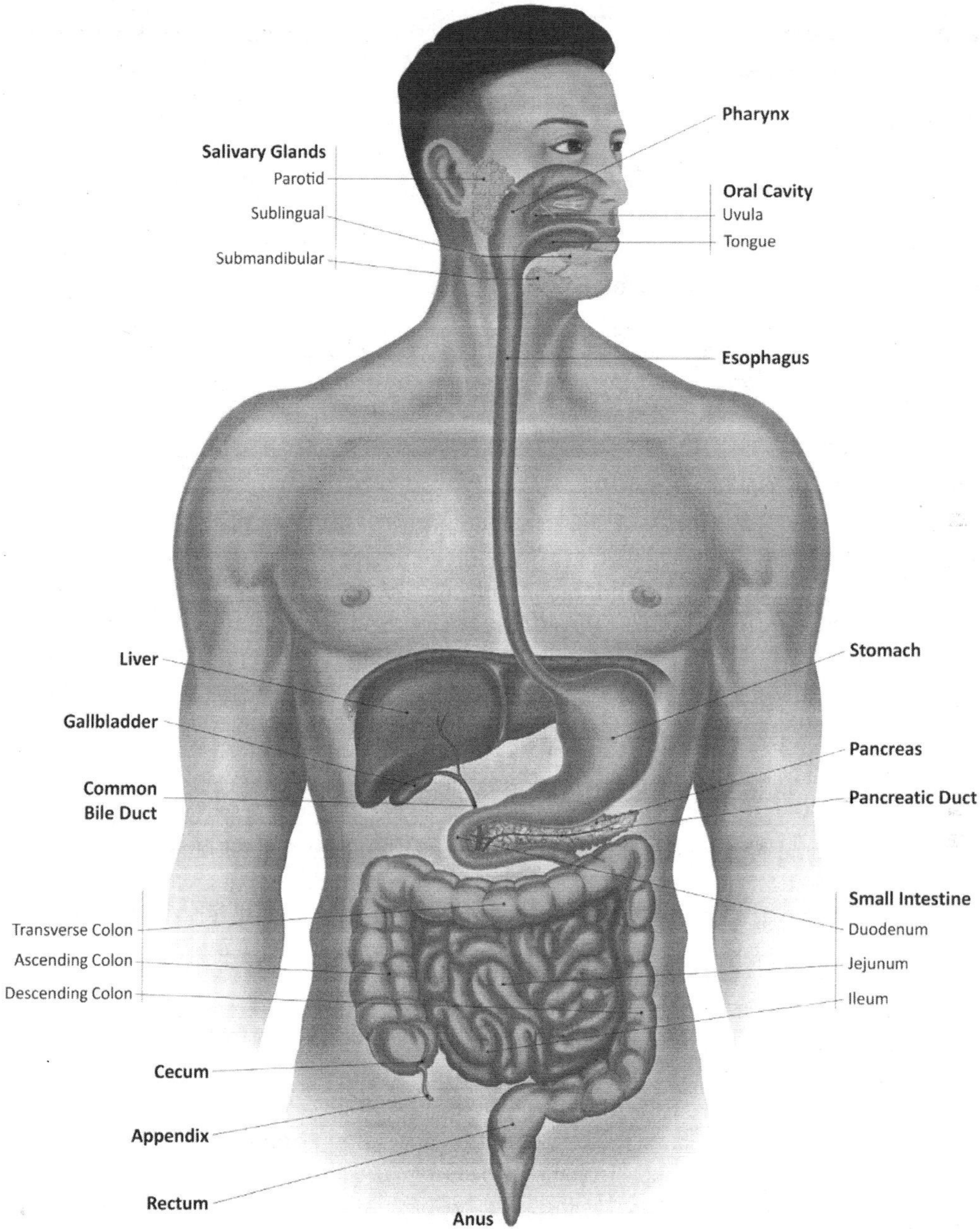

Elements of the **gastrointestinal tract**:

- **Mouth**: Chews, moistens, begins carbohydrate hydrolysis (the breakdown of food by enzymes), creates a bolus of food. Connected to the esophagus by the pharynx.
- **Esophagus**: Transports a bolus through the lower esophageal sphincter (which prevents backflow up the esophagus) to the stomach by peristalsis (wavelike contractions)
- **Stomach**: Churns, secretes acids and enzymes, begins hydrolysis of proteins, and creates chyme (a more fluid substance)
- Small intestine (about 20 feet long):

- Duodenum: Accepts chyme and digests food to prepare for absorption
- Jejunum: Absorbs most of the nutrients from the food, including vitamin B_{12}; accepts bile from the liver and gallbladder to digest fats and pancreatic enzymes from the pancreas to digest proteins, fats, and carbohydrates
- Ileum: Contains the ileocecal valve, which controls the flow of chyme into the large intestine

- Large intestine (about 5 feet long):
    - Cecum: Reabsorbs fluids and electrolytes
    - Appendix: Is believed to store useful gut bacteria
    - Ascending, transverse, descending colon: Reabsorbs water, vitamin K, and electrolytes to form feces
- **Rectum**: Stores feces
- **Anus**: Contains sphincters that control the expelling of feces

Review Video: Gastrointestinal System
Visit mometrix.com/academy and enter code: 378740

Abdominal Assessment

Inspection and Auscultation of the Abdomen

With the patient's abdomen exposed, observing and inspecting his/her abdominal area can provide information about the patient's medical condition(s). During inspection, the transport team member should make note of any skin abnormalities on the abdomen. Additionally, the team member should determine whether the abdomen looks swollen. Abdominal contours are typically best seen by standing at the patient's feet and looking up in the direction of the patient's head. If the abdomen appears distended, the transport team member should note whether the distension is symmetrical. Inspection can also offer information about whether the patient is comfortable moving and/or whether he/she is able to lie still. Auscultation should be performed before percussion and palpation. Note quality and frequency of sounds.

Percussion and Palpation of the Abdomen

Percussion should be performed before palpation, as patients with peritonitis will have pain even with percussion. To percuss the abdomen, the examiner should place one hand on the abdominal wall so that his/her middle finger is against the patient's skin. Using the tip of the middle finger of his/her other hand, the examiner should strike the joint two or three times of the middle finger of the hand that is on the patient. This process should be repeated in each quadrant of the abdomen. The transport team member should note whether tympanitic (drum-like) or dull sounds are heard; he/she should also note any pain felt by the patient during percussion. The examiner should then lightly palpate each quadrant of the patient's abdomen to identify areas of tenderness. Deeper palpation can be performed to identify abdominal masses and/or areas of extreme tenderness. It is most effective to watch the patient's face during palpation, as the patient's expressions tend to change when tenderness is encountered. A tympany sound may indicate a distended bowel while a dull sound may indicate a solid mass. In palpation, start with the abdominal quadrant with the least pain. Note tender areas, guarding, and rebound tenderness.

Gastrointestinal Bleeding

Gastrointestinal bleeding may occur anywhere within the GI system but is most common from the upper GI. Bleeding may range from slow and insidious to massive hemorrhage. Causes include esophageal inflammatory bowel disease (IBD), HIV/CMV infection, polyps, cancer, hemorrhoids, diverticulosis, ulcers, varices (associated with liver disease), Meckel's diverticulum, anticoagulation, and overuse of NSAIDS, such as aspirin and ibuprofen, so history can provide important clues. Output may help to differentiate upper GI bleeding from lower:

- Hematemesis/Coffee ground emesis: Upper GI
- Melena (dark, tarry, foul-smelling stool): Upper GI

- Hematochezia (bright bloody stool)/Clots: Lower GI or massive upper GI
- Bright blood about outside of stool: Hemorrhoids, lower GI

Interventions: Assess vital signs and oxygen saturation, abdominal tenderness, and signs of hypovolemic shock (pallor, hypotension, tachycardia, cool/clammy skin, loss of consciousness). With rectal bleeding, place absorbent pads on stretcher. Start two large-bore IVs and begin resuscitation with 1-2 L of crystalloid (NS/Lactated Ringer's) with signs of hypovolemia. Provide supplemental oxygen as needed to maintain oxygen saturation above 94%. Monitor ECG readings. With upper GI bleeding, vomiting, and abdominal distention, insertion of an NG tube may be indicated. Provide blood transfusions if indicated and available.

Ecchymosis

Ecchymosis occurs when bleeding into the skin or mucous membranes is present. Characterized by large, flat areas on the skin where blood has pooled under the tissue, ecchymoses tend to be greater than a centimeter in diameter. Ecchymoses can be quite dangerous and should always be evaluated. In order to appropriately treat an ecchymosis, it is important to recognize the difference between the condition and general skin redness or inflammation. To determine whether a patient has an ecchymosis or skin redness, slight pressure can be applied to the site of the discoloration. An ecchymosis will not blanch (turn pale and then return to its original color) when pressure is applied; conversely, inflammations of the skin will blanch when pressure is applied.

Acute Abdomen

Acute abdomen is an acute intra-abdominal disorder that occurs with abrupt onset and usually requires emergency surgical intervention, although some patients may respond to other treatments, such as antibiotics. Acute abdomen may result from infection (peritonitis, pancreatitis, cholecystitis, appendicitis, diverticulitis), perforation, rupture of an internal organ (such as the spleen), aortic aneurysm, obstruction, or infarction (necrotic tissue resulting from a blood clot or obstructed blood supply). If the blood supply is interrupted, gangrene may occur within 6 hours. Acute abdomen is characterized by inflammation, distension (often including guarding and rigidity), and acute pain (moderate to severe of fewer than 7 days duration). Abdominal pain is especially concerning in pediatric and geriatric patients and those with impaired immune systems (such as HIV/AIDS patients and those receiving chemotherapy). Acute abdomen in infants and children may indicate conditions not commonly found in adults such as pyloric stenosis, volvulus, and necrotizing enterocolitis.

Interventions: Obtain a medical history regarding the quality, location, and duration of pain as well as referred pain; place the patient in a comfortable position; administer oxygen; and provide rapid transport.

Diverticulitis and Appendicitis

Diverticulitis is inflammation of diverticula, which are bulging herniations in the intestinal wall, most commonly in the sigmoid colon, although they can occur anywhere within the GI tract from pharynx to anus. Diverticulitis may result in bowel obstruction, infection, perforation, or hemorrhage as undigested food and bacteria accumulate in diverticula, forming a fecalith (hard mass) that can impair circulation. Symptoms include acute pain (usually LLQ), abdominal distension, nausea, flatus, fever, constipation, and irregular bowel habits.

Appendicitis is inflammation of the appendix resulting from bacterial infection and obstruction. Appendicitis is most common in adolescents and young adults. Typical symptoms include abdominal pain (often initially around the umbilicus [navel] and then localizing to the RLQ). Nausea and vomiting are common. With rupture, high fever and intense pain are common as the patient develops signs of peritonitis. Any movement may increase the pain and the patient may develop shock.

Interventions: Take a complete medical history, and position the patient for comfort with his or her knees flexed. Provide pain management, antiemetics, supplemental oxygen as needed, and an IV access line.

Bowel Obstruction

Bowel obstruction occurs when there is a mechanical obstruction of the passage of intestinal contents because of constriction of the intestine, occlusion, or a lack of muscular contractions (paralytic ileus). Obstructions may be caused by congenital or acquired abnormalities/disorders. Small bowel obstruction may be caused by adhesions, surgical manipulation, cancer, or Crohn's disease, and large bowel obstruction may be caused by cancer, diverticulitis, or volvulus. Small bowel obstructions are usually corrected nonsurgically with a nasogastric (NG) tube and suction, whereas large bowel obstruction usually requires surgical intervention. Symptoms include abdominal pain, distension, and rigidity; nausea and vomiting; diminished or absent bowel sounds; severe constipation; respiratory distress from the diaphragm pushing against the pleural cavity; shock; and sepsis. Untreated bowel obstruction may lead to infarction (ischemia and necrosis). Infarction has a high mortality rate even with surgery.

Interventions: Provide IV access and insert an NG tube (according to protocol). Provide pain management and a position of comfort. Monitor vital signs and provide supplemental oxygen/ventilation as necessary.

Acute Pancreatitis

Acute pancreatitis is related to chronic alcoholism or cholelithiasis in 90% of patients, but it may also be caused by viral infections, cysts, cystic fibrosis, drugs, trauma, and metabolic disorders. Pain is usually acute and is midepigastric, left upper abdominal, or more generalized and may radiate to the back. Nausea and vomiting and abdominal distension are common. Pancreatitis may result from direct injury to pancreatic cells or activation of pancreatic enzymes that essentially autodigest pancreatic tissue, resulting in edema, necrosis, and hemorrhage. Vasodilation and increased capillary permeability may result in hypovolemia as fluid shifts to the retroperitoneal space. Complications may include shock, acute respiratory distress syndrome, and multiorgan failure. Pancreatitis may range from mildly edematous to necrotizing. Chronic pancreatitis may develop over years, resulting in extensive tissue damage with symptoms occurring intermittently initially and then continuously. Oily, foul-smelling stools may occur.

Interventions: Take a complete medical history of the patient's complaints, provide pain management, antiemetics, and supplemental oxygen/ventilation as needed. Start an IV access line and provide shock treatment per protocol if necessary.

Hepatitis and Fulminant Hepatitis

Hepatitis, inflammation of the liver, is caused by bacteria, viruses, or exposure to toxic chemicals, including alcohol or drugs. However, viral infection is most common and may be foodborne or bloodborne, although only bloodborne diseases, hepatitis B and C, cause chronic liver disease. Symptoms include jaundice (yellowing of the skin and eyes) and clay-colored stool from impaired excretion of bile, dark urine, abdominal pain, flu-like symptoms, nausea and vomiting, loss of appetite, itching, and increased risk of bleeding.

Fulminant hepatitis is an acute inflammation of the liver that may be caused by viruses, toxic substances, or overdose with acetaminophen and can result in encephalopathy, liver failure, and death within 1 to 72 days. Vaccinations are available for hepatitis A virus (HAV) and hepatitis B virus (HBV). Treatment for accidental exposure to HAV is prophylaxis with HAV immune globulin, and that for HBV is initiating vaccinations if the patient is unvaccinated or HBV immune globulin.

Interventions: Use standard precautions, provide supportive care as needed, manage the patient's airway/ventilation, and provide IV fluids if necessary.

Types of Hepatitis

Type of hepatitis	Transmission	Characteristics
Hepatitis A (HAV)	Foodborne/oral-fecal and oral-anal sex	Usually mild infection (may be asymptomatic) lasting about 2 months.
Hepatitis B (HBV)	Bloodborne/blood, body fluids/sex, and needle sharing	Most common bloodborne hepatitis and very infectious. Most recover within 6 months, but up to 10% develop chronic disease, which can lead to liver failure or liver cancer, and they become carriers.
Hepatitis C (HCV)	Bloodborne/blood and body fluids/sex/needle sharing	Causes chronic infection and is the most common cause of liver transplantation. May be asymptomatic for 20 years.
Hepatitis D (HDV)	Bloodborne/blood and body fluids/sex/needle sharing	Co-infection with HBV and increases the risk of developing fulminant hepatitis and cirrhosis.
Hepatitis E (HEV)	Foodborne/oral-fecal and oral-anal sex	Usually found in travelers from South Asia or Africa from areas with poor sanitation. It is a mild form similar to HAV.
Hepatitis G (HGV-C)	Bloodborne/blood and body fluids/sex/needle sharing	Believed to be a variation of type C and can be a co-infection of HBV and HBC. Usually a mild infection, but it may be chronic.

Gastric Decompression Via NG/OG Tube

An **NG/OG tube** is indicated when gastric insufflation or vomiting impedes the patient's ability to breathe or the paramedic's ability to ventilate the patient. Under some protocols, an NG/OG tube is placed prior to intubation and ventilation. Procedure:

1. Select appropriate size NG/OG tube (usually double lumen for adults) and measure from xyphoid process to the angle of the jaw and then to the corner of the mouth for an OG tube or to the corner of the nose for an NG tube.
2. Lubricate the tube with water soluble gel.
3. Insert into the largest nostril (usually right) or midline in the mouth and guide to the appropriate length. Encourage the patient to swallow as the tube passes through the esophagus, to help guide the tube to the stomach.
4. Check placement by placing the stethoscope over the gastric area and injecting 20 to 60 mL of air into the suction port and listening for the sound of the air.
5. Aspirate gastric contents for additional confirmation.
6. Remove tube if incorrectly placed and secure with gastric placement.
7. Connect to low suction or manually aspirate air/gastric contests to decompress the stomach.

NG/OG tube is contraindicated with esophageal varices because of the risk of hemorrhage. An NG tube is contraindicated with head injury, mid-face injury, or basilar skull fracture.

Confirming Placement

A chest x-ray can confirm when a nasogastric (NG) tube has successfully been placed in a patient's stomach. However, if it is not possible to obtain a chest x-ray, an irrigation syringe can be used to aspirate the contents of the patient's stomach. If a salem sump tube is correctly positioned, if you instill 30 cc of warm water via syringe and area able to immediately suction back most of the water, the sump is most likely correctly placed. If the patient coughs, chokes, and/or develops a bluish skin tone, a condition known as cyanosis, while attempting to talk, the tube has likely passed through the larynx. Finally, improper tube placement may also be detected by placing the open end of the tube in water; if the tube has passed through the larynx, the water will bubble. Placement should always be verified by radiology before instilling medications or formulas due to risk of placement in bronchial tree. On arrival to a facility, notify and document that new caregivers were made aware that the tube was only clinically confirmed, but will need x-ray confirmation before anything should be instilled. Transport nurses should also be aware that during long interfacility transports, previously confirmed tubes can become dislodged and that their placement should be reconfirmed if needed.

Electrolyte Imbalances

Sodium

Sodium (**Na**) regulates fluid volume, osmolality, acid-base balance, and activity in the muscles, nerves, and myocardium. It is the primary **cation** (positive ion) in extracellular fluid (ECF), necessary to maintain ECF levels that are needed for tissue perfusion:

- Normal range: 135-145 mEq/L
- Hyponatremia: <135 mEq/L
- Hypernatremia: >145 mEq/L

Hyponatremia may result from inadequate sodium intake, excess sodium loss through diarrhea, vomiting, or NG suctioning, or illness, such as severe burns, fever, SIADH, and ketoacidosis.

- **Symptoms**: Irritability to lethargy and alterations in consciousness, cerebral edema with seizures and coma, dyspnea to respiratory failure.
- **Treatment**: Identify and treat underlying cause and provide Na replacement.

Hypernatremia may result from renal disease, diabetes insipidus, and fluid depletion.

- **Symptoms**: Irritability to lethargy to confusion to coma; seizures; flushing; muscle weakness and spasms; thirst.
- **Treatment**: Identify and treat underlying cause, monitor Na levels carefully, and give IV fluid replacement.

Potassium

Potassium (**K**) is the primary **electrolyte** in intracellular fluid (ICF) with about 98% inside cells and only 2% in ECF, although this small amount is important for neuromuscular activity. Potassium influences activity of the skeletal and cardiac muscles. Its level is dependent upon adequate renal functioning because 80% is excreted through the kidneys and 20% through the bowels and sweat:

- Normal range: 3.5-5.5 mEq/L
- Hypokalemia: <3.5 mEq/L. Critical value: <2.5 mEq/L
- Hyperkalemia: >5.5 mEq/L. Critical value: >6.5 mEq/L

A healthy NPO patient will need about 40 mEq of K per day to maintain serum K levels. (expect alterations in renal disease and other disease processes).

Hypokalemia is caused by loss of potassium through diarrhea, vomiting, gastric suction, and diuresis, alkalosis, decreased intake with starvation, and nephritis.

- **Symptoms**: Lethargy and weakness; nausea and vomiting; paresthesia and tetany; muscle cramps with hyporeflexia; hypotension; dysrhythmias with EKG changes: PVCs or flattened T-waves.
- **Treatment**: Treatment involves identifying and treating the underlying cause and replacing K. When possible, oral replacement is preferable to IV, as it allows slower adjustment of K levels. When given IV, K should be given no faster than 20 mEq/hour via central line if possible. If given peripherally, 10 mEq/hour is preferable for patient comfort.

Hyperkalemia is caused by renal disease, adrenal insufficiency, metabolic acidosis, severe dehydration, burns, hemolysis, and trauma. It rarely occurs without renal disease but may be induced by treatment (such as NSAIDs and potassium-sparing diuretics). Untreated renal failure results in reduced excretion. Those with Addison's disease and deficient adrenal hormones suffer sodium loss that results in potassium retention.

- **Symptoms**: The primary symptoms relate to the effect on the cardiac muscle: ventricular arrhythmias with increasing changes in EKG lead to cardiac and respiratory arrest, weakness with ascending paralysis and hyperreflexia, diarrhea, and increasing confusion.
- **Treatment**: Treatment includes identifying the underlying cause and discontinuing sources of increased K. Calcium gluconate to decrease cardiac effects. Sodium bicarbonate shifts K into the cells temporarily. Insulin and hypertonic dextrose shift K into the cells temporarily. Cation exchange resin (Kayexalate®) to decrease K. Peritoneal dialysis or hemodialysis to remove excess K.

Note: When a tourniquet is on, a patient opening and closing their hand can lead to falsely elevated K levels.

Calcium

More than 99% of calcium (**Ca**) is in the skeletal system with 1% in serum, but it is important for transmitting nerve impulses and regulating muscle contraction and relaxation, including the myocardium. Calcium activates enzymes that stimulate chemical reactions and has a role in coagulation of blood:

- Normal range: 8.2 to 10.2 mg/dL
- Hypocalcemia: <8.2. Critical value: <7 mg/dL
- Hypercalcemia: >10.2 mg/dL. Critical value: >12 mg/dL

Hypercalcemia may be caused by acidosis, kidney disease, hyperparathyroidism, prolonged immobilization, and malignancies. Crisis carries a 50% mortality rate.

- **Symptoms**: Increasing muscle weakness with hypotonicity; anorexia; nausea and vomiting; constipation; bradycardia and cardiac arrest.
- **Treatment**: Identify and treat underlying cause, loop diuretics, IV fluids, phosphate.

Hypocalcemia may be caused by a damage to the parathyroid resulting in hypoparathyroidism (directly decreasing calcium production), vitamin D resistance or inadequacy, or liver/kidney disease.

- **Symptoms**: Muscle cramping or spasms; seizures; numbness or tingling of the feet, hands, or lips; tetany if severe.
- **Treatment**: Identify and treat underlying cause, replace calcium by administering IV calcium gluconate in acute circumstances or increasing oral Vitamin D and calcium in chronic cases.

Phosphorus

Phosphorus, or phosphate, (**PO_4**) is necessary for neuromuscular and red blood cell function, the maintenance of acid-base balance, and provides structure for teeth and bones. About 85% is in the bones, 14% in soft tissue, and <1% in ECF.

- Normal range: 2.4-4.5 mEq/L
- Hypophosphatemia: <2.4mEq/L
- Hyperphosphatemia: >4.5 mEq/L

Hypophosphatemia occurs with severe protein-calorie malnutrition, excess antacids with magnesium, calcium, or aluminum, hyperventilation, severe burns, and diabetic ketoacidosis.

- **Symptoms**: Irritability, tremors, seizures to coma; hemolytic anemia; decreased myocardial function; respiratory failure.
- **Treatment**: Identify and treat underlying cause and replace phosphorus.

Hyperphosphatemia occurs with renal failure, hypoparathyroidism, excessive intake, and neoplastic disease, diabetic ketoacidosis, muscle necrosis, and chemotherapy.

- **Symptoms**: Tachycardia; muscle cramping; hyperreflexia and tetany; nausea and diarrhea.
- **Treatment**: Identify and treat underlying cause, correct hypocalcemia, and provide antacids and dialysis.

Magnesium

Magnesium (**Mg**) is the second most common intracellular electrolyte (after potassium) and activates many intracellular enzyme systems. Mg is important for carbohydrate and protein metabolism, neuromuscular function, and cardiovascular function, producing vasodilation and directly affecting the peripheral arterial system:

- Normal range: 1.7-2.2 mg/dL
- Hypomagnesemia critical value: <1.2 mg/dL
- Hypermagnesemia critical value: >4.9 mg/dL

Hypomagnesemia occurs with chronic diarrhea, chronic renal disease, chronic pancreatitis, excess diuretic or laxative use, hyperthyroidism, hypoparathyroidism, severe burns, and diaphoresis.

- **Symptoms**: Neuromuscular excitability or tetany; confusion, headaches, dizziness; seizure and coma; tachycardia with ventricular arrhythmias; respiratory depression.
- **Treatment**: Identify and treat underlying cause, provide magnesium replacement. IV magnesium is a vasodilator, 2 g over 60 mins.

Hypermagnesemia occurs with renal failure or inadequate renal function, diabetic ketoacidosis, hypothyroidism, and Addison's disease.

- **Symptoms**: Muscle weakness, seizures, and dysphagia with decreased gag reflex; tachycardia with hypotension.
- **Treatment**: Identify and treat underlying cause, IV hydration with calcium, and dialysis.

Review Video: Fluid and Electrolytes
Visit mometrix.com/academy and enter code: 384389

Metabolic and Endocrine

Endocrine System Organs and Glands

The endocrine system consists of the following organs and glands:

- **Hypothalamus**: Links the endocrine and nervous systems; produces hormones that are stored in the posterior lobe of the pituitary gland; stimulates the pituitary to release hormones
- **Pineal gland**: Secretes melatonin and dimethyltryptamine, which control sleep cycles and dreaming

- **Pituitary gland**: The posterior lobe secretes oxytocin (it stimulates uterine contractions/lactation) and vasopressin (aka antidiuretic hormone, which raises BP and promotes water reabsorption); the anterior lobe secretes hormones that control cell growth (somatotropin), body growth (growth hormone), release of hormones by the thyroid (thyrotropin), release of steroids from the adrenal glands (corticotropin), and reproductive functions (follicle-stimulating hormone and luteinizing hormone)
- **Thyroid gland**: Secretes hormones that control protein production, basal metabolic rate, and oxygen consumption (T3, T4, and calcitonin)
- **Parathyroid glands**: Secretes parathyroid hormone, which controls the use of calcium
- **Adrenal glands**: Produce cortisol (roles in metabolism), aldosterone (water and sodium levels), and androgens (male hormones)
- **Ovaries**: Secrete female hormones (estrogen and progesterone)
- **Testes**: Secrete androgens (testosterone)

Review Video: Endocrine System
Visit mometrix.com/academy and enter code: 678939

Diabetic Conditions

Diabetes mellitus is a group of metabolic disorders that involve hyperglycemia (increased blood glucose [sugar]) because of defective production and/or action of insulin. Insulin metabolizes glucose to produce energy as fuel for body cells.

- **Type 1**: Autoimmune destruction of beta cells in the pancreas results in no or deficient insulin production. Treatment is with insulin. Symptoms include rapid onset, increased thirst, frequent urination, increased hunger, delayed healing, weight loss, frequent infections, and blurred vision.
- **Type 2**: Insulin baseline may be normal or deficient, but there is no or an inadequate increase in response to a meal, so the glucose level rises but there is decreased uptake by the tissues. Insulin resistance occurs because there is decreased sensitivity to insulin by the tissues. Type 2 diabetes is often related to older age and obesity. Treatment is with oral diabetic agents. Symptoms include slow onset, increased thirst, increased urination, candidal (fungal) infections, delayed healing, and weight gain.
- **Gestational**: Beta cells in the pancreas are unable to produce adequate insulin during pregnancy, but normal production resumes after delivery. Treatment varies. Symptoms include increased thirst, urinary frequency, or sometimes no symptoms at all.

Review Video: Diabetes Mellitus
Visit mometrix.com/academy and enter code: 501396

Hyperglycemia and Diabetic Ketoacidosis

Hyperglycemia is high blood glucose (sugar) with a level >126 mg/dL after fasting for 8 hours or >180 mg/dL 2 hours after eating. Hyperglycemia may occur in undiagnosed diabetic patients, diabetic patients who have taken inadequate insulin, those who have eaten a diet too high in carbohydrates (sugars), or those who are ill, such as with an infection. It can also be induced by certain medications, such as steroids, statins, thiazide diuretics, and some antipsychotics. Initial signs include polyuria (increased urine), polyphagia (hunger), polydipsia (increased thirst), headaches, lethargy, fatigue, and blurred vision, but if the blood sugar is very high (>250 mg/dL), then patients may become increasingly somnolent, and he or she may develop diabetic ketoacidosis from the buildup of ketones as fat is broken down by the body for energy because sugar/glucose cannot be used. The patient may exhibit Kussmaul's breathing (fruity-smelling breath from ketones), lapse into a coma, and die if left untreated.

Interventions: Question the patient about diabetes and the use of diabetes medications. Check the patient's blood sugar level, and monitor the vital signs and oxygen saturation. Manage the airway and assisted ventilation as needed, and provide an IV access line and crystalloid fluids and regular insulin if indicated. Rapid transport is required with altered levels of consciousness.

Hyperglycemic Hyperosmolar Nonketotic Syndrome (HHNS) or Coma (HHNK)

Hyperglycemic hyperosmolar nonketotic syndrome (HHNS) or coma (HHNK) occurs in people without a history of diabetes or in people with mild type 2 diabetes but with insulin resistance resulting in persistent hyperglycemia, which causes osmotic diuresis. Fluid shifts from intracellular to extracellular spaces to maintain osmotic equilibrium, but the increased glycosuria and dehydration result in hypernatremia and increased osmolality (concentration). This condition is most common in persons 50–70 years old, and it often is precipitated by an acute illness such as a stroke, medications such as thiazides, or dialysis treatments. HHNS differs from ketoacidosis because although the insulin level is not adequate, it is high enough to prevent the breakdown of fat. Symptoms include polyuria, dehydration, hypotension, tachycardia, blood glucose >500 mg/dL, changes in mental status, hallucinations, seizures, and hemiparesis.

Interventions: Question the patient about his or her history of diabetes and use of diabetes medications. Check the patient's blood sugar level, monitor the vital signs and oxygen saturation, and provide supportive care and an IV access line as needed. Rapid transport is needed for altered levels of consciousness.

Hypoglycemia

Hypoglycemia (low blood sugar/glucose) is most often caused by an insulin reaction (too much insulin for the amount of glucose/sugar intake) or an overdose of oral diabetes medications, which stimulate the overproduction of insulin. Hypoglycemia may occur if patients took insulin but skipped a meal, vomited, or exercised too strenuously, depleting the body of sugar/glucose while insulin levels remain high. Increased insulin levels cause glucose levels to fall to ≤70 mg/dL, initially resulting in tremors, headache, blurred vision, dizziness, and pallor leading to confusion, bizarre behavior, lack of coordination, combative behavior, personality changes, tachycardia, and irregular heartbeat. Severe hypoglycemia may lead to seizures, coma, and death. Hypoglycemia is life threatening if untreated. Infants may have dehydration and seizures; geriatric patients may have dehydration and stroke.

Interventions: Ask the patient about his or her diabetes status and use of diabetes medications. Check the patient's glucose level, and administer oral glucose tablets, one tablespoon of sugar, or a glass of orange juice if the patient is able to swallow. Provide rapid transport for altered levels of consciousness.

Diabetes Treatment

Insulin

Insulin is used to metabolize glucose when the pancreas does not produce insulin in cases of type 1 diabetes mellitus. Patients may need to take a combination of insulins (short and long acting) to maintain glucose control. The duration of action may vary according to the individual's metabolism, intake, and level of activity:

Insulin Type/Brand	Onset	Peak	Duration	Miscellaneous Notes
Rapid-Acting: Lispro (Humalog), aspart (Novolog), glulisine (Apidra)	3-15 min	45-75 min	2-4 hr	
Short-Acting Human: Regular (R) (Humulin, Novolin)	30 min	2-4 hr	5-8 hr	Regular insulin is clear and should be drawn up before cloudy insulin (NPH).
Short-Acting Human: Velosulin	30-60 min	1-2 hr	2-3 hr	Velosulin is used for insulin pumps.
Intermediate-Acting Human: NPH (N)	2 hr	4-12 hr	8-18 hr	NPH is cloudy and should be drawn up after clear (regular).

Insulin Type/Brand	Onset	Peak	Duration	Miscellaneous Notes
Long-Acting Analog: Glargine (Lantus/Basaglar)	2 hr	No peak	20-24 hr	
Long-Acting Analog: Detemir (Levemir)	2 hr	3-9 hr	6-24 hr	
Ultralong-Acting Analog: Degludec (Tresibal)	2 hr	No peak	>40 hr	
Combined/Premixed: NPH/Regular (70/30, 50/50, various other combinations)	15-30 min	2-12 hr	16-24 hr	Peak time depends on the combination.

Oral Antidiabetic Drugs for Type 2 Diabetes Mellitus

Oral antidiabetic drugs are generally recommended for type 2 diabetics when lifestyle changes are insufficient.

Sulfonylureas

- The oldest and most widely used medications for treatment of Type 2 DM.
- These increase the production of insulin by the pancreas. They are more effective early in treatment, but they become less effective over time.
- **First generation**: Tend to cause more hypoglycemia than second generation. Includes acetohexamide (Dymelor), chlorpropamide (Diabinese), tolazamide (Tolinase), and tolbutamide (Orinase).
- **Second generation**: Have largely replaced first generation—they are more potent, can be administered in lower doses, and are preferred when there is poor kidney function. Includes glipizide (Glucotrol), glyburide (Diabeta/Glynase/Micronase), glimepiride (Amaryl).

Meglitinides

- These increase the production of insulin by the pancreas. They are faster acting than sulfonylureas. They are taken 30 minutes prior to a meal up to the time of the meal so that they increase insulin production during and after the meal.
- Includes repaglinide (Prandin) and nateglinide (Starlix).

Biguanides

- These reduce glucose production by the liver. They are often taken as part of combination therapy with another drug.
- Metformin is the first line oral antidiabetic recommended in the treatment of type 2 diabetes.
- Includes metformin (Glucophage).

Alpha-Glucosidase Inhibitors

- These slow the absorption of carbohydrates by the intestines. They are not effective for people with fasting hyperglycemia.
- Includes acarbose (Precose) and miglitol (Glyset).

Thiazolidinediones

- These improve insulin sensitivity, transport, and utilization. They are most effective for people with insulin resistance, but they do not increase the production of insulin, although they may be combined with another drug.
- Includes pioglitazone (Actos) and rosiglitazone (Avandia). Both drugs increase the risk of heart failure.

Diabetes Insipidus

Diabetes insipidus (DI) may be central (characterized by decreased levels of antidiuretic hormone [ADH]), or nephrogenic (characterized by renal ADH resistance). DI may be also psychogenic from fluid intake >5L day. Central DI, transient or permanent, is most common in critical care, especially with traumatic brain injury, surgery in the area of the pituitary or hypothalamus, brain tumors, and encephalitis/meningitis. Primary symptoms of DI are polydipsia and polyuria (3–20 L output daily). Symptoms include dry skin, fatigue, and hair loss. If unable to drink adequate fluids, patients may become dehydrated and develop hypernatremia. With hypernatremia, the patient should receive D_5W IV at 500-750 mL per hour to decrease Na levels by 0.5 mEq/L per hour. The drug of choice for central DI is desmopressin: intranasal 10-40 mcg daily in one or divided doses; oral 0.1-1.2 in divided doses 2-3 times daily; IV/SC 2-4 mcg daily in divided doses. Administering desmopressin immediately before transport may delay the need to urinate if the patient is not catheterized.

SIADH

Syndrome of inappropriate secretion of antidiuretic hormone (SIADH) is related to hypersecretion of the posterior pituitary gland. This causes the kidneys to reabsorb fluids, resulting in fluid retention, and triggers a decrease in sodium levels (dilutional hyponatremia), resulting in production of only concentrated urine. This syndrome may result from central nervous system disorders, such as brain trauma, surgery, or tumors. It may also be triggered by other disorders, such as tumors of various organs, pneumothorax, acute pneumonia, and other lung disorders. Some medications (vincristine, phenothiazines, tricyclic antidepressants, and thiazide diuretics) may also trigger SIADH.

Interventions: (treat underlying cause)

- Correct fluid volume excess and electrolytes.
- Monitor urine output continuously: <0.5-1 mL/kg/hour is cause for concern.
- Seizure precautions.
- With SIADH expect low serum sodium and serum osmolality with high urine osmolality.

Hyperthyroidism, Thyrotoxicosis, and Thyroid Storm

Hyperthyroidism is a pathologic disorder in which excess thyroid hormone is produced by the thyroid gland. **Thyrotoxicosis** refers to the clinical syndrome of excess circulating thyroid hormones, regardless of the source. The most common cause of hyperthyroidism is **Graves' disease**, an autoimmune disorder that stimulates excess production of thyroid hormones. Important causes of thyrotoxicosis include thyroiditis, iodine-induced, and drug-induced thyroid dysfunction from ingestion of excess thyroid medications. Symptoms of hyperthyroidism vary and include anxiety, tachycardia (90-160 bpm), atrial fibrillation, tremor, exophthalmos (bulging eyes), heat intolerance, dry itching skin (especially in geriatric patients), progressive weakness, and altered mental status progressing to coma. Treatment is with radioactive iodine or surgical removal of the thyroid.

Thyroid storm represents the extreme manifestation of thyrotoxicosis and is characterized by compromised organ function. It is precipitated by stress, such as injury, diabetic ketoacidosis, infection, heart failure, or surgery, in those untreated or inadequately treated for hyperthyroidism. If it is not promptly treated, it is fatal. Symptoms are similar to hyperthyroidism but more severe. Hyperthermia may be present (>38.5 °C) with tachycardia (>130) and nausea, vomiting, and diarrhea.

Interventions: Initiate cooling procedures, provide an IV access line, manage the airway/ventilation/intubation/supplemental oxygen as necessary, provide cardiac monitoring, and provide rapid transport.

Hypothyroidism

Hypothyroidism occurs when the thyroid gland produces inadequate levels of thyroid hormones. Conditions may range from mild to severe myxedema (an extreme complication of hypothyroidism in which patients display multiple organ abnormalities and progressive mental deterioration). Myxedema is a term used interchangeably with hypothyroidism and myxedema coma. It also refers to the swelling of the skin and soft tissue that occurs in patients who are hypothyroid. There are a number of causes, including the following:

- Chronic lymphocytic thyroiditis (Hashimoto's thyroiditis)
- Excessive treatment for hyperthyroidism
- Atrophy of the thyroid gland
- Medications such as lithium and iodine compounds
- Radiation to the area of the thyroid gland
- Diseases that affect the thyroid, such as scleroderma
- Iodine imbalances

Symptoms may include chronic fatigue, weight gain, constipation, menstrual disturbances, hoarseness, cold intolerance and subnormal temperature, bradycardia (slow pulse), hypotension, thinning hair, thickening skin. It may also interfere with pregnancy and be an underlying cause of miscarriage in women. Some dementia may occur with advanced conditions, resulting in misdiagnosis of Alzheimer's disease. Myxedema may be characterized by changes in respiration with hypoventilation and carbon dioxide retention resulting in coma. Treatment involves hormone replacement with synthetic levothyroxine.

Interventions: Manage the patient's airway/ventilation/supplemental oxygen and intubation if necessary. Monitor oxygen saturation and carbon dioxide levels, provide an IV access line, and administer a vasopressor or atropine for severe bradycardia if necessary.

Addison's Disease and Addisonian Crisis

Adrenocortical insufficiency (**Addison's disease**) is caused by damage to the adrenal cortex, related to a variety of causes, such as autoimmune diseases, genetic disorders, infections, surgical removal of the gland, idiopathic atrophy, or tumor. Addison's disease may occur secondary to hypothalamus or pituitary malfunction if adrenocorticotropic hormone (ACTH) is not available to stimulate the adrenal cortex. Whatever the cause, the glucocorticoids, mineralocorticoids, and androgens normally produced by the adrenal cortex are deficient or absent. With Addison's disease, serum glucose and sodium levels decrease and serum potassium increases. This can lead to severe dehydration and **Addisonian crisis**, characterized by circulatory shock, altered mental status, tachycardia, cardiac dysrhythmias, tachypnea, and hypotension. Addisonian crisis is life threatening.

Interventions: Manage the patient's airway/ventilation/supplemental oxygen as needed, provide IV access and IV fluids, and provide rapid transport because the administration of hydrocortisone is time critical. Calcium chloride and albuterol (per nebulizer) may help reduce potassium levels.

Cushing's Syndrome/Disease

Cushing's syndrome is characterized by excessive production of the steroid hormone cortisol (a "fight or flight" hormone). The most common cause is a tumor of the pituitary gland, but it can also result from adrenal tumors, alcoholism, and steroid use (such as long-term steroid treatment for patients with COPD).

Cushing's disease occurs when the following physical changes occur because of the increased cortisol level: Moon facies (round face), excessive weight gain and abdominal girth, excessive hair growth, abdominal stretch marks, bruising of the skin, generalized weakness, hypertension, severe insulin-dependent diabetes mellitus, decreased fertility, vision loss or impaired vision, and mood/behavioral or psychiatric problems. Treatment options may include surgery, radiation, or a change in medication, depending on the cause.

Interventions: Monitor patient's vital signs and general condition; if he or she is in diabetic ketoacidosis, provide an IV access line and insulin (per protocol). Manage the patient's airway/ventilation/supplemental oxygen as needed.

Hematology

Components of the Blood

Blood cells are produced in the bone marrow. Blood is a viscous, dark-red fluid comprised of cells, gases, and plasma. Blood components include the following:

- **Erythrocytes** (red blood cells [RBCs]): RBCs carry hemoglobin, which transports oxygen. If the RBC count is low (such as from blood loss) or the oxygen-carrying capacity is impaired (such as with anemia), the patient may experience hypoxemia (low oxygen). The life cycle of RBCs is normally 120 days.
- **Leukocytes** (white blood cells [WBCs]): WBCs defend the body against invading organisms (viruses, bacteria, fungi, and parasites), and in the bloodstream and tissues they respond to allergies. WBCs include lymphocytes (B, T, natural killer, and null cells), monocytes, eosinophils, basophils, and neutrophils.
- **Thrombocytes** (platelets): Platelets release clotting factors and have an active role in forming blood clots.
- **Plasma** (55% of blood): Plasma carries water, proteins, electrolytes, lipids (fats), blood cells, and glucose as well as clotting factors.

The primary blood types are A, B, AB, and O. Blood is either Rh– or RH+, and patients must receive transfusions of blood that are type and Rh compatible.

Hematological Conditions

Hematological conditions include:

- **Anemia**: Anemia occurs when there are deficient numbers of RBCs or the hemoglobin doesn't bind to sufficient oxygen to meet body demands. Anemia results in a decrease in oxygen transportation and decreased perfusion throughout the body, causing the heart to compensate by increasing cardiac output. The types include iron-deficiency (inadequate iron), blood-loss, hemolytic (red cells destroyed), aplastic (bone marrow damaged), and pernicious (vitamin B_{12} deficiency) anemia.
- **Leukopenia**: A low WBC count (<4000) makes the patient vulnerable to infection. Causes include chemotherapy, autoimmune disorders, cancer, viral infections, medications (such as antibiotics), radiation, HIV/AIDS, and TB.
- **Lymphomas**: Cancer of the lymphocytes (the WBCs involved in the immune response). Two main types are Hodgkin's and non-Hodgkin's lymphoma.
- **Polycythemia**: Excessive RBC count, resulting in viscous (thick) blood and an increased risk of clots.
- **Multiple myeloma**: Cancer of the plasma cells, resulting in tumor in the bone marrow, bone pain, anemia, kidney failure, and infection.
- **Thrombocytopenia**: Low platelet count, increasing the risk of bruising and bleeding.

Sickle Cell Disease

Sickle cell disease is a recessive genetic disorder of chromosome 11, causing hemoglobin to be defective so that the red blood cells (RBCs) are sickle-shaped and inflexible, resulting in their accumulating in small vessels and causing painful blockages. Although normal RBCs survive for 120 days, sickled blood cells may survive only 10–20 days, stressing the bone marrow that can't produce RBCs fast enough and resulting in anemia. Different types of **crises** occur (aplastic, hemolytic, vaso-occlusive, and sequestering), which can cause infarctions in organs, severe pain, damage to organs, and rapid enlargement of the liver and spleen. Vaso-occlusive crisis is common in adolescents and adults, and it can be triggered by sickness, stress, dehydration, temperature changes, and high altitude. Young children are prone to splenic sequestration (RBCs trapped in the spleen, causing it to enlarge and sometimes rupture), which is characterized by pain in the left abdomen.

Interventions: Manage the patient's airway, ventilation, and oxygen supplementation and circulation, provide emotional support, and provide rapid transport for severe symptoms.

Clotting Disorders

Clotting disorders include the following:

- **Hemophilia** is an inherited disorder in which the person lacks adequate clotting factors, which results in bleeding with trauma, bruising, spontaneous hemorrhage (often in the joints), and epistaxis. There are three primary types: A (80–90%), B, and C.
- **Disseminated intravascular coagulation (DIC)** (consumption coagulopathy) is a secondary disorder that is triggered by another event, such as trauma, congenital heart disease, necrotizing enterocolitis, sepsis, and severe viral infections. DIC triggers coagulation (clotting) and hemorrhage through a complex series of events, with clotting and hemorrhage occurring simultaneously, putting the patient at risk of death.
- **Von Willebrand's disease** is a group of congenital bleeding disorders (inherited from either parent) affecting 1-2% of the population, associated with deficiency or lack of von Willebrand factor (vWF), a glycoprotein.

Interventions: Monitor for signs of bleeding, and manage the patient's airway/ventilation/oxygen supplementation. Provide rapid transport for hemorrhage or acute blood loss resulting in hypotension.

Transfusion Components

Blood components that are commonly used for transfusions include:

- **Packed red blood cells**: RBCs (250-300 mL per unit) should be warmed >30 °C (optimal temperature is 37 °C) before administration to prevent hypothermia and may be reconstituted in 50-100 mL of normal saline to facilitate administration. RBCs are necessary if blood loss is about 30% (1,500-2,000 mL) (Hgb ≤7). Above 30% blood loss, whole blood may be more effective. RBCs are most frequently used for transfusions.
- **Platelet concentrates**: Transfusions of platelets are used if the platelet count is <50,000 cells/mm^3. One unit increases the platelet count by 5,000-10,000 cells/mm^3. Platelet concentrates pose a risk for sensitization reactions and infectious diseases. Platelet concentrate is stored at a higher temperature (20-24 °C) than RBCs. This contributes to bacterial growth, so it is more prone to bacterial contamination than other blood products and may cause sepsis. Temperature increase within 6 hours should be considered an indication of possible sepsis. ABO compatibility should be observed but is not required.
- **Fresh frozen plasma** (FFP) (obtained from a unit of whole blood frozen ≤6 hours after collection) includes all clotting factors and plasma proteins, so each unit administered increases clotting factors by 2-3%. FFP may be used for deficiencies of isolated factors, excess warfarin therapy, and liver-disease related coagulopathy. It may be used for patients who have received extensive blood transfusions but continue to hemorrhage. It is also helpful for those with antithrombin III deficiency. FFP should be warmed to 37 °C prior to administration to avoid hypothermia. ABO compatibility should be observed if possible, but it is not required. Some patients may become sensitized to plasma proteins.
- **Cryoprecipitate** is the precipitate that forms when FFP is thawed. It contains fibrinogen, factor VIII, von Willebrand, and factor XIII. This component may be used to treat hemophilia A and hypofibrinogenemia.

TRANSFUSION-RELATED COMPLICATIONS

There are a number of transfusion-related complications, which is the reason that transfusions are given only when necessary. **Complications** include:

- **Infection**: Bacterial contamination of blood, especially platelets, can result in severe sepsis. A number of infective agents (viral, bacterial, and parasitic) can be transmitted, although increased testing of blood has decreased rates of infection markedly. Infective agents include HIV, hepatitis C and B, human T-cell lymphotropic virus, CMV, WNV, malaria, Chagas' disease and variant Creutzfeldt-Jacob disease (from contact with mad cow disease).
- **Transfusion-related acute lung injury (TRALI)**: This respiratory distress syndrome occurs ≤6 hours after transfusion. The cause is believed to be antileukocytic or anti-HLA antibodies in the transfusion. It is characterized by non-cardiogenic pulmonary edema (high protein level) with severe dyspnea and arterial hypoxemia. Transfusion must be stopped immediately and the blood bank notified. TRALI may result in fatality but usually resolves in 12-48 hours with supportive care.
- **Graft vs. host disease**: Lymphocytes cause immune response in immunocompromised individuals. Lymphocytes may be inactivated by irradiation, as leukocyte filters are not reliable.
- **Post-transfusion purpura**: Platelet antibodies develop and destroy the patient's platelets, so the platelet count decreases about 1 week after transfusion.
- **Transfusion-related immunosuppression**: Cell-mediated immunity is suppressed, so the patient is at increased risk of infection and transfusions may correlate with tumor recurrence in cancer patients. This condition relates to transfusions that include leukocytes. RBCs cause a less pronounced immunosuppression, suggesting a causative agent is in the plasma. Leukoreduction is becoming more common to reduce transmission of leukocyte-related viruses.
- **Hypothermia**: This may occur if blood products are not heated. Oxygen utilization is halved for each 10 °C decrease in normal body temperature.

Renal

ACUTE KIDNEY INJURY

Acute kidney injury is an abrupt and almost complete failure of kidney function, occurring over a period of hours or days. It most commonly occurs in hospitalized patients, but it may occur in others as well. Causes include MI, heart failure, sepsis, anaphylaxis, burns, trauma, infections, transfusion reactions, medications (NSAIDs and ACE inhibitors), and obstruction. Symptoms include reduced or absent urinary output, increased nocturia (nighttime urination), altered mental status, tinnitus, a metallic taste in the mouth, tremors, seizures, flank pain, abdominal pain, hypertension, increased bruising.

CHRONIC RENAL FAILURE

Chronic renal failure occurs after years of disease that damages the kidneys, often being essentially asymptomatic until the damage is severe. Early symptoms may include anorexia, general malaise, headaches, itching, and weight loss. Later symptoms include fluid retention (pulmonary edema, peripheral edema, ascites), headache, bruising, dry skin, muscle cramping, bone pain, weakness, breath odor, excessive thirst, frequent hiccups, dyspnea, vomiting (especially in the morning), and hypertension.

Interventions: Manage the patient's airway/ventilation/oxygen, provide an IV access line (if the patient is hypotensive or if there is evidence of pulmonary edema), and transport.

END-STAGE RENAL DISEASE (ESRD)

Acute kidney injury and chronic renal failure may progress to end-stage renal disease (ESRD) when the kidneys are no longer able to function and the patient needs dialysis or a kidney transplant. The patient may develop uremic syndrome, which results in decreased production of red blood cells and platelets, electrolyte imbalances, bone disease, multiple endocrine disorders, cardiac problems (especially congestive heart failure), anorexia, and malnutrition. Symptoms include altered mental status, hallucinations, and confusion from the accumulation of waste products in the blood; increasing edema and shortness of breath from accumulated fluids; chest and bone pain; severe pruritus; nausea, vomiting, and diarrhea; tremors, muscle twitching, and seizures; and increased bruising and discoloration of the skin.

Review Video: End Stage Renal Disease
Visit mometrix.com/academy and enter code: 869617

Interventions: Manage the patient's airway/ventilation/oxygen, start an IV access line (if the patient is hypotensive or if there is evidence of pulmonary edema), and transport

Medication Considerations

Because patients with end-stage-renal disease (ESRD) are unable to adequately remove body fluids through urination, intravenous fluids should be restricted in these patients, although a fluid bolus may be needed for hypovolemia or hypotension. If a patient is in a state of fluid overload already (such as right before a scheduled hemodialysis treatment), IV fluids may result in pulmonary edema. The patient's residual urinary output (if any) should be determined, and the dosage of some common drugs excreted through the kidneys reduced to avoid toxicity or overdose. Some medications, such as loop diuretics, may be ineffective if a patient has no urinary output. Many drugs are excreted by the kidneys (antibiotics, beta-blockers, lithium, digoxin, and ranitidine) and must be administered with caution. If a patient is receiving hemodialysis, this process may decrease serum levels of some medications, such as anticonvulsants, especially immediately after dialysis, so dosages may need to be increased.

Assessing Dialysis Sites

When assessing dialysis sites (usually AV fistula or graft) for patients with ESRD, the transport nurse should assess the skin to determine if it appears normal and without swelling, erythema, or discharge indicative of infection. The site should be palpated for indications of swelling (aneurysm/pseudoaneurysm), thrombosis, or stenosis. A thrill should be felt only at the arterial anastomosis; a marked thrill elsewhere may indicate stenosis. The bruit should be low pitched and continuous on auscultation. A high-pitched discontinuous bruit may indicate stenosis. The pulse should be soft and easy to compress. Circulation should also be assessed in the extremity distal to the fistula or graft. Swelling or lack of pulse many indicate obstruction. The dialysis access site and the extremity containing the dialysis access site should not be used for IVs, blood draws, or blood pressure readings. Because patients may have had previous access sites and may have extensive scarring, finding a vein to use can be challenging. The patient may be able to provide guidance.

Treating Hypotension and Dehydration

Hypotension is a common problem associated with hemodialysis because up to 400 mL of blood is outside of the body during the process and excess fluid is removed rapidly. Hypotension can also result from eating during hemodialysis. Symptoms include nausea and vomiting, dizziness, impaired perfusion, confusion, chest pain, seizures, and arrhythmias. Hypotension during treatment is usually treated with a bolus of fluid and lowering the patient's head. If hypotension persists, the patient may require further fluid resuscitation and supportive care.

Dehydration can occur from dialysis removing too much body fluid, toxin buildup, inadequate fluid intake, or excessive loss of body fluids, such as may occur with strenuous exercise or exposure to high environmental temperatures, especially shortly after dialysis. Patients are usually limited to fluid intake of 32–50 ounces daily, depending on age, size, and activity level. Symptoms include nausea, tachycardia, thirst, dry mouth, itching, and anxiety. Treatment includes careful administration of IV fluids and treatment of hypernatremia.

Treating Hyperkalemia and Bleeding

Hyperkalemia (>5.5 mEq/L with a critical value >6.5 mEq/L) is common in dialysis patients and can be related to constipation and excessive intake of potassium. Symptoms include ventricular arrhythmias leading to cardiac arrest, weakness, hyperreflexia, diarrhea, and confusion. Treatment includes ECG monitoring, calcium carbonate (to decrease cardiac abnormalities), sodium bicarbonate, insulin, and hypertonic dextrose (to temporarily shift potassium into cells), sodium polystyrene sulfonate (Kayexalate®) retention enema (to decrease potassium), and a dialysis treatment.

Bleeding may result from the heparin required for hemodialysis and thrombocytopenia. Patients may develop bruising, bleeding of gums, nosebleeds, and prolonged bleeding after removal of needles. Patients are at risk for internal bleeding (GI, intracranial). Outflow stenosis of the AV shunt may also cause prolonged bleeding after needle removal, so the shunt should be carefully assessed. Treatment depends on the severity of bleeding and ranges from applying pressure to transfusions to heparin antidote (protamine sulfate1%).

Infectious and Communicable Diseases

Infection Control Measures

Standard Precautions

Standard precautions should be utilized for all patients because all body fluids (sweat, urine, feces, blood, sputum) and non-intact skin and mucous membranes may be infected:

Hand hygiene	Wash hands before and after each patient contact and after any contact with body fluids and contaminated items. Use soap and water for visible soiling.
Protective equipment	Use personal protective equipment (PPE), such as gloves, gowns, and masks, eye protection, and/or face shields, when anticipating contact with body fluids or contaminated skin.
Respiratory hygiene/ Cough etiquette	Utilize source control measures, such as covering cough, disposing of tissues, using surgical mask on person coughing or on staff to prevent inhalation of droplets, and properly disposing of dressings and used equipment. Wash hands after contacting respiratory secretions. Maintain a distance of >3 feet from coughing person when possible.

Soiled articles of clothing and linens should be handled as little as possible, and disposable items should be placed in leak-proof bags that can be burned.

Transmission-Based Precautions

The **2007 CDC isolation guidelines** include both standard precautions that apply to all patients and transmission-based precautions for those with known or suspected infections as well as those with excessive wound drainage, other discharge, or fecal incontinence. Transmission-based precautions include:

Contact	Use personal protective equipment (PPE), including gown and gloves, for all contacts with the patient or patient's immediate environment.
Droplet	(Appropriate for influenza, streptococcus infection, pertussis, rhinovirus, and adenovirus and pathogens that remain viable and infectious for only short distances.) Use mask while caring for the patient. Maintain patient in > 3 feet away from other patients (with curtain separating in an emergency department. Use patient mask when transporting patient.
Airborne	(Appropriate for measles, chickenpox, tuberculosis, SARS because pathogens remain viable and infectious for long distances.) Use ≥N95 respirators (or masks) while caring for patient. Patient should be placed in an airborne infection isolation room in an emergency department.

Droplet Transmission

When a person with an infectious disease coughs or sneezes, he/she sends droplets containing germs into the air. If a non-infected individual is within approximately three feet or less of the infected individual, the germ-carrying droplets can come in contact with the non-infected individual; the infectious disease germs are likely to cause symptoms of the illness in the non-infected individual if the droplets come in contact with that person's nose, mouth, or eyes. While particles are considerably smaller than droplets, their potential for transmitting infectious disease such as tuberculosis is quite large. Particles can carry germs that cause infectious diseases, and they can carry them through the air for extended periods of time; additionally, particles can travel in air currents. Consequently, if a non-infected individual inhales air that contains germs from an infectious disease, that individual will likely develop the disease.

Managing Fever in a Patient

A fever can accompany almost any kind of infection or illness. When a patient's core body temperature is at or above 100.4 °F (38 °C), the patient is said to have a fever. Many times, a fever is simply the body's way of fighting an infection and may not pose a serious medical risk to the patient. However, a high fever may develop into further complications such as convulsions if left untreated. Certain medications including acetaminophen, aspirin, and ibuprofen are often effective at reducing a patient's fever. Additionally, the patient can be sponged with lukewarm water to assist in bringing his/her core body temperature back down to normal range. Patients with fevers should be encouraged to consume as much fluid as possible as well; clear fluids such as water and diluted juices are best.

SIRS and Sepsis

Systemic inflammatory response syndrome (SIRS), a generalized inflammatory response affecting may organ systems, may be caused by infectious or non-infectious agents, such as trauma, burns, adrenal insufficiency, pulmonary embolism, and drug overdose. If an infectious agent is identified or suspected, SIRS is an aspect of sepsis. SIRS includes 2 of the following:

- Elevated (>38 °C) or subnormal rectal temperature (<36 °C).
- Tachypnea (>20/min) or $PaCO_2$ <32 mmHg.
- Tachycardia >90/min.
- Leukocytosis (>12,000) or leukopenia (<4000) or >10% bands.

Sepsis is presence of infection either locally or systemically in which there is a generalized life-threatening inflammatory response (SIRS). It includes all the indications for SIRS as well as one of the following:

- Changes in mental status.
- Hypoxemia (<72 mmHg) without pulmonary disease.
- Elevation in plasma lactate.
- Systolic BP <90 mmHg or ≥40 mmHg below baseline.
- Decreased urinary output <5 mL/kg/wt for ≥1 hour.

If organs are affected, sepsis is classified as severe sepsis; and with hypotension, septic shock. MODS occurs with evidence of failure of 2 or more organs.

Denver Sepsis Protocol

About a million cases of sepsis occur in the United States annually with incidence increasing, and about 25% of those with sepsis die, so rapidly identifying and treating sepsis is critical if the patient is to survive. The Denver

Sepsis Protocol was developed to try to better respond to sepsis. The protocol is utilized if patients are 18, not pregnant, and have:

- SIRS: At least 2 criteria AND temperature >38 °C (100.4 °F) or <36 °C (96 °F), heart rate >90, respiration >20.
- Infection: Suspected/Documented.
- Hypotension or hypoperfusion with SBP <90, MAP <65, and lactate >4 mmol/L. (Utilizing portable lactate testing.)

Protocol:

- Administer high flow oxygen with a non-rebreather mask.
- Insert two large-bore angiocaths and draw blood samples for baseline values.
- Administer IV fluid bolus at 20 mL/kg in rapid infusion.
- Reassess BP and respirations after infusion of 500 mL and contact physician if SBP <90 mmHg.
- Monitor vital signs (auscultate BP), ECG, pulse oximetry, capnography, glucose, and respirations regularly.

Patients should reach destination within 15 minutes and should receive antibiotics within one hour.

Managing Patients with Highly Infectious Diseases

Patients diagnosed with or suspected of having highly infectious diseases, such as tuberculosis or meningitis, should be cared for utilizing the standard contact isolation procedures (gowns, gloves) as well as an airborne isolation procedures, which require the use of N95 respirators and eye protection during patient care. The patient should be transported to an airborne infection (negative pressure) isolation room in a receiving facility. Personal protective equipment (PPE) must be donned (beginning with mask, eye protection, gown, and gloves last) prior to patient contact. The patient should be masked before transport and air should be circulated continuously if possible. Disposable equipment should be used when possible as well as a closable emesis basins. The receiving facility should be made aware of the patient's infectious status. Any possible exposure should be reported immediately following protocols. In special circumstances, such as transport of Ebola patients, CDC guidelines for personal protection and isolation procedures must be followed exactly.

Inter-Facility Transfer and Post-Transport Cleaning

Before inter-facility transfer of a patient with a highly infectious disease, the transport nurse should ensure that all necessary equipment is available in transport vehicles and that medical transport team members are all aware of the patient's status and necessary isolation and decontamination procedures. Post-transport cleaning should correspond to CDC guidelines and should involve careful cleaning of all surfaces in proximity to the patient with removal of dust, body fluids, and debris before decontamination. The recommended decontamination agent for highly infectious agents is sodium hypochlorite (bleach) in a 1:100 dilution or pre-mixed wipes with one minute of contact needed to adequately kill organisms. Special cleaning supplies, such as Ambu-Stat®, an atomized cold sterilant solution, are also available. This type of fogger fills the vehicle with a sterilant and is used after surface cleaning. Critical and non-critical items should be cleaned and sterilized according to manufacturer's guidelines. Equipment left at the receiving facility must be properly cleaned or placed in a red bag before being returned to the transportation provider.

Cleaning Solutions for Decontamination

Bleach in a 1:10 mL solution can decontaminate items composed of plastic. If areas such as the transport vehicle floor and stretcher mattresses do not have any dirt or dried blood, they can be cleaned with a bleach solution as well. A drawback to using bleach is its ability to discolor fabrics on items such as stretcher mattresses. Alcohol can be highly effective at decontaminating areas; however, it is flammable and extremely drying if it comes into contact with skin. As with bleach solution, alcohol should be used only on surfaces that do not have any dirt or dried blood present. Glutaraldehyde diluted with water is effective at decontaminating items made of plastic or vinyl. One drawback to using glutaraldehyde is that its acidic nature can cause corrosion; as such, it should not be used around electronic equipment on the transport vehicle and/or on items containing stainless steel.

Disposal of Biohazard Waste

Biohazard bags should be used to collect dry solid waste such as medical gloves worn when treating a patient with an infectious disease. Leak-proof biohazard bags can also be used to collect waste that contains blood or other bodily fluids. Puncture-resistant containers designated for sharp items should be used to collect "sharps" such as needles. Potentially contaminated fluids suctioned from patients during transport should be enclosed in sealed containers; unnecessary handling of such fluids should be avoided during transport, particularly if a risk of splashing exists. Biohazard bags, sharps containers, and sealed containers should be properly disposed of at the destination facility according to the facility's local disposal requirements.

Environmental and Toxicological Emergencies

Temperature-Related Emergencies

Measuring Core Body Temperature

The hypothalamus is a mechanism in the brain responsible for controlling a person's core body temperature. The normal body temperature for a human is 98.6 °F (37.1 °C). Core body temperature is most effectively measured by taking a patient's temperature rectally, which is the most common method of measuring temperature in a neonatal patient. However, if an adult patient is able to breathe through his/her nose without difficulty, temperature can also be measured orally by placing a thermometer underneath the patient's tongue. If an adult patient is not able to breathe through his/her nose due to illness or injury, temperature must be measured rectally, in an axillary position, or in the ear. When taking a neonatal patient's temperature rectally, it is best to place the patient face down in order to carefully insert the thermometer a little over one centimeter into the anal canal.

Hypothermia

Hypothermia occurs when a person is not able to maintain a core body temperature at or above 95 °F (35 °C). Subjective data to look at when determining whether a patient may be suffering from the condition can include: the geographic location of the patient and the corresponding temperature of the surroundings in which he/she is located; how appropriately the patient is dressed in relation to the temperature of his/her surroundings; the length of time the patient was exposed to conditions that may contribute to the development of hypothermia; and whether or not the patient has medical risk factors for developing the condition. Risk factors for hypothermia can include: 1) patient age (older and very young patients may be more susceptible to hypothermia); 2) certain medical conditions such as Parkinson's disease and stroke; and 3) mental impairment such as Alzheimer's disease and alcohol or drug use.

Mild, Moderate, and Severe Hypothermia

- Mild hypothermia occurs when a patient has a core body temperature less than 95 °F (35 °C) and greater than 89.6 °F (32 °C); patients with mild hypothermia have a very low risk of dying from the condition.
- Moderate hypothermia occurs when a patient has a core body temperature less than 89.6 °F (32 °C) and greater than 82.4 °F (28 °C).
- Severe hypothermia occurs when a patient has a core body temperature at or below 82.4 °F (28 °C); patients with severe hypothermia are at an increased risk of dying from the condition than those with mild or moderate forms of hypothermia.

Restoring Core Body Temperature

In patients whose core body temperature is too high or too low, it is important to monitor the patient's airway, breathing, and circulation periodically during transport. To help restore a patient's core body temperature when it has dropped too low, the patient can be wrapped in insulated blankets during transport. Warm gel packs can also be applied to areas of the body to help elevate the core body temperature. If the patient has any articles of clothing on his/her body that appear to be wet, it is best to remove those articles to prevent a further decrease in temperature. If available, warm fluids can be administered to the patient as well.

Frostbite Symptoms

Upon physical examination, a patient with frostbite may present with pale or bluish colored skin. A patient with bluish colored skin may be displaying signs of not having enough oxygen in his/her blood. Necrosis may occur when not enough blood is being pumped to the area(s) where the frostbite is located. Necrosis occurs when portions of tissue or portions of an organ stop functioning; bluish or purplish regions on the body may indicate this condition. Edema may also be present in patients with frostbite. At the area(s) where the frostbite is located, the patient may not be as sensitive to touch, due to decreased sensation in and around those areas.

Treatment for frostbite includes rapid rewarming with a warm water bath (40–42 °C, 104–107.6 °F) for 10–30 minutes or until the frostbitten area is erythematous and pliable as well as treatment for generalized hypothermia. After warming, treatment includes debridement of clear blisters but not hemorrhagic blisters. Frostbite most often affects the nose, ears, and distal extremities. As frostbite develops, the affected part feels numb and aches or throbs, becoming hard and insensate as the tissue freezes, resulting in circulatory impairment, necrosis of tissue, and gangrene. Three zones of injury include:

- Coagulation (usually distal): severe irreversible cellular damage
- Hyperemia (usually proximal): minimal cellular damage
- Stasis (between other two zones): severe but sometimes reversible damage

Cardiac Arrhythmia Secondary to Hypothermia

During early stages of hypothermia, when the condition would be classified as mild, patients almost always experience an increase in heart rate for a brief period of time. As the core body temperature of the patient decreases, as it does when hypothermia progresses from mild to moderate to severe stages, the patient's heart rate also begins to decrease. At core body temperatures lower than 91.4 °F (33 °C), the heart can decrease to a rate of 20 beats per minute. When a patient's heart rate fluctuates as it commonly does when hypothermia sets in, the fluctuation can lead to cardiac arrhythmia, which is a condition characterized by an irregular or abnormal heart rate.

Heatstroke

In patients whose core body temperature is too high or too low, it is important to monitor the patient's airway, breathing, and circulation periodically during transport. To help restore a patient's core body temperature when it is too high, it is often helpful to dampen the patient's skin with cool water using a misting technique. If a cooling blanket is available during the transport process, place the patient on the device. Additionally, cold packs may be applied to the patient's neck, groin area, and/or under the arms. Administer fluids to the patient in a manner that prevents fluid overload, which could lead to pulmonary edema. The patient's urine production should be closely monitored during transport, as it is necessary for heat stroke patients to produce more urine than usual to avoid the risk of developing acute renal failure.

Decompression Sickness

Decompression sickness occurs when a patient is exposed to an abrupt decrease in either the water or air pressure around him/her. The condition can be characterized by symptoms including limb pain, decreased respiratory functioning, skin reactions, and it can lead to problems related to the central nervous system such as headaches, confusion, and diminished motor skills. Patients should be treated at a hyperbaric compression chamber. To prevent circulatory collapse, the patient must be transported to the chamber within a period of six hours or less from the onset of the condition. During transport, the patient should be administered 100 percent oxygen to relieve the deprivation of oxygen to the tissues, a condition known as tissue hypoxia.

Envenomation

Envenomation can occur from a variety of animal bites including certain types of fish such as jellyfish and stingrays, poisonous snakes such as pit vipers, and spiders such as Black Widows. Common signs of envenomation in a patient include swelling at the site of venom injection, redness and pain at the site, gastrointestinal problems, and neurological issues. Gastrointestinal-related symptoms may include diarrhea and/or nausea/vomiting as well as abdominal discomfort or pain. Neurological symptoms may include dizziness, numbness at the injection site, and lethargy. Envenomation may also cause hypotension and bradycardia.

Management

Once it has been determined that the patient has been envenomated, the injured body part should be immobilized, which can help limit the amount of venom that circulates throughout the patient's bloodstream. In all envenomation cases, the transport team should make every effort to help the patient remain calm, which also helps decrease venom circulation throughout the bloodstream. Additionally, the patient's airway, breathing, and overall circulation should be consistently and closely monitored during transport to ensure that the reaction to the snake bite remains local and not systemic. A large-bore IV line should be established in the patient, away from the location of the bite, if possible. Analgesia can be given to the patient for pain. Treatment is largely dependent on the type of envenomation sustained. Severe local pain and edema (signs of mild envenomation) around the bite site are indications for antivenin (5 vials). Because some bites are "dry" and antivenin is expensive, not readily available, and can have significant side effects, it is not given on request or without evidence of envenomation. Fang marks and some pain and local tenderness are common from trauma without envenomation. Moderate envenomation may include swelling beyond the area of bite, mild coagulopathy, and systemic manifestation with increasing symptoms with severe or life-threatening envenomation. Treatment may include 5–25 vials of antivenin, depending on the grade of envenomation and symptoms.

Exposure to Toxic Substances

When a patient intentionally exposes him/herself to a toxic substance or substances, the result is known as an overdose. Patients can also be exposed to toxic substances inadvertently. Unintentional exposure to toxic substances is usually caused by medication errors, food poisoning, environmental sources, and/or bites or stings from animals or insects that transfer toxins into the patient's bloodstream. Medication errors occur when a patient or caregiver incorrectly reads a label and ingests too much of a particular medication. Pediatric patients are often victims of unintentional exposure to toxic substances, as medication bottles often pique their curiosity, and, subsequently, cause medical complications if they ingest the medication.

N-acetylcysteine is the antidote for acetaminophen toxicity and is most effective in protecting the liver if given within 8 hours. Toxicity is plotted on the Rumack–Matthew nomogram with serum levels of more than 150 mg requiring an antidote. The 72-hour N-acetylcysteine protocol includes 140 mg/kg initially and 70 mg/kg every 4 hours for seventeen more doses.

Hydroxocobalamin is the preferred treatment of choice for cyanide toxicity with the dose of 70 mg/kg IV. Nitrites (found in some cyanide treatment kits) displace oxygen on the hemoglobin molecules, forming methemoglobin, thereby reducing the ability of hemoglobin to carry sufficient oxygen, and may result in unstable hemodynamic status.

Medical Management for Toxic Ingestion

The first component of managing of a patient who has ingested a toxic substance is to evaluate his/her airway, breathing, and circulation. The patient's heart and lungs should also be evaluated to ensure that the cardiopulmonary system is functioning properly. It is important to manage the symptoms of the toxic substance ingestion as well as managing the toxic substance itself by attempting to prevent the substance from being absorbed into the stomach. Absorption can potentially be prevented by using activated charcoal, by performing whole bowel irrigation, or through nasogastric aspiration. Activated charcoal effectively absorbs most toxic substances. For substances that are not absorbed by charcoal, flushing out the gastrointestinal tract through whole bowel irrigation may be necessary. Placing a tube down a patient's nose into his/her stomach and suctioning out the contents, a procedure known as nasogastric aspiration, may also be necessary for substances that cannot be absorbed by charcoal.

Treatment for Toxic Ingestion

Treatment for toxic ingestions is related to the type of toxin and whether or not it is identified:

- Administration of reversal agent if substance is known and an antidote exists. Antidotes for common toxins include:
    - Opiates: Naloxone (Narcan).
    - Toxic alcohols: Ethanol infusion and/or dialysis.
    - Acetaminophen: N-acetylcysteine.
    - Calcium channel blockers, beta-blockers: Calcium chloride, Glucagon.
    - Tricyclic antidepressants: Sodium bicarbonate.
    - Ethylene glycol: fomepizole.
    - Iron: deferoxamine
- GI decontamination at one time was standard procedures (Ipecac® and gastric lavage followed by activated charcoal). It is no longer advised for routine use although selective gastric lavage may be appropriate if done within 1 hour of ingestion.
- Activated charcoal (1 g/kg/wt) orally or per NG tube binds to many toxins if given within one hour of ingestion. It may also be used in multiple doses (q 4-6 hrs) to enhance elimination

Forced diuresis with alkalinization of urine (>7.5) may prevent absorption of drugs that are weak bases or acids.

Activated Charcoal Indications and Contraindications

Activated charcoal is often administered to a patient who has ingested a toxic substance or overdosed on a drug. It is intended to absorb the substance or drug and safely eliminate it from the patient's body before it reaches the stomach. While activated charcoal can be effective against certain forms of poisoning, it is ineffective at absorbing others; therefore, its use is not advisable when such poisons are involved. The use of activated charcoal is not advised when a patient has ingested acids, alkalis, iron, lithium, alcohols, and/or products containing petroleum such as cleaning agents, coal or fuel oil, and paint thinner. Gastrointestinal decontamination is most effective if done within 1 hour of ingestion, although activated charcoal may have some protective effects if given within 4 hours of ingestion.

Drug Overdose

Given the vast number of drugs available, symptoms of drug overdose vary widely and depend on the specific drug. The pupils of a drug overdose patient may not appear normal; they may appear enlarged/dilated or extremely small like pin points, or they may also appear unchanging and stay their normal size when exposed to light. Sweating, shakiness, and convulsions can also be symptoms of a drug overdose. A patient's behavior can provide further indications of a possible drug overdose. Patients who overdose often act delusional or paranoid, and they tend to become agitated and aggressive relatively easily. They may also have hallucinations as a result of the substance abuse. Patients who act unusually drowsy and/or who have an unstable gait may be exhibiting symptoms of an overdose as well. Breathing difficulties such as rapid breathing, shallow breathing, or labored breathing can also be indications of a drug overdose.

Mild to Moderate Symptoms of Substance Use Withdrawal

Patients who experience symptoms of withdrawal when they stop using alcohol or other substances often experience both physical and psychological symptoms. Similar to drug overdose symptoms, symptoms of withdrawal vary widely depending on the patient and depending on the substance in question. Mild to moderate physical symptoms of withdrawal can include headaches, nausea and/or vomiting, appetite loss, clammy and/or pale skin, heart palpitations, abnormal pupil size, difficulty sleeping, and sweating. While they may have a difficult time actually sleeping, fatigue is another common symptom of withdrawal. Psychological withdrawal symptoms that would be considered mild or moderate may include feelings of anxiety, depression, excitability, nervousness, irritability, and swift changes from one emotion to another. Additionally, patients going through withdrawal often have a difficult time thinking clearly.

Delirium Tremens

Chronic abuse of ethanol (alcoholism) is associated with alcohol withdrawal syndrome *(delirium tremens)* with abrupt cessation of alcohol intake, resulting in hallucinations, tachycardia, diaphoresis, and sometimes-psychotic behavior. It may be precipitated by trauma or infection and has a high mortality rate, 5-15% with treatment and 35% without treatment. Management includes:

- Monitor vital signs and blood gases.
- Use the Clinical Instrument for Withdrawal for Alcohol (CIWA) to measure symptoms of withdrawal.
- Assess and monitor level of consciousness, orientation, alterations in sensory impressions, agitation, and anxiety.
- Provide an environment with minimal sensory stimulus (lower lights, close blinds).
- Implement fall and seizure precautions.
- Provide nutritional support and monitor intake and output.
- Implement measures to assure proper sleep and stress management.
- Express acceptance and reassurance.
- Maintain body temperature.

People easily aroused can usually safely sleep off the effects of ingesting too much alcohol but if semi-conscious or unconscious, emergency medical treatment (such as IV fluids and medications, intubation, and/or dialysis) may be necessary.

Exposure to Hazardous Materials

Management

The patient who has been exposed to a dangerous substance should be moved to a location where the air is fresh and not contaminated. If oxygen is available, the patient should be supplied with oxygen. In cases where a patient is not breathing, cardiopulmonary resuscitation efforts should be initiated. If the patient's skin and/or eyes have been exposed to the dangerous substance, they should be flushed thoroughly with water. The flushing process should continue until it is evident that the dangerous substance no longer poses a threat to the patient's skin and/or eyes. Any clothing worn by the patient when he/she was exposed to the dangerous substance should be considered contaminated and should be properly removed and stored.

Decontamination Process

Patients exposed to a hazardous material should always be considered potentially contaminated. Any clothing the patient was wearing at the time of contamination should be removed in a designated location and stored there until disposal. Contaminated patients and the personnel assisting them, should be washed at least two times with water and/or water mixed with a mild soap. Personal protective equipment (PPE) worn by personnel during the decontamination process should also be removed and stored with the contaminated clothing. Anyone involved in the decontamination process should be evaluated for medical repercussions. Contaminated materials should be properly disposed of, and contaminated equipment should be decontaminated appropriately and thoroughly cleaned.

Any **exposure/contamination** should be reported at hand-off and to the appropriate infection control person, following protocols, and follow-up care should be sought if necessary. When reporting exposures/contamination, note the type of exposure, the date and time of exposure, circumstances, actions taken to decontaminate, and any other required information.

Mental Health Considerations

Behavioral Alterations

Behavioral alterations may include agitation, anger, throwing temper tantrums (children), acting aggressively (adolescents/adult), exhibiting poor judgment, and acting inappropriately. Behavioral alterations may result from psychiatric disorders (e.g., depression, schizophrenia, bipolar disorder) and psychiatric medications as well as numerous other causes, including the following:

- Hypoglycemia/low blood sugar (insulin reaction)
- Lack of adequate oxygen interfering with brain function
- Shock (low BP; a rapid pulse results in inadequate blood supply to the brain)
- Mind-altering substances (cocaine, methamphetamine, LSD, Rohypnol [date-rape drug])
- Brain infection (meningitis, encephalitis, brain abscess)
- Seizure disorders (epilepsy, other causes of seizures)
- Poisoning/Overdose (lead poisoning, drug overdose)
- Malnutrition resulting in inadequate nourishment of brain tissue
- Substance abuse (drug or alcohol abuse/withdrawal)
- Heat extremes (hypothermia/hyperthermia)

Indications of being a danger to self or others include severe agitation, hallucinations, delusional thinking, paranoia, self-destructive behavior (e.g., cutting, drug/alcohol abuse, promiscuity, risk-taking activities), depression, and suicide attempts. A patient may pose a risk to others if he or she is behaving in a threatening or violent manner and has a weapon (e.g., gun, knife, baseball bat).

Assessment of Psychiatric Patients

Assessment of patients with psychological/psychiatric symptoms should begin with a history that includes the patient's age and cultural/spiritual background and whether the patient has experienced similar symptoms previously or has a history of a psychiatric disorder as well as any history of substance abuse. Assessment includes the following:

- **General appearance:** Note hygiene, grooming, appropriate dress, eye contact, unusual movements (twitching, posturing, repetitive movements), and the appearance and condition of the skin.
- **Speech**: Note speech cadence and abnormal word use, such as neologisms (invented words), clang associations (rhyming), word salad (string of random words), and associative looseness (ideas shifting from one to another).
- **Posture/Gait:** Note automatisms (purposeless behaviors, such as drumming fingers), slowed motions, waxy flexibility (maintaining an awkward position for extended periods of time), ability to walk, and abnormalities of gait.
- **Mental status**: Note the patient's state of being alert versus non-alert, responsive versus unresponsive, and coherent versus incoherent; clarity of ideas; suicidal ideation; and desire for self-harm.
- **Mood and affect**: Note facial expressions, expressed emotions, and affect (blunted, broad, flat, inappropriate, restricted).
- **Memory/Intellectual processes**: Note if memory and intellectual processes are intact or impaired. Is the patient disoriented and confused or alert and responsive?
- **Attention**: Note if the patient's attention is focused or unfocused.

Assessing For Risk of Suicide

Suicidal ideation occurs frequently in those with mood disorders or depression (common in geriatric patients). Although females are more likely to attempt suicide, males actually successfully commit suicide three times more often, primarily because females tend to take overdoses from which they can be revived, whereas males choose more violent means (jumping from a high place, shooting, or hanging). This holds true for adolescents and adults. Risk factors include psychiatric disorders (schizophrenia, bipolar disorder, post-traumatic stress disorder [PTSD], and substance abuse), physical disorders (HIV/AIDS, diabetes, traumatic brain injury, spinal cord injury), and social problems (bullying). Passive suicidal ideation involves wishing to be dead or thinking about dying without making plans, whereas active suicidal ideation involves making plans. Patients at risk should be questioned about their feelings, problems, plans for suicide, and access to weapons. High-risk findings include the following:

- Violent suicide attempt (knives, gunshots) or access to a weapon
- History of a suicide attempt and a suicide attempt with a low chance of rescue
- Ongoing psychosis or disordered thinking
- Ongoing severe depression and feelings of helplessness
- Lack of a social support system

Schizophrenia and Psychosis

Schizophrenia, a thought disorder, causes psychotic episodes and distortion of reality and the inability to determine the line between fantasy and reality. The onset may be acute or more insidious. Symptoms are positive (delusions, hallucinations, disorganized or catatonic behavior, disorganized speech) or negative (flat affect/decreased emotional range, social isolation, poverty of speech, lack of interest and drive). Patients may have bizarre delusions (thought broadcasting) or hear voices (which they may try to drown out by turning the TV, radio, or music volume up loud). Patients may isolate themselves socially, exhibit poor hygiene, exhibit catatonia (a stiff, unmoving position), and have odd speech. Treatment is with typical and atypical antipsychotics and antidepressants (such as selective serotonin reuptake inhibitors [SSRIs]).

Psychosis is not a disease but a description of a condition and may apply to various diagnoses (such as schizophrenia and bipolar disease). Psychosis is characterized by marked derangement of the personality and a distorted view of reality. Patients may experience hallucinations (seeing/hearing something not present), delusions (false or distorted beliefs), and illusions (false impressions).

Delirium

Delirium is an acute sudden change in consciousness, characterized by reduced ability to focus or sustain attention, language and memory disturbance, disorientation, confusion, audiovisual hallucinations, sleep disturbance, and psychomotor activity disorder. **Delirium** differs from disorders with similar symptoms in that delirium is fluctuating. Delirium occurs in 10%–40% of hospitalized older adults and about 80% of patients who are terminally ill. Delirium may result from drugs such as anticholinergics and numerous conditions including infection, hypoxia, trauma, dementia, depression, vision and hearing loss, surgery, alcoholism, untreated pain, fluid/electrolyte imbalance, and malnutrition. Delirium increases the risks of morbidity and death, especially if untreated. Asking the patient to count backward from 20 to 1 and spell his or her first name backward can identify an attention deficit.

Interventions: Ensure the patient's safety, manage the patient's airway, ventilation, and oxygen supplementation, and reorient the patient frequently.

Agitated/Excited Delirium

Patients with agitated/excited delirium are often very combative, aggressive, violent, and uncooperative, and they may exhibit shouting, threaten violence, and behave bizarrely. The patient may experience hallucinations, disorientation, paranoia, and panic. Patients may be exceptionally strong and seem insensitive to pain. They are often hyperthermic (high temperature). Agitated or excited delirium may be associated with hypoglycemia, brain damage, chemical imbalance, and substance abuse (methamphetamine, cocaine, phencyclidine [PCP, angel dust], and LSD). Patients often require restraints for their own or for others' safety, but they are at risk of death by asphyxiation or restraint (positional) because they fight desperately against the restraints.

Interventions: The transport nurse should use active listening and try to establish rapport while assessing the patient's intellectual functioning, orientation, judgment and thought processes, language, mood, and appearance to determine if law enforcement or other assistance is needed. The patient may refuse care, but implied consent is legal for patients with abnormal behavior. The patient must be transported safely for treatment. The transport nurse should look for medications or drugs on site and take them to the receiving facility.

Calming Patients with Behavioral Emergencies

Patients with behavioral emergencies are often agitated and may be confused, fearful, and/or aggressive, so the paramedic must remain calm and approach the patient slowly; remain at a safe distance; and avoid fast movements, threatening postures, or attempts at physical contact, acknowledging the patient's agitation and offering assistance ("I can see that you're upset, and I want to help") and maintaining eye contact (unless the person is violent and reacts aggressively). The transport nurse should encourage the patient to talk about what is causing the behavior and should answer questions honestly while avoiding threatening, arguing, or challenging the patient. If the patient is suffering hallucinations or delusional thinking, the transport nurse should avoid playing along ("I don't see what you do") but should also avoid contradicting the patient directly when responding. Family or friends may assist with intervention. The transport nurse should not leave the patient unattended and should try to lower distressing stimuli (such as lights and noise) and consider contacting law enforcement. Restraints should be avoided if possible.

Restraints

If a combative patient poses a risk to him- or herself or transport personnel, **restraints** may be necessary to safely assess, treat, and transport the patient, keeping in mind that the altered state of consciousness may result from drug or alcohol use; traumatic injury; or from a mental or physical disorder, such as schizophrenia, dementia, or hypoglycemia (insulin reaction). Protocols for use of restraints must be followed, and restraints should be applied under medical direction. If possible, the police should be present and there should be one transport personnel for each limb, staying beyond the limb's range of motion until ready to secure the limb, with one transport team member talking to the patient and explaining the procedure. The transport nurse should avoid unnecessary force, which may result in increased combativeness and injury to the patient or others. Patients should not be restrained in the prone (face-down) position. Documentation must include the reason for restraining the patient, the time, and the method of restraint.

Types of Restraints

Patients needing restraints are often agitated, confused, and refuse care, but implied consent is legal for patients with abnormal behavior. **Types of restraints** include the following:

- **Verbal:** Try to calm the patient while being firm.
- **Nonverbal:** Use body language and a show of force (with a number of transport personnel being present) to convince the patient.
- **Physical:** Use standard precautions; one person is assigned to each limb, while a fifth person reassures and tries to calm the patient. Apply multiple restraints as necessary, including across the trunk, being careful not to restrict the patient's breathing.
- **Chemical:** Use as a last resort (usually after physical restraints). Includes benzodiazepines (lorazepam) and neuroleptics (haloperidol).
- **Tasers/electrical stun guns:** These may be used by law enforcement to subdue a severely agitated patient. They may cause burns, dart injuries, fall injuries, or cardiac arrest. Stun guns require direct contact, but Tasers may be shot from 20 feet away.

Document the reason for restraint, the types of restraints, the restraint technique, and the time the patient is restrained. Monitor the patient's condition continuously, including the heart rate, airway, ventilation, oxygen supplementation, and circulation.

Types of Physical Restraints

Common types of physical restraints include the following:

- **Soft:** Padded cuffs (often leather) that fasten about the wrists and ankles and are attached to a long board. These are the most commonly used restraints.
- **Stretcher/Spinal board straps:** These may be strapped across the chest (not too tight), abdomen, or legs to help restrict movement.
- **Long board/Spinal board:** Patient should be restrained to the long board and then placed on a wheeled stretcher and never tied to or fastened to the stretcher.
- **Spit sock:** This is a hood that fits over the patient's head to prevent him or her from biting or spitting.
- **Cervical collar:** This is used to protect the patient's cervical spine and to prevent him or her from biting.

The transport nurse should not place the patient in handcuffs or hard plastic ties. If these were placed on a patient by a law enforcement officer and must stay in place, such as with a criminal suspect or an extremely violent patient, then a law enforcement officer must stay with the patient at all times.

Special Populations

Obstetrical Patients

Anatomical Structures of Pregnancy

The anatomical structures involved with pregnancy and fetal development are contained within the female **uterus** (womb). The **placenta** is attached to the walls of the uterus; it includes the **umbilical cord**, which provides blood, nutrients, and oxygen to the fetus. The fetus is inside an **amniotic sac**, which contains amniotic fluid that cushions the fetus. The opening to the uterus is the **cervix**, which thins and dilates for delivery. The cervix opens into the **vagina**, which acts as the birth canal.

Initial Assessment of the Pregnant Patient

Initial assessment of a pregnant patient should determine if the patient's emergency is related to the pregnancy (bleeding, cramping, pain, contractions), to an accident (fall or other injury), or to an unrelated illness:

- Assess patient's vital signs, including oxygen saturation. Monitor ECG.
- Assess pain using the 1-10 numeric scale.
- Determine the patient's week of gestation, singleton vs multiples, gravida, and parity.
- Determine if the patient has had prenatal care.
- If the patient is having contractions, determine the onset, frequency, and duration.
- If the patient is bleeding, determine if it is associated with trauma and estimate the amount, observe the character (dark, bright, scant, flowing, massive), and ask patient about onset and number of pads used in an hour.
- If BP is elevated, ask the patient about headaches, weight gain, seizures, and visual disturbances as these may indicate preeclampsia.
- If patient has supine hypotension, position patient on the left side with a blanket or roll under the left hip.
- Ask about medications including illegal drugs and history of substance abuse.

Vaginal Bleeding During Pregnancy

Vaginal bleeding may occur during any part of a pregnancy and may be related to any of the structures within the uterus. Vaginal bleeding during the **first trimester** of pregnancy may indicate spontaneous abortion, ectopic pregnancy, or infection, although light occasional spotting may be normal. All vaginal bleeding during pregnancy should be assessed by a physician, and a large amount of bleeding may indicate a medical emergency. Bloody show near term may indicate that delivery is near.

Interventions: Use standard precautions and position the patient on her left side. Place a sanitary pad over the vaginal opening and save any soaked pads in a plastic bag so the physician can estimate the amount of blood loss. Manage the patient's airway, ventilation, and oxygen supplementation and provide emotional support. Provide an IV access line and fluids if indicated.

Ectopic Pregnancy

Ectopic pregnancy: Pregnancy in which the egg fertilizes and attaches outside of the uterus (usually in the fallopian tubes), resulting in abdominal pain, absent menstrual periods, and vaginal bleeding. There is a risk of the fallopian tube rupturing, resulting in internal hemorrhage, which is a life-threatening emergency.

Interventions: In the case of a rupture, start an IV and provide fluids. Monitor vital signs and level of consciousness. This patient will be rushed in for immediate surgery.

Premonitory Signs of Labor

Premonitory signs of labor include:

- **Lightening**: As the fetal head engages and moves toward the birth canal, the fundal pressure on the diaphragm lessens, so the mother can breathe more easily, but pressure in the pelvic area increases, causing urinary frequency. The lower abdomen may protrude more than previously. Increased circulatory impairment may cause venous stasis and ankle edema as well as increased vaginal secretions as the vaginal mucous membranes become congested. Pressure on the nerves may result in leg cramps or increased pelvic, back and leg pain.
- **Braxton Hicks (BH)**: BH contractions are short in duration, occur at irregular intervals in the lower abdomen, and do not change the cervix. They are often relieved by activity or mild analgesia. The intensity and frequency of BH contractions often increase immediately prior to the onset of true labor.
- **Cervical changes**: The cervix ripens (softens) to allow for effacement (thinning) and dilation.
- **Bloody show**: A mucous plug from pooled secretions forms at the opening of the cervical canal during pregnancy; when the cervix begins to efface, this mucous plug is expelled, exposing capillary vessels that bleed. Bloody show typically appears as pink mucus and usually occurs within 24 to 48 hours of the onset of labor.
- **Ruptured membranes**: Rupture of the membranes occurs in about 12% of women prior to the onset of labor, which usually then occurs within 24 hours. Before rupture, the membranes typically bulge through the dilating cervix; fluid comes in a gush, although it may come in smaller spurts in some cases. If the membranes rupture before engagement of the fetal head, the umbilical cord may prolapse with the fluid, increasing the risk to the fetus, so mothers should always seek medical attention after rupture. If the mother is at term and labor does not start within 24 hours of rupture, labor may be induced.

Stages of Labor

The stages of labor proceed as follows:

- First stage (dilation stage): Consists of three phases
  - **Latent phase**: The cervix begins to dilate from 0-3 cm; contractions are mild to moderate and occur every 3-30 minutes and are of short duration.
  - **Active phase**: The cervix dilates from 4-7 cm; contractions are every 1-5 minutes, lasting 20-40 seconds. Pain is increased.
  - **Transitional phase**: The cervix dilates from 8-10 cm; contractions come every 1.5-2.0 minutes, lasting 60-90 seconds. There is increased pain, hyperventilation, crying, moaning, vomiting, and rectal pressure.
- **Second stage (expulsion stage)**: Starts when the cervix is fully dilated and ends with delivery of the baby. The patient feels an uncontrollable urge to push, the perineum begins to bulge, and the fetal head crowns as the mother begins to bear down and birth is imminent. Pressure on the rectum and anus may cause stool to be expelled. Birth occurs head first if it is a normal delivery, feet first if it is a breech delivery.
- **Third stage (placental stage)**: Delivery of the placenta should occur 5-30 minutes after birth. There are two phases: placental separation and placental expulsion. Normal blood loss as a result of placental separation is 300-500 mL. Retained placenta may occur if more than 30 minutes elapse.
- **Fourth stage**: The period of 1-4 hours after birth, which involves 250-400 mL blood loss, moderate hypotension (low BP), and tachycardia (rapid pulse).

COMPLICATIONS OF PREGNANCY AND LABOR

<table>
<tr><th>Complication</th><th>Characteristic</th><th>Interventions</th></tr>
<tr><td>Preterm labor</td><td>Labor between weeks 20 and 37 weeks; presents a risk to the fetus.</td><td rowspan="3">Provide supportive care in the left lateral position.
Manage the patient's airway, ventilation, and oxygen supplementation (100%).
Transport rapidly if there is severe bleeding or a risk of imminent preterm delivery.
Start an IV access line and give NS for placental abruption.</td></tr>
<tr><td>Premature rupture of membranes</td><td>Membranes rupture before the onset of labor; this may lead to preterm labor and risk to the fetus.</td></tr>
<tr><td>Substance abuse</td><td>May result in damage to the fetus and preterm labor. Many drugs restrict blood flow to the fetus, resulting in growth restriction and low oxygen. Some drugs, such as cocaine, affect the fetal nervous system. Sudden withdrawal of opiates may trigger preterm labor. Alcohol may result in fetal alcohol syndrome, characterized by facial abnormalities, growth restriction, and neurological defects.</td></tr>
<tr><td>Placental abruption</td><td>The placenta prematurely detaches, partially or completely, from the uterus. Risk factors: maternal hypertension, traumatic injury, cigarette smoking, and cocaine use. Partial detachment interferes with the functioning of the placenta, causing intrauterine growth restriction. Severe bleeding occurs with total detachment.</td><td>Provide supportive care in the left lateral position.
Manage the patient's airway, ventilation, and oxygen supplementation (100%).
Transport rapidly if there is severe bleeding or a risk of imminent preterm delivery.
Start an IV access line and give NS for placental abruption.</td></tr>
<tr><td>Placenta previa</td><td>The placenta implants over or near the internal cervical opening. Implantation may be complete (covering the entire opening), partial, or marginal (to the edge of the cervical opening). Results in increased incidences of hemorrhage in the third trimester. Symptoms include painless bleeding after the 20th week of gestation.</td><td rowspan="2">Provide supportive care in the left lateral position.
Manage the patient's airway, ventilation, and oxygen supplementation (100%). IV access line and NS. Transport rapidly if there is severe bleeding, high BP ≥160/110, seizures, or altered mental status. Provide ECG monitoring. Administer magnesium sulfate for preeclampsia/ eclampsia.</td></tr>
<tr><td>Pregnancy-induced hypertension/ Preeclampsia/ Eclampsia</td><td>Hypertension >140/90 associated with increased protein in the urine and edema (peripheral or generalized) or increase of ≥ 5 pounds of weight in one week after the 20th week of gestation. Severe preeclampsia is BP ≥ 160/110. Symptoms include headache, abdominal pain, and visual disturbances. May progress to eclampsia (seizures) and death.</td></tr>
</table>

Complication	Characteristic	Interventions
Cephalic (vertex) presentation	Military: Head straight, neck not flexed. Brow: Neck extended, brow presents first, can cause birth trauma, so episiotomy or cesarean section (C-section) is usually required. Face: Severely extended neck with face presentation, may prolong labor, increase swelling of the fetus, and cause neck trauma.	Provide supportive care. Manage the patient's airway, ventilation, and oxygen supplementation (100%). Transport rapidly.
Breech presentation	Frank breech (buttocks presentation with legs extended upward) is the most common, but single- or double-footling breech (incomplete breech) or buttocks presentation with legs flexed (complete breech) can also occur. Breech presentation is most common with placenta previa, hydramnios, fetal anomalies, and multiple gestations. Cord prolapse is more likely. Head trauma may occur because molding does not occur, and the head can become entrapped.	

Prolapse of the Umbilical Cord

A prolapse of the umbilical cord occurs when the umbilical cord precedes the fetus in the birth canal and becomes entrapped by the descending fetus. With an **occult cord prolapse**, the umbilical cord is beside or just ahead of the fetal head. With a **nuchal cord prolapse**, the cord tightly wraps about the fetal neck. About half of the time, prolapses occur in the second stage of labor and relate to premature delivery, multiple gestations, or other complications. As contractions occur and the head descends, pressure to the umbilical cord occludes the blood flow, causing hypoxia and bradycardia. The decrease in blood flow through the umbilical vessels can cause impaired gas exchange, and if pressure on the cord is not relieved, the fetus can suffer severe neurological damage or death.

Interventions: Elevate the presenting part off the cord, pull the cord off of the fetus's neck if possible, elevate the mother's knees to the chest to relieve pressure on the cord, provide 100% oxygen, and transport rapidly.

Hyperemesis Gravidarum (HG) and Rh Incompatibility

About 60–80% of pregnant woman suffer from nausea and vomiting (N/V), especially during the first trimester, but only about 2% suffer **hyperemesis gravidarum** (HG). Symptoms of HG include severe (sometimes intractable) N/V, weight loss, and dehydration.

Interventions: Provide intravenous fluids with 5% glucose in NS or Ringer's lactate; administer antiemetic drugs, including promethazine (Phenergan), prochlorperazine (Compazine), or chlorpromazine (Thorazine).

Rh incompatibility occurs if the mother is Rh-negative and the father is Rh-positive, putting their infant at risk for hemolytic disease of the newborn (HDN). The blood from an Rh-positive baby can mix with the Rh-negative blood of the mother, causing the mother's immune system to make antibodies to destroy the Rh factor. This immune response is called Rh sensitization and can occur during C-section or vaginal delivery, miscarriage, abortion, placental abruption, amniocentesis, chorionic villus sampling, ectopic pregnancy, toxemia, and trauma during pregnancy. Women who are Rh-negative with an Rh-positive mate receive the serum RhoGAM, containing anti-Rh (anti-D) immunoglobulin in order to agglutinate any fetal red blood cells that pass over into the mother's circulatory system and thus prevent the mother from forming antibodies against them that will attack the infant and sensitize her for future pregnancies.

Multiple Gestations

In vitro fertilization and ovulation-inducing drugs have increased the incidence of high-order **multiple gestations** over the past 30 years. The trend of delayed childbearing has led to an increase in twin/multiple gestations. Infants born from multiple gestations are more likely to be born prematurely and with low birth weights. The incidence of premature birth and low birth weight is proportional to the number of fetuses. There may be growth restriction/growth discordance, oligohydramnios, and restriction of movement of one or more fetuses. Approximately 50% of twins and 90% of triplets are born premature, compared to 10% of singletons. With this increase in prematurity and proportion of infants born with low birth weight, there are increased morbidities, such as cerebral palsy and intellectual disabilities. The risk for genetic disorders, such as neural tube defects and GI and cardiac abnormalities, is twice that of single gestations.

Shoulder Dystocia

Shoulder dystocia is a condition whereby a baby's shoulders are not able to progress through the birth canal after his/her head emerges. The condition oftentimes occurs with babies who are very large. Due to cord compression, time is a vital consideration in cases of shoulder dystocia; as such, delivery of the shoulders should be attempted prior to suctioning the baby's nose and mouth. Emptying a distended bladder may also be helpful. If an episiotomy incision has not already been made to enlarge the opening of the vagina for delivery, such an incision may assist in delivering the baby's shoulders. Performing the McRoberts maneuver, a technique that involves flexing the patient's legs up towards her chest in order to increase the diameter of the pelvis, may also assist in delivery. Additionally, the application of suprapubic pressure in an attempt to manually dislodge one of the baby's shoulders can be an effective strategy for delivering the baby. If possible, and cord isn't being compressed or other emergencies are not present, rapid transport to a facility with OB emergency care.

Early, Variable, and Late Decelerations

Early decelerations in a fetal heart rate (FHR) mimic the pattern of contraction; they tend to start at the beginning of a contraction and end when the contraction ends. This type of deceleration is harmless and is caused by head compression, which stimulates the vagus nerve. Early decelerations are most often seen when women are dilated between four and seven centimeters in active labor. Variable decelerations are caused by cord compression and can be seen at any time during the course of a contraction. They are characterized by a "V" or "W" shape on the fetal heart monitor. They are not typically associated with poor fetal outcome. Late decelerations generally begin after a contraction begins. After the onset of a late deceleration, the FHR gradually decelerates and then returns to baseline once the contraction ends. Late decelerations indicate that the baby is not receiving a sufficient amount of oxygen.

Interventions for Fetal Distress

The patient should be placed in a left lateral recumbent position, which means she should be lying down on her left side. Placing the patient on her left side prevents compression of the inferior vena cava, which is a large vein that supplies blood to the heart from the lower half of the body; however, if placing the patient on her left side makes it difficult to provide appropriate care in the transport vehicle, it is acceptable to have her lie down on her right side.

Using a mask, provide oxygen to the patient. Correct the problem(s) that led to the fetal distress if known. Keep monitoring the fetal heart rate (FHR), and follow appropriate protocols for abnormal FHR. IV fluids for the mother if there is questionable dehydration. Protect the umbilical cord from being compressed by the fetus's head if this is applicable and transport the patient to facility.

Delivery of a Newborn

If the fetal head is obvious at the vaginal opening (crowning), delivery is imminent. Steps to delivery include the following:

1. Wash hands and don PPE for standard precautions and obtain an OB kit and supplies.
2. Position the patient on her back with hips and knees flexed, feet flat on the stretcher, and legs apart.
3. Position one person at the mother's head to support and care for the mother, while the other person delivers the baby.
4. Provide oxygen to the mother, and if time allows, provide an IV access line and NS, cardiac monitoring, and analgesia as needed.
5. As the infant's head is crowning, support the perineum with the palm of your hand, also supporting the baby's head as it delivers.
6. Palpate the neck to determine if the umbilical cord has wrapped around the neck. If there is a nuchal cord, carefully attempt to slip it over the infant's head.
7. Once the body delivers, make note of the time of birth.
8. If the infant is not vigorous, stimulate by drying with a towel, and possibly suctioning the mouth and nose with a bulb syringe. Blow-by oxygen or bag-mask ventilation is utilized if the infant is not breathing.
9. If the infant is stable, place the baby skin to skin on mom's chest.
10. After about 2 minutes, place a cord clamp about 4 cm from the neonate's abdomen, and another cord clamp or hemostat a few centimeters down, then cut the cord in between the clamps.
11. Monitor the baby and assign an Apgar score at one and five minutes after birth.
12. Placental separation and delivery usually occur within 10-20 minutes after birth. Never pull on the umbilical cord as it may cause uterine inversion or placental tearing.
13. Place a sanitary pad over the vaginal opening to contain any bleeding. Observe for hemorrhage.
14. The uterus should be massaged to promote contractions and control excessive bleeding.

Management of Preterm Labor

Tocolytic Therapy for Preterm Labor

Tocolytic therapy is the use of medication to suppress the contractions of a patient in preterm labor, which is defined as labor that occurs before the 37th week of pregnancy. Tocolytic therapy should not be employed if the gestational age of the fetus is greater than 37 weeks or if the fetus weighs more than 2,500 grams. If the fetus is in acute distress, medication should not be administered to delay labor. If chorioamnionitis (inflammation of the membranes of the amniotic sac) is present, tocolytic therapy should not be employed. Additionally, if the patient has pregnancy-induced hypertension, eclampsia, active vaginal bleeding, or cardiac disease, labor should be allowed to progress without introducing tocolytic therapy to suppress the patient's contractions.

Delivery of the Preterm Infant

A preterm infant is one born prior to 37 weeks gestational age. In the United States, preterm birth is the most important factor influencing infant mortality, accounting for 75-80% of all neonatal morbidity and mortality. Preterm birth is often associated with comorbidities. The original cause of the preterm birth (such as maternal infection) may also play an integral role in the likely health problems associated with the infant's prematurity. Findings may include the following:

- Respiratory distress syndrome because of inadequate surfactant production (hyaline membrane disease)
- Hypothermia because of inadequate subcutaneous fat, small amounts of brown fat, and large skin surface area to mass ratio
- Hypoglycemia secondary to poor nutritional intake, poor nutritional stores, and increased glucose consumption associated with sepsis
- Skin trauma or infection secondary to fragile, transparent, immature skin with less subcutaneous fat

- Periods of apnea because of an immature respiratory center in the brain
- Intraventricular hemorrhage
- Large trunk and short extremities

Interventions: Attempt resuscitation with signs of life, suction, ventilate/oxygenate, give compressions if indicated, administer epinephrine for bradycardia, and maintain body temperature.

Antepartum Hemorrhage

Antepartum hemorrhage is bleeding from the genital tract (above the cervix) that occurs from week 20 of pregnancy to before delivery. Because some bleeding may be internal, the patient should be assessed for indications of shock (hypotension, nausea, pallor, dyspnea, and tachycardia) as well as estimation of blood loss:

- Spotting: Streaks of blood
- Minor hemorrhage: <50 mL blood.
- Major hemorrhage: 50 mL to 1,000 mL without clinical evidence of shock.
- Massive hemorrhage: >1,000 mL with clinical evidence of shock.

Causes may include placenta previa (separation of placenta that is over or near the cervical opening), placental abruption (premature detachment of placenta), and vasa previa (rupture of vessels below the presenting part of fetus because of aberrant insertion of cord into the placenta, resulting in fetal exsanguination). Diagnosis must be differentiated from bloody show, which is a small amount of blood with mucus discharge that may precede the onset of labor by as much as 72 hours and is a normal occurrence with cervical dilatation and effacement.

Interventions: Ensure airway and ventilation, provide oxygen at high concentration, assess vital signs and oxygen saturation, assess fetal heart tone with Doppler if possible, assess contractions (presence, frequency, duration, intensity), insert large-bore IV access and administer IV NS or lactated Ringer's, and administer packed red blood cells as indicated.

Considerations for the Pregnant Trauma Patient

Considerations for the pregnant trauma patient include:

- **Spinal immobilization**: Pregnant patients have impaired venous return when flat during the third trimester and increased risk of nausea and vomiting, so spinal immobilization should be used only with indications of neurological impairment. Once the patient is secured, the spinal board should be tilted 15-30° to the left (and head elevated if possible) to improve circulation to the placenta and avoid supine hypotensive syndrome.
- **Hypoxia/Shock**: With hypoxia, maternal blood is shunted from the fetal blood circulation to the mother's vital organs, and this can result in fetal distress, so it is critical to keep the mothers oxygen saturation level close to 100%.
- **Cardiopulmonary resuscitation**: Perform high quality chest compressions (2:30) as in non-pregnant patients and administer shock as soon as possible, administer 2 minutes of CPR between shocks

Interventions: Administer 100% oxygen with non-rebreather mask at ≥15L/min. Use bag-mask ventilation with CPR. Insert two large-bore IV lines, infuse NS, and maintain continuous ECG monitoring.

Uterine Massage After Delivery

Once the baby and the placenta have both been delivered, the fundus of the uterus should be manually massaged to aid with contraction. The uterine fundus should be massaged every 10 minutes during the first postpartum hour; the massage process can be repeated as many times as necessary during the second postpartum hour. After each massage session, the uterus should be palpated to ensure that it remains properly contracted and does not become relaxed and/or soft. Bleeding should also be assessed each time uterine massage is performed.

Uterine Inversion

Uterine inversion occurs when the uterus turns inside out and protrudes through the cervix; in some cases, the top of the uterus comes out of the vagina. The condition is a potentially life-threatening one that can lead to severe hemorrhaging and shock. One way to manage uterine inversion is to attempt to manually return the uterus to its proper positioning; this attempt can be made by applying pressure to the top of the uterus with the fingertips and palm of the hand in order to push it back through the cervix. Once it has been repositioned, it is best to continue to apply pressure to the uterus with one hand inside the vagina and one hand on the patient's abdomen; pressure should be applied in this manner until the uterus firms up. If the uterus is not easily put back in place, surgical intervention may be necessary.

Risk Factors for Emergency Delivery

The labor and delivery process tends to progress more rapidly when certain conditions exist. Patients who have given birth before, particularly those patients who have had a rapid delivery in the past, generally have faster deliveries with each successive pregnancy. Patients with certain connective tissue diseases, which are disorders involving abnormalities in the patient's collagen and elastin, are more likely to have fast deliveries. Pregnant women who have either sustained an injury and/or have been seriously ill during their pregnancy often have an increased risk of going into premature labor, which would necessitate an emergency delivery. Additionally, women with cervical incompetence, a condition whereby the cervix lacks the ability to stay closed when it should stay closed, generally have rapid deliveries.

Risks for Delivery During Transport

Several signs can help determine whether a pregnant patient may need to deliver her baby during transport. The patient should be considered to be in active labor if she is experiencing contractions in a regular pattern about three minutes apart that last approximately one minute each. If the patient is experiencing rectal pressure or a feeling similar to the urge to have a bowel movement, these sensations may indicate that the baby's head is in the birth canal and that the baby needs to be delivered. Additionally, if the transport team member can see the baby's head in the birth canal and/or if the birth canal appears to be bulging, the patient is at risk for delivering during transport. An uncontrollable desire to push is another strong indicator that delivery needs to occur promptly.

Neonatal/Pediatric

Initial Care of the Newborn

Dr. Virginia Apgar developed the **APGAR assessment** in 1952. APGAR stands for **a**ppearance, **p**ulse, **g**rimace, **a**ctivity, and **r**espiration. The APGAR is the first test given to a newborn. It is used as a quick evaluation of a newborn's physical condition to determine if any emergency medical care is needed, and it is administered 1 minute and 5 minutes after birth. The test is administered more than once because the baby's condition may change rapidly. It may be administered for a third time 10 minutes after birth if needed. The baby is rated on the five subscales, and scores are added together. A total score of ≥7 is a sign of good health.

Sign	0	1	2
Appearance (skin color)	Cyanotic or pallor over entire body	Acrocyanosis	Pink
Pulse (heart rate)	Absent	<100 bpm	>100 bpm
Grimace (reflex irritability)	Unresponsive	Grimace	Infant sneezes, coughs, and recoils
Activity (muscle tone)	Absent	Flexed limbs	Infant moves freely

Sign	0	1	2
Respiration (breathing rate and effort)	Absent	Slow, irregular; weak cry	Vigorous cry

Review Video: Newborn APGAR Score
Visit mometrix.com/academy and enter code: 253451

ROUTINE CARE OF THE NEWBORN

Infants have poor temperature regulation ability, particularly preterm infants who lack brown fat, which is one of the body's tools to regulate body temperature, so providing warmth is critical as a component of resuscitation. An infant who is just seconds old and wet will need aggressive measures to keep him or her warm while any resuscitation efforts are being initiated. Infants lose heat through their heads, so one of the first steps should be to place a hat on the head or cover the head in some way. The infant should be vigorously dried with warmed blankets. Often, this stimulation, drying and warming, is all that is needed to establish a regular respiration pattern in the neonate. Preterm infants weighing <1500 grams should be placed in a plastic bag (made specifically for this purpose), if available, up to the height of the shoulders to prevent cold shock. A term infant with no distress can be placed on the mother's chest and covered with a warm blanket.

ABCS OF RESUSCITATION OF THE NEONATE

The ABCs of resuscitation should begin immediately after delivery with assisted ventilation begun within 60 seconds if required.

- **Airway:** An airway should be established as the very first thing tended to; if there is no airway, air cannot be moved during resuscitation attempts. This step includes using a bulb syringe to clear the mouth, then the nose of secretions and properly positioning the infant's head in the sniffing position.
- **Breathing**: This step involves initiating breathing after the airway has been established; this can be done with stimulation, supplemental oxygen, or through artificial ventilation if there is apnea, gasping, or heart rate below 100 bpm. Attach pulse oximeter, consider cardiac monitor, and give PPV at 40-60 breaths per minute.
- **Circulation**: Start compressions if heart rate is <60 bpm after 30 seconds of PPV with chest movement. Check HR every 60 seconds. Compress one-third of the anterior-posterior diameter of the chest, using two thumbs or two fingers. Give 3 compressions to 1 breath every 2 seconds (90 compressions to 30 ventilations per minute). Increase oxygen to 100% during compressions. If the HR remains <60 bpm after 60 seconds of CPR, administer epinephrine by IV or ET. Volume expanders (isotonic crystalloid at 10 mL/kg) can be given IV if the neonate is hypovolemic.

ESTABLISHING AN AIRWAY

To establish an airway, the infant is placed supine with the head slightly extended in the sniffing position. A small neck roll may be placed under the shoulders to maintain this position in a very small premature infant. Once the proper position is established, the mouth and nose are suctioned (suction the mouth first to prevent reflex inspiration of secretions when the nose is suctioned) with a bulb syringe or catheter if necessary. The infant's head can be turned momentarily to the side to allow secretions to pool in the cheek where they can be more easily suctioned and removed to establish the airway. Stimulating the newborn is often all that is needed to initiate spontaneous respirations. This tactile stimulation can be accomplished by gently rubbing the back or trunk of the infant. Another technique that is used to provide stimulation is flicking or rubbing the soles of the feet. Slapping neonates as stimulation is no longer practiced and should NOT be used.

Managing Airway and Ventilation

Airway management is based on the severity of respiratory distress:

- **Blow-by oxygen**: Provide if the newborn is cyanotic and heart rate is >100 bpm and respiratory effort is adequate. Provide warm oxygen at 5 L/min. with a direct flow on the face. Avoid oral airways.
- **Bag-valve mask (BVM)**: Provide if the newborn is apneic, the heart rate <100, and/or there is inadequate respiratory effort. Use an appropriate size and avoid excess pressure, which may cause pneumothorax, although initial ventilation requires higher pressure to expand the lungs. Disable the pop-off valve.
- **Intubation**: Provide if other measures are ineffective and the heart rate is <60. Use a straight-blade laryngoscope size #1 for full term and size #0 for preterm with ETT 2.5-4.0 mm, depending on the weight of newborn. Confirm placement through visualization, auscultation (lateral, superior chest wall, epigastric region), improvement in respirations, $ETCO_2$ detector, and pulse oximetry. Secure the ETT. Provide PEEP as indicated at 5 cmH_2O. Gastric decompression may be necessary if the abdomen is distended. Provide CPR as needed.

Neonatal Assessment

Rapid Assessment

The infant should be given a rapid assessment within seconds of birth to determine if the infant is at term, if the amniotic fluid is clear, if there is muscle tone, and if there are respirations or crying. If any of these conditions is not met, then the child should be placed under radiant heat and further resuscitation done. The basic steps to resuscitation include:

- Warming the infant after drying
- Positioning the infant and clearing the airway if necessary
- Stimulating and repositioning the infant

The child should be evaluated throughout the initial procedures:

- Respirations: Rate and character of respirations should be noted as well as observation of chest wall movement. Respiratory rate should be 35-60 breaths per minute, which should be counted over a full minute.
- Heart rate: Should be >100 bpm, assessed with stethoscope or at the base of the umbilical cord.

Normal Neonatal Cardiac Rates

Normal cardiac rates can vary widely from one neonate to another, so it's important to understand the normal range in order to determine if the infant has an abnormal pulse. Rates will also vary depending upon whether the infant is awake, sleeping, or active. Pulse rate should be taken with a stethoscope, because the pulse may be difficult to palpate or count accurately manually. The neonatal **point of maximal intensity (PMI)** is located at the intersection between the 4th intercostal space and the midclavicular line (versus the adult PMI located at the 5th intercostal). Additionally, this allows for assessment of heart murmurs.

Newborn Infant	Awake/Alert: 100-205 Asleep: 90-160
1-12 Weeks	Awake/Alert: 100-180 Asleep: 90-160

Monitoring of heart rate is particularly important as alterations of heart rate occur with periods of apnea. A period of apnea is usually followed by decreased heart rate, as well as decreased oxygen saturation. Respiratory rates should be monitored as well as heart rate. **Color** should be noted. Pink coloring indicates good perfusion. Generalized mottling or central cyanosis should be investigated further.

NEONATAL BLOOD PRESSURE

Normal blood pressure values for a **term infant**:

- Systolic-56-77 mmHg
- Diastolic 33-50 mmHg
- MAP 42-60 mmHg
- Hypertension: Systolic >90 and diastolic >60

In a **preterm infant**, normal systolic and diastolic values will vary depending on the gestational age and size of the infant. A preterm infant should have an MAP that is at least as high as the gestational age (in weeks) of that infant. For example, an infant born at 28 weeks gestation should have an MAP of at least 28. A preterm infant is considered hypertensive with systolic >80 and diastolic >50.

Proper **fit of the blood pressure cuff** is imperative to obtain an accurate reading. One must measure the width of the infant's arm in the area that the cuff will be applied. Once this measurement is obtained, the cuff should be approximately 25% wider than this measurement. A cuff too small results in BP reading too high and too large results in BP reading too low.

NEONATAL HEART SOUNDS

S1

S1 is the heart sound heard as the mitral and tricuspid valves close at the beginning of the contraction of the ventricle (systole). S1 is easiest to hear if the stethoscope is placed at the fourth intercostal space while the infant is supine and calm. If the S1 heard is louder than normal, that means **cardiac output** and **blood flow** are higher than normal. The conditions that can cause this are:

- Patent ductus arteriosus
- Ventricular septal defect
- Tetralogy of Fallot

If the S1 heard is softer or quieter than normal, this is an indication of **lowered cardiac output**, which could cause these problems:

- Congestive heart failure
- Myocarditis

S2

S2 is the sound heard when the pulmonic valve and the aortic valve close at the end of the contraction of the ventricles (systole). S2 is easiest to hear at the upper left border of the sternum. S2 is normally split, as the aortic valve closes slightly ahead of the pulmonic valve. In the presence of a cardiac defect, the S2 split becomes wider (the difference in time between the closing of the aortic and pulmonic valve becomes greater). Conditions that cause a **widened S2 split** include:

- Atrial septal defect
- Tetralogy of Fallot
- Pulmonary stenosis
- Ebstein anomaly

Conditions that cause **no split** in the S2 (the two valves close at the same time, or one is not closing) include:

- Pulmonary or aortic atresia
- Aortic or pulmonary stenosis
- Persistent pulmonary hypertension

Neonatal Complications

Condition	Characteristics	Interventions
Meconium in amniotic fluid	The infant is at risk for aspiration with complete obstruction (causing atelectasis and/or right-to-left shunt through the foramen ovale) or incomplete obstruction (causing pneumothorax or pneumonitis). The infant may be hypoxic, hypercapnic, and acidotic.	Avoid stimulating respirations. If there are no signs of distress, suction the mouth, nose, and throat. If there is respiratory distress, intubate and suction the trachea and ventilate with 100% oxygen.
Apnea	This is failure to breathe spontaneously or respiration pauses for >20 seconds. It usually results from hypothermia or hypoxia, but it may result from other causes, such as narcotics in the system.	Stimulate, ventilate, suction, and/or intubate as indicated.
Bradycardia	It usually results from hypoxia, so the airway must be assessed for obstruction.	Suction, BVM with 100% oxygen, intubation, chest compressions as indicated. Administer IV epinephrine.
Hypoglycemia	Blood glucose is <30 mg/dL in the first 24 hours of life and <45 mg/dL thereafter. The infant exhibits twitching, limpness, lethargy, seizures, eye rolling, apnea, cyanosis, irregular respirations, and a high-pitched cry.	Manage the airway, ventilation, circulation. When possible, feed the newborn breastmilk or formula. Administer dextrose 10% (D10).

CHEAP TORCHES and TORCH Panel

CHEAP TORCHES is the acronym used to recall common causes of congenital and neonatal infections. Many congenital infections are present for at least a month prior to birth and remain present at birth, such as the following:

C = Chickenpox (varicella)
H = Hepatitis (B, C, and E)
E = Enterovirus (RNA viruses, including coxsackievirus, echovirus, and poliovirus)
A = AIDS (HIV)
P = Parvovirus (B19)
T = Toxoplasmosis
O = Other (group B streptococcus, Candida, Listeria, TB, lymphocytic choriomeningitis)
R = Rubella (measles)
C = Cytomegalovirus
H = Herpes simplex virus
E = Every other STD (chlamydia, gonorrhea, Ureaplasma, papillomavirus)
S = Syphilis

Exposure to these pathogens in utero may cause a miscarriage or congenital defect, especially if the exposure was during the first trimester. Symptoms may include being small for gestational age, an enlarged liver and spleen, thrombocytopenia, skin rash, jaundice, seizures, or encephalitis. The **TORCH panel,** which tests for toxoplasmosis, rubella, cytomegalovirus, and herpes simplex virus, is commonly used to screen pregnant women for infectious diseases.

Brief, Resolved, Unexplained Event and Sudden Infant Death Syndrome

Brief, resolved, unexplained event (BRUE) refers to a group of alarming symptoms that can occur in infants. They involve a sudden appearance of apnea, altered responsiveness, and change in color or muscle tone. The event lasts <1 minute in an infant <1 year of age, in which there is no underlying cause, and there is a quick spontaneous return to their baseline state of health. With **sudden infant death syndrome (SIDS)**, which is almost always related to respiratory arrest, the child cannot be resuscitated. There are numerous proposed causes for SIDS, so a careful history, including familial history of SIDS, and physical examination or postmortem examination can provide important information, such as indications of child abuse or metabolic/infectious disorders.

Interventions: Continue resuscitative efforts (airway, ventilation, oxygen supplementation, and compressions as indicated) and stabilize the infant if possible. The child with BRUE should be hospitalized for observation, further studies, and apnea monitoring because these children are at increased risk for SIDS. For SIDS patients, the transport nurse should provide support and information to the family. The protocol for reporting SIDS varies by state, but it usually involves notifying the coroner's office.

Growth and Development of Pediatric Patients

Normal growth and development by age, in the first two years of life, is as follows:

- **0–2 months**: Sleeps up to 16 hours per day but should rouse easily. Cries for a reason; persistent crying may indicate illness. Limited head control. Gazes at faces.
- **2–6 months**: Smiles voluntarily and makes eye contact, uses both hands, begins to hold his or her head up, rolls over, and sleeps through the night.
- **6–12 months**: Sits, crawls, has pincer grasp, mouths objects (increasing risk of poisoning and aspiration), babbles, and speaks first words by 12 months. Exhibits separation anxiety from parents.
- **12–18 months**: Begins to walk; imitates others; knows body parts and 4-6 words; lacks molars for grinding food, increasing the risk of aspiration; and has increased mobility.
- **18–24 months**: Begins to run and climb, knows 100 words (24 months), clings to parents, attaches to special objects, labels objects, and begins to understand cause and effect.
- **2–5 years**: Walks, runs, throws, catches, is toilet trained, has magical thinking and irrational fears, learns acceptable behavior, has temper tantrums, and develops modesty.
- **6–12 years**: Loses baby teeth; thinks logically; becomes self-conscious; understands the finality of death; attaches importance to school, popularity, and peers.
- **12–20 years**: Puberty begins, reasons (imperfectly), is self-conscious, seeks independence and peer approval, and takes risks.

Pediatric Considerations

Pediatric patients have the following physiologic considerations:

- Proportionately greater body surface area to body mass ratio, so they are at greater risk of fluid and heat loss, burns, and absorption of toxins
- Higher respiratory rates and heart rates than adults, resulting in higher oxygen demand
- Immature blood/brain barrier, resulting in more neurological symptoms
- Immature immune system, resulting in a higher risk of infection
- Narrower and shorter airway and smaller jaw, so the tongue may easily obstruct the airway
- Soft tracheal cartilage that increases the risk of airway collapse, and a large epiglottis
- More pliable ribs, which provide less protection for abdominal organs, which are more forward
- Liver and spleen that are proportionately larger and at risk of injury
- Bones that are softer with open growth plates (an open growth plate injury can impair growth)
- Less protection for the brain and spinal cord (increasing the risk of injury) and less subarachnoid space
- Cerebral blood flow needs twice that of adults, increasing the risk of hypoxia
- Limited glucose stores and risk of hypothermia (especially in the first month)
- Anterior fontanel that closes by 12 months and posterior fontanel that closes by 3-4 months

Infant Assessment

Information Gathered by Observation of an Infant

An infant in distress will likely show signs and symptoms of the distress even prior to a physical examination. An infant's nutritional state and fluid level can typically be observed without an examination as well. For example, an infant who looks emaciated may not be getting an adequate supply of calories, and an infant whose eyes look sunken may be insufficiently hydrated. The infant's overall shape can provide information about whether he/she may be suffering any injuries or has sustained any trauma. Skin tone and overall color can provide clues about the infant's temperature regulation and circulation. An infant's respiratory effort and his/her ability to cry may offer information about his/her airway and breathing. Additionally, the infant's posture provides indications of his/her gross motor skills functioning. Finally, the activity level and behavioral state of an infant can also provide information about the infant's state prior to a physical examination.

Moro and Step Reflexes

The Moro reflex can be tested by placing an infant in a supported position on a surface. With the examiner supporting the infant behind his/her neck with one hand and grasping the infant's hands with the other hand, the infant should feel relaxed and secure. When the infant's hands are suddenly released and the hand supporting his/her neck is relaxed, the infant should respond by throwing his/her arms outward. Additionally, an infant should clench his/her fists and look startled when the Moro reflex is tested. The Moro reflex tends to disappear around six months of age. The step reflex can be tested by supporting the infant under the arms and placing the soles of his/her feet on a surface; if the infant's step reflex is intact, he/she will making stepping motions even before the infant displays the ability to walk. The step reflex typically disappears by three months of age.

Pediatric Assessment

The pediatric assessment should include the following:

- Pediatric assessment triangle:
  - *Appearance* (abnormal tone, decreased interactivity, decreased consolability, abnormal look/gaze, and abnormal speech or cry)
  - *Work of breathing* (abnormal sounds [wheezing, stridor], position, retractions [sternum], flaring [nostrils], and apnea/gasping)
  - *Circulation* (pallor, mottling, and cyanosis)
- **Assess airway, breathing, and circulation (heart rate/pulse)**: Place in the shock position and provide a warming blanket for signs of shock.
- **Ventilation/oxygenation**: Administer oxygen and assist with ventilation if it is abnormal.
- **Determine the patient's level of consciousness**: Use the alert, voice, pain, unresponsive (AVPU) assessment. Note movement of the extremities and whether the pupils are normal, dilated, constricted, reactive, or fixed.
- **Prevent hypothermia**: Cover with a warming blanket, cover the head, and avoid unnecessary exposure of the skin.
- **Obtain the medical history from the caregiver/parent**: Include the type and duration of symptoms, fever, level of activity, recent foods/fluids, medications, medication allergies, past or chronic illnesses, and events leading to the current problem.
- **Head-to-toe physical examination**: Note any bruising, swelling, drainage, loose teeth, unusual odors, bleeding, rashes, deformities, and pain on movement.

Common Fears of Toddlers, Preschoolers, and School-Age Children

For toddlers, a major fear is separation from their parents, guardians, or caretakers. At the toddler stage, fears about having their bodily orifices invaded begin to develop. Experiencing bodily injuries and/or pain are also common fears of toddlers. Additionally, toddlers fear losing control over objects in or aspects of their lives. At the preschool level, fears related to imaginary things such as monsters begin to surface as preschoolers' imaginations develop further. Fears about people such as kidnappers and robbers begin to develop as well at the preschool age as preschoolers become more aware of the world around them. Like toddlers, the fear of experiencing bodily injuries is common among preschool-age children. For school-age children, common fears include experiencing bodily injuries, losing control over objects in or aspects of their lives, not being able to live up to others' expectations, and death.

Assessing Pediatric Cardiopulmonary Functioning

Pediatric Advanced Life Support (PALS), is an assessment model that helps to quickly recognize and treat conditions that may be life threatening. First, a quick general assessment is done using the pediatric assessment triangle (PAT), which observes appearance, breathing and circulatory status. Appearance includes TICLS- tone, interactiveness, consolabilty, look, and speech/cry. Breathing notes obvious airway sounds, positioning used to aid breathing and accessory muscle use. Circulatory status is rapidly assessed by noting cyanosis or pallor. During this rapid assessment, obvious compromise can be recognized and treated. A child with an alteration in 2–3 of these areas is likely close to experiencing arrest. After this quick general assessment, the transport nurse should rapidly assess airway, breathing, circulation, disability, and exposure.

The patient's airway is assessed initially and categorized as either: 1) clear, 2) able to be maintained once the patient is repositioned, or 3) not able to be maintained without intubation or removal of a foreign object. Next the child's breathing is assessed. Respiratory rate, effort, breath sounds, and skin color are all appropriate measures of the patient's ability or inability to breathe. To determine circulation, the patient's heart rate, pulse, blood pressure, level of alertness, skin color, and temperature are monitored. Disability uses the APVU scale, GSC scale, and pupil response. Exposure assesses temperature, skin, and trauma evidence.

Transporting Pediatric Patients with Spinal Cord Injuries

Steps must be taken when caring for a pediatric patient with spinal injury to ensure that the injury is not exacerbated. Cervical spine motion should be restricted, and movement of the patient's head and neck should be avoided, if possible. When assessing the patient's airway, the head should not be tilted per regular airway management protocol; rather, the patient's airway should be opened and maintained by thrusting the jaw. Due to the imperative nature of establishing an airway, the head-tilt maneuver may be utilized in situations where a jaw thrust is not feasible. Oftentimes, due to the disproportionate size of a child's head in relation to the rest of his/her body, the patient's torso must be elevated in order to prevent the transport backboard from imposing flexion on the cervical spine.

Pediatric Trauma Score

The Pediatric Trauma Score (PTS) is the most commonly used scoring method used in the assessment of pediatric trauma patients. A child with a score lower than 8 is at increased risk of morbidity, disability, and mortality.

Factor	+2	+1	-1
Weight	<20 kg	10-20 kg	<10 kg
Airway	Normal	Oral or nasal airway	Intubation or cricothyroidotomy
Systolic BP (mmHg) and pulse character	>90, good peripheral pulses	50-90, able to palpate carotid/femoral pulses.	<50, weak or absent pulses.
Level of consciousness	Awake	Obtunded, any loss of consciousness	Comatose
Cutaneous injury	No injury	Minor with contusion or laceration <7 cm and not through fascia	Major with penetrating wound through fascia
Fractures	None	Single closed	Multiple open

Intubation of the Pediatric Patient

Specific considerations for ETT placement in pediatric patients include:

- Some anatomy structures of children can make intubation and airway management in general more challenging. Their oropharyngeal structures are larger in comparison and their epiglottis tends to be large and floppy in nature. These anatomic structures can make intubation of children more difficult because visualizing the vocal cords is more challenging. Because the trachea is shorter, the ETT is more prone to be displaced.
- Children usually have a shorter time that they can tolerate apnea during RSI due to their decreased functional residual capacity and higher oxygen metabolism. They should be preoxygenated and monitored during RSI and provided bag mask ventilation as needed. As studies have proven that intubation success is higher with more training, and opportunities for intubation experience with pediatric patients is limited, providers should seek simulation training and other opportunities to gain experience. For a provider who does not feel that they have had sufficient experience, use of an LMA may be appropriate, as its placement is more likely to be correct in this situation.

Causes of Deterioration in the Intubated Pediatric Patient

One of the most common causes for deterioration in the condition of an intubated pediatric patient is that the endotracheal tube has become dislodged or displaced from the patient's trachea. This can often be identified even before there is a change in a patient's condition as there will be a loss of end-tidal CO_2. Another common problem that can cause a patient's condition to worsen occurs when the tube becomes obstructed in some manner. Common causes of obstruction of the ETT include touching an internal mucosal surface, kinks in the tube, or secretions. It is also possible for equipment to fail while the patient is intubated, which would cause his/her condition to deteriorate. When a patient experiences a change in condition, equipment should be assessed and patient should be given oxygen by Ambu bag until the problem is identified and solved. Barotrauma, especially pneumothorax, which occurs when air or gas collects outside the patient's lungs, can also cause deterioration in his/her condition leading to a thoracostomy. Signs of pneumothorax can include shortness of breath, bluish skin tone, and an increased heart rate.

Pediatric Seizures

Febrile seizure is a generalized seizure associated with fever, usually >38.8 °C (101.8 °F) from any type of infection (upper respiratory, urinary tract) but without intracranial infection or other cause, occurring between 6 months and 5 years of age. Seizures usually last <15 minutes and are without subsequent neurological deficit.

Interventions: Provide fever control (acetaminophen OR ibuprofen) and a tepid-water bath.

Other types of seizures may result from pathology, such as meningitis, cerebral edema, brain trauma, or brain tumors, but most seizures in children >3 are related to idiopathic epilepsy, which predisposes the child to recurrent seizures, usually of the same type. Seizures are characterized as focal (localized), focal with rapid generalization (spreading), and generalized (widespread). In most children, seizures become generalized with loss of consciousness. Seizure disorders with onset younger than 4 years of age usually cause more neurological damage than those with onset at older than 4 years of age.

Interventions: Place the patient on the floor or on a safe surface, loosen clothes, and protect him or her from injury during seizure. Afterward, place the patient in the recovery position, monitor the airway/ventilation, and provide oxygen supplementation (the patient may need assisted ventilation if he or she is cyanotic), and suction if needed.

PALS Algorithm for Bradycardia

Poor Perfusion with Pulse Present

In the pediatric patient with bradycardia (<60 bpm) and a pulse and signs of poor perfusion, attempt to identify cause. Signs of compromise include hypotension, sudden change in GCS, or signs of shock. Maintain airway, assist with ventilation as necessary, IV access, ECG, cardiac monitor and vital signs should be monitored. If this fixes the signs of poor perfusion, continue to observe will supporting ABC's and transporting for definitive care. However, if the heart rate remains less than 60 beats/minute with signs of cardiopulmonary compromise after implementing the above, start CPR. If bradycardia persists, epinephrine (0.01 mg/kg every 3-5 minutes IV) or atropine (0.02 mg/kg IV) can be given or pacing initiated. If the patient becomes pulseless, begin regular cardiac arrest protocol. If transport team personnel are able to determine causes for the patient's lack of responsiveness, attempts should be made to reverse those causes, if they are reversible.

Symptomatic with a Pulse

According to the Pediatric Advanced Life Support (PALS) bradycardia algorithm for symptomatic patients, the patient's airway, breathing, and circulation should be supported first, and oxygen should be administered. A defibrillator should then be set up and attached to the patient. If the patient's heart rate continues to remain lower than 60 beats per minute with poor perfusion, cardiopulmonary resuscitation (CPR) should be performed. If the patient is still showing signs of persistent symptomatic bradycardia, epinephrine should be administered through an intravenous line or an endotracheal tube every 3–5 minutes. A dose of atropine may be delivered if the patient's vagal tone is increased. Additionally, external cardiac pacing may be considered as an option to stimulate the heart and surrounding muscles to contract and help return the heart rate to normal range.

Pediatric CPR

For children between 1 and puberty, after assessing scene safety, if the patient is unresponsive, assess breathing while checking carotid pulse (only assess for 10 seconds). If there is no pulse, begin CPR. Do chest compressions using the heel of one hand in the center of the chest.

- One Rescuer: Begin cycles of 30 compressions and 2 breaths.
- Two Rescuers: Begin cycles of 15 compressions and 2 breaths.

After the victim is connected to a defibrillator, check rhythm after 5 cycles (about 2 minutes) of CPR. If a defibrillator shows shockable rhythm, give shock and resume CPR immediately for two minutes. If possible, interruptions to the delivery of chest compressions should be minimized; transport team personnel should continue chest compressions after completing a rhythm check while the defibrillator is charging for another round of shock. Five cycles of CPR should be administered to the patient, lasting approximately two minutes each, and then the patient's rhythm should be checked once again. Continue CPR and defibrillation until return of spontaneous circulation.

For infants less than one, compressions may be either done with two fingers or with two thumb-encircling hands technique.

Manual Defibrillation of the Pediatric Patient

When using a manual defibrillator on a pediatric patient, hand held paddles or adhesive electrode pads can be used, with electrode pads having more advantages. Electrode pads can be used to monitor heart rhythm, are not associated with sparks, have less chance of pad misplacement, and are safer for the rescuer. The electrodes should be as large as possible to fit on the patient's chest wall without having them touch. For pediatric patients who weigh more than 10 kilograms, adult electrodes sized 12 centimeters are usually the most effective ones to use. For pediatric patients who weigh less than 10 kilograms, infant-sized electrodes are most effective during defibrillation. The pads may either be placed anterior/apex or anterior/posterior.

The first shock for a pediatric patient in ventricular fibrillation or pulseless ventricular tachycardia should be at 2 J/kg. When indicated, second shock should be at 4 J/kg and subsequent shocks at greater than equal to 4 J/kg with maximum energy 10 J/kg or the adult dosage.

Manual defibrillators are preferred but AEDs may be used when manual defibrillators are unavailable. If possible when using an AED for children less than 8 years old, use a pediatric dose attenuator system, however if this is not available use the AED without an attenuator for a shockable rhythm.

Considerations for Managing Pediatric Shock

One essential consideration when managing a pediatric shock patient is the patient's size. It is imperative to consider the patient's size when treating him/her to ensure that proper length-based resuscitation protocols are followed and that the right size equipment is used. Another consideration that needs to be made when working with a pediatric shock patient is the patient's increased risk for hypothermia and/or dehydration. Risks for such conditions are elevated in pediatric patients due to their immature systems and to the increase in their surface area to overall body mass ratio. While pediatric shock patients tend to experience a prolonged compensatory stage of shock, their state also tends to deteriorate faster than adults once they enter into the progressive stage.

Geriatric

Special Considerations for Geriatric Patients

Geriatric patients have the following special considerations and characteristics:

- Decreased sensory input (hearing, vision, touch, pain), impaired depth perception and night vision, and decreased ability to differentiate colors
- Hypertension, increasing the risk of heart attack and stroke
- Decreased breathing capacity and decreased cough, increasing the risk of infection
- Difficulty chewing and swallowing, digestive problems, and reflux when lying flat, which increases the risk of aspiration
- Short-term memory deficit and slower reflexes
- Decreased bone density, increasing the risk of breaks; loss of muscle tone
- Increased risk of infection and less obvious symptoms of infection
- Arthritis in the neck, interfering with airway assessment
- Dentures that can obstruct the airway (leave them in place if possible, during ventilation)
- Skin that is fragile and tears easily
- Irregular pulse from underlying heart problems
- Dementia (incidence increases with age), making history taking and treatment difficult
- Atypical symptoms for illnesses, even if severely ill
- Multiple comorbidities and multiple medications
- Shock with BP greater than 100

Polypharmacy and Pharmacokinetic Changes

Geriatric patients are at risk of polypharmacy, the simultaneous use of many drugs, some of which may duplicate or interact with other drugs. Patients may have similar prescriptions from different physicians and may take multiple OTC drugs. Patients taking 5 different drugs have a 50% risk of interactions and 100% risk with 10 drugs. Additionally, aging affects pharmacokinetics:

- **Absorption**: While the percentage of drug absorbed changes little with age for most drugs, the rate of absorption slows, delaying response. Decreased gastric acidity may reduce absorption of some drugs.

- **Distribution**: Body water content, lean body mass, and protein binding sites decrease, and fat content increases, resulting in (1) increased storage of lipid-soluble drugs resulting in decreased plasma level and response, (2) decreased volume for water-soluble drugs resulting in intensified response, and (3) decreased protein binding resulting in increased free drug and intensified response.
- **Metabolism**: Decreased hepatic metabolism may result in increased half-life of drugs.
- **Excretion**: Decreased renal function may result in drug accumulation and adverse effects.

Bariatric

Physical Assessment of the Bariatric Patient

The bariatric patient poses a number of physical examination challenges. Equipment must be appropriate for the patient's size to ensure correct results. For example, the inflatable bladder of a BP cuff should encircle at least 80% of the arm. If no adequate BP cuff is available, a thigh cuff may be substituted. Lung assessment should be done with auscultation on bare skin because of diminished breath sounds. Cardiovascular assessment should be done if possible with the patient leaning forward so the heart is in closer proximity to the chest wall, and the carotid pulse should be assessed along with the apical pulse. If the patient is supine, the patient should raise the arms above the head. Taking VS after exertion may result in elevated results, so patients should be allowed a few minutes rest first or VS should be reassessed. A tongue depressor may be necessary to view the posterior oropharynx. The liver scratch test may be utilized to assess the liver margin.

Transporting Bariatric Patients

The first considerations when transporting bariatric patients are the ability to safely handle the patient and the availability of adequate personnel to facilitate transport. Transport equipment must be appropriate for the patient's size and weight (so it's important to ascertain the patient's weight), and the transport vehicle must be able to accommodate the patient. Loading the patient head first. Patients may require extra padding to prevent pressure during transport. Obese patients have increased risk of fat emboli and should receive 100% oxygen for at least 15 minutes before transport if possible. Patients may need light sedation if they experience claustrophobia because of the tight space in many vehicles.

Airway Management and Drug Dose Considerations

The bariatric patient is at increased risk of obstructive sleep apnea and hypoxemia when in supine position, so the patient should be transported with the head in semi-Fowler's position or upright to relieve pressure of the abdominal organs on the diaphragm if possible. Obesity makes it difficult to position the patient or to view the glottis for endotracheal intubation. Preoxygenation for 3–5 minutes before intubation per nasal cannula or non-invasive positive pressure ventilation may improve oxygenation. Two people should be used for bag-mask ventilation, which may be facilitated with insertion of an oropharyngeal or nasopharyngeal tube. The stacking maneuver (elevating the shoulders and head to raise the chin) rather than the sniffing position may facilitate ET intubation. When administering drugs based on ideal weight, the patient may receive inadequate medication, but administration based on actual weight may result in overdose, so weight is sometimes adjusted to 40% of actual weight minus ideal weight, but each medication should be checked in a drug-dosing reference table. If unsure, dosage is usually based on ideal weight.

How to Overcome Test Anxiety

Just the thought of taking a test is enough to make most people a little nervous. A test is an important event that can have a long-term impact on your future, so it's important to take it seriously and it's natural to feel anxious about performing well. But just because anxiety is normal, that doesn't mean that it's helpful in test taking, or that you should simply accept it as part of your life. Anxiety can have a variety of effects. These effects can be mild, like making you feel slightly nervous, or severe, like blocking your ability to focus or remember even a simple detail.

If you experience test anxiety—whether severe or mild—it's important to know how to beat it. To discover this, first you need to understand what causes test anxiety.

Causes of Test Anxiety

While we often think of anxiety as an uncontrollable emotional state, it can actually be caused by simple, practical things. One of the most common causes of test anxiety is that a person does not feel adequately prepared for their test. This feeling can be the result of many different issues such as poor study habits or lack of organization, but the most common culprit is time management. Starting to study too late, failing to organize your study time to cover all of the material, or being distracted while you study will mean that you're not well prepared for the test. This may lead to cramming the night before, which will cause you to be physically and mentally exhausted for the test. Poor time management also contributes to feelings of stress, fear, and hopelessness as you realize you are not well prepared but don't know what to do about it.

Other times, test anxiety is not related to your preparation for the test but comes from unresolved fear. This may be a past failure on a test, or poor performance on tests in general. It may come from comparing yourself to others who seem to be performing better or from the stress of living up to expectations. Anxiety may be driven by fears of the future—how failure on this test would affect your educational and career goals. These fears are often completely irrational, but they can still negatively impact your test performance.

Elements of Test Anxiety

As mentioned earlier, test anxiety is considered to be an emotional state, but it has physical and mental components as well. Sometimes you may not even realize that you are suffering from test anxiety until you notice the physical symptoms. These can include trembling hands, rapid heartbeat, sweating, nausea, and tense muscles. Extreme anxiety may lead to fainting or vomiting. Obviously, any of these symptoms can have a negative impact on testing. It is important to recognize them as soon as they begin to occur so that you can address the problem before it damages your performance.

The mental components of test anxiety include trouble focusing and inability to remember learned information. During a test, your mind is on high alert, which can help you recall information and stay focused for an extended period of time. However, anxiety interferes with your mind's natural processes, causing you to blank out, even on the questions you know well. The strain of testing during anxiety makes it difficult to stay focused, especially on a test that may take several hours. Extreme anxiety can take a huge mental toll, making it difficult not only to recall test information but even to understand the test questions or pull your thoughts together.

Effects of Test Anxiety

Test anxiety is like a disease—if left untreated, it will get progressively worse. Anxiety leads to poor performance, and this reinforces the feelings of fear and failure, which in turn lead to poor performances on subsequent tests. It can grow from a mild nervousness to a crippling condition. If allowed to progress, test anxiety can have a big impact on your schooling, and consequently on your future.

Test anxiety can spread to other parts of your life. Anxiety on tests can become anxiety in any stressful situation, and blanking on a test can turn into panicking in a job situation. But fortunately, you don't have to let anxiety rule your testing and determine your grades. There are a number of relatively simple steps you can take to move past anxiety and function normally on a test and in the rest of life.

Physical Steps for Beating Test Anxiety

While test anxiety is a serious problem, the good news is that it can be overcome. It doesn't have to control your ability to think and remember information. While it may take time, you can begin taking steps today to beat anxiety.

Just as your first hint that you may be struggling with anxiety comes from the physical symptoms, the first step to treating it is also physical. Rest is crucial for having a clear, strong mind. If you are tired, it is much easier to give in to anxiety. But if you establish good sleep habits, your body and mind will be ready to perform optimally, without the strain of exhaustion. Additionally, sleeping well helps you to retain information better, so you're more likely to recall the answers when you see the test questions.

Getting good sleep means more than going to bed on time. It's important to allow your brain time to relax. Take study breaks from time to time so it doesn't get overworked, and don't study right before bed. Take time to rest your mind before trying to rest your body, or you may find it difficult to fall asleep.

Along with sleep, other aspects of physical health are important in preparing for a test. Good nutrition is vital for good brain function. Sugary foods and drinks may give a burst of energy but this burst is followed by a crash, both physically and emotionally. Instead, fuel your body with protein and vitamin-rich foods.

Also, drink plenty of water. Dehydration can lead to headaches and exhaustion, especially if your brain is already under stress from the rigors of the test. Particularly if your test is a long one, drink water during the breaks. And if possible, take an energy-boosting snack to eat between sections.

Along with sleep and diet, a third important part of physical health is exercise. Maintaining a steady workout schedule is helpful, but even taking 5-minute study breaks to walk can help get your blood pumping faster and clear your head. Exercise also releases endorphins, which contribute to a positive feeling and can help combat test anxiety.

When you nurture your physical health, you are also contributing to your mental health. If your body is healthy, your mind is much more likely to be healthy as well. So take time to rest, nourish your body with healthy food and water, and get moving as much as possible. Taking these physical steps will make you stronger and more able to take the mental steps necessary to overcome test anxiety.

Mental Steps for Beating Test Anxiety

Working on the mental side of test anxiety can be more challenging, but as with the physical side, there are clear steps you can take to overcome it. As mentioned earlier, test anxiety often stems from lack of preparation, so the obvious solution is to prepare for the test. Effective studying may be the most important weapon you have for beating test anxiety, but you can and should employ several other mental tools to combat fear.

First, boost your confidence by reminding yourself of past success—tests or projects that you aced. If you're putting as much effort into preparing for this test as you did for those, there's no reason you should expect to fail here. Work hard to prepare; then trust your preparation.

Second, surround yourself with encouraging people. It can be helpful to find a study group, but be sure that the people you're around will encourage a positive attitude. If you spend time with others who are anxious or cynical, this will only contribute to your own anxiety. Look for others who are motivated to study hard from a desire to succeed, not from a fear of failure.

Third, reward yourself. A test is physically and mentally tiring, even without anxiety, and it can be helpful to have something to look forward to. Plan an activity following the test, regardless of the outcome, such as going to a movie or getting ice cream.

When you are taking the test, if you find yourself beginning to feel anxious, remind yourself that you know the material. Visualize successfully completing the test. Then take a few deep, relaxing breaths and return to it. Work through the questions carefully but with confidence, knowing that you are capable of succeeding.

Developing a healthy mental approach to test taking will also aid in other areas of life. Test anxiety affects more than just the actual test—it can be damaging to your mental health and even contribute to depression. It's important to beat test anxiety before it becomes a problem for more than testing.

Study Strategy

Being prepared for the test is necessary to combat anxiety, but what does being prepared look like? You may study for hours on end and still not feel prepared. What you need is a strategy for test prep. The next few pages outline our recommended steps to help you plan out and conquer the challenge of preparation.

Step 1: Scope Out the Test

Learn everything you can about the format (multiple choice, essay, etc.) and what will be on the test. Gather any study materials, course outlines, or sample exams that may be available. Not only will this help you to prepare, but knowing what to expect can help to alleviate test anxiety.

Step 2: Map Out the Material

Look through the textbook or study guide and make note of how many chapters or sections it has. Then divide these over the time you have. For example, if a book has 15 chapters and you have five days to study, you need to cover three chapters each day. Even better, if you have the time, leave an extra day at the end for overall review after you have gone through the material in depth.

If time is limited, you may need to prioritize the material. Look through it and make note of which sections you think you already have a good grasp on, and which need review. While you are studying, skim quickly through the familiar sections and take more time on the challenging parts. Write out your plan so you don't get lost as you go. Having a written plan also helps you feel more in control of the study, so anxiety is less likely to arise from feeling overwhelmed at the amount to cover.

Step 3: Gather Your Tools

Decide what study method works best for you. Do you prefer to highlight in the book as you study and then go back over the highlighted portions? Or do you type out notes of the important information? Or is it helpful to make flashcards that you can carry with you? Assemble the pens, index cards, highlighters, post-it notes, and any other materials you may need so you won't be distracted by getting up to find things while you study.

If you're having a hard time retaining the information or organizing your notes, experiment with different methods. For example, try color-coding by subject with colored pens, highlighters, or post-it notes. If you learn better by hearing, try recording yourself reading your notes so you can listen while in the car, working out, or simply sitting at your desk. Ask a friend to quiz you from your flashcards, or try teaching someone the material to solidify it in your mind.

Step 4: Create Your Environment

It's important to avoid distractions while you study. This includes both the obvious distractions like visitors and the subtle distractions like an uncomfortable chair (or a too-comfortable couch that makes you want to fall asleep). Set up the best study environment possible: good lighting and a comfortable work area. If background music helps you focus, you may want to turn it on, but otherwise keep the room quiet. If you are using a computer to take notes, be sure you don't have any other windows open, especially applications like social media, games, or anything else that could distract you. Silence your phone and turn off notifications. Be sure to keep water close by so you stay hydrated while you study (but avoid unhealthy drinks and snacks).

Also, take into account the best time of day to study. Are you freshest first thing in the morning? Try to set aside some time then to work through the material. Is your mind clearer in the afternoon or evening? Schedule your study session then. Another method is to study at the same time of day that you will take the test, so that your brain gets used to working on the material at that time and will be ready to focus at test time.

Step 5: Study!

Once you have done all the study preparation, it's time to settle into the actual studying. Sit down, take a few moments to settle your mind so you can focus, and begin to follow your study plan. Don't give in to distractions or let yourself procrastinate. This is your time to prepare so you'll be ready to fearlessly approach the test. Make the most of the time and stay focused.

Of course, you don't want to burn out. If you study too long you may find that you're not retaining the information very well. Take regular study breaks. For example, taking five minutes out of every hour to walk briskly, breathing deeply and swinging your arms, can help your mind stay fresh.

As you get to the end of each chapter or section, it's a good idea to do a quick review. Remind yourself of what you learned and work on any difficult parts. When you feel that you've mastered the material, move on to the next part. At the end of your study session, briefly skim through your notes again.

But while review is helpful, cramming last minute is NOT. If at all possible, work ahead so that you won't need to fit all your study into the last day. Cramming overloads your brain with more information than it can process and retain, and your tired mind may struggle to recall even previously learned information when it is overwhelmed with last-minute study. Also, the urgent nature of cramming and the stress placed on your brain contribute to anxiety. You'll be more likely to go to the test feeling unprepared and having trouble thinking clearly.

So don't cram, and don't stay up late before the test, even just to review your notes at a leisurely pace. Your brain needs rest more than it needs to go over the information again. In fact, plan to finish your studies by noon or early afternoon the day before the test. Give your brain the rest of the day to relax or focus on other things, and get a good night's sleep. Then you will be fresh for the test and better able to recall what you've studied.

Step 6: Take a Practice Test

Many courses offer sample tests, either online or in the study materials. This is an excellent resource to check whether you have mastered the material, as well as to prepare for the test format and environment.

Check the test format ahead of time: the number of questions, the type (multiple choice, free response, etc.), and the time limit. Then create a plan for working through them. For example, if you have 30 minutes to take a 60-question test, your limit is 30 seconds per question. Spend less time on the questions you know well so that you can take more time on the difficult ones.

If you have time to take several practice tests, take the first one open book, with no time limit. Work through the questions at your own pace and make sure you fully understand them. Gradually work up to taking a test under test conditions: sit at a desk with all study materials put away and set a timer. Pace yourself to make sure you finish the test with time to spare and go back to check your answers if you have time.

After each test, check your answers. On the questions you missed, be sure you understand why you missed them. Did you misread the question (tests can use tricky wording)? Did you forget the information? Or was it something you hadn't learned? Go back and study any shaky areas that the practice tests reveal.

Taking these tests not only helps with your grade, but also aids in combating test anxiety. If you're already used to the test conditions, you're less likely to worry about it, and working through tests until you're scoring well gives you a confidence boost. Go through the practice tests until you feel comfortable, and then you can go into the test knowing that you're ready for it.

Test Tips

On test day, you should be confident, knowing that you've prepared well and are ready to answer the questions. But aside from preparation, there are several test day strategies you can employ to maximize your performance.

First, as stated before, get a good night's sleep the night before the test (and for several nights before that, if possible). Go into the test with a fresh, alert mind rather than staying up late to study.

Try not to change too much about your normal routine on the day of the test. It's important to eat a nutritious breakfast, but if you normally don't eat breakfast at all, consider eating just a protein bar. If you're a coffee drinker, go ahead and have your normal coffee. Just make sure you time it so that the caffeine doesn't wear off right in the middle of your test. Avoid sugary beverages, and drink enough water to stay hydrated but not so much that you need a restroom break 10 minutes into the test. If your test isn't first thing in the morning, consider going for a walk or doing a light workout before the test to get your blood flowing.

Allow yourself enough time to get ready, and leave for the test with plenty of time to spare so you won't have the anxiety of scrambling to arrive in time. Another reason to be early is to select a good seat. It's helpful to sit away from doors and windows, which can be distracting. Find a good seat, get out your supplies, and settle your mind before the test begins.

When the test begins, start by going over the instructions carefully, even if you already know what to expect. Make sure you avoid any careless mistakes by following the directions.

Then begin working through the questions, pacing yourself as you've practiced. If you're not sure on an answer, don't spend too much time on it, and don't let it shake your confidence. Either skip it and come back later, or eliminate as many wrong answers as possible and guess among the remaining ones. Don't dwell on these questions as you continue—put them out of your mind and focus on what lies ahead.

Be sure to read all of the answer choices, even if you're sure the first one is the right answer. Sometimes you'll find a better one if you keep reading. But don't second-guess yourself if you do immediately know the answer. Your gut instinct is usually right. Don't let test anxiety rob you of the information you know.

If you have time at the end of the test (and if the test format allows), go back and review your answers. Be cautious about changing any, since your first instinct tends to be correct, but make sure you didn't misread any of the questions or accidentally mark the wrong answer choice. Look over any you skipped and make an educated guess.

At the end, leave the test feeling confident. You've done your best, so don't waste time worrying about your performance or wishing you could change anything. Instead, celebrate the successful completion of this test. And finally, use this test to learn how to deal with anxiety even better next time.

Review Video: Test Anxiety
Visit mometrix.com/academy and enter code: 100340

Important Qualification

Not all anxiety is created equal. If your test anxiety is causing major issues in your life beyond the classroom or testing center, or if you are experiencing troubling physical symptoms related to your anxiety, it may be a sign of a serious physiological or psychological condition. If this sounds like your situation, we strongly encourage you to seek professional help.

Online Resources

Due to our efforts to try to keep this book to a manageable length, we've created a link that will give you access to all of your online resources:

mometrix.com/resources719/ctrn

It's Your Moment, Let's Celebrate It!

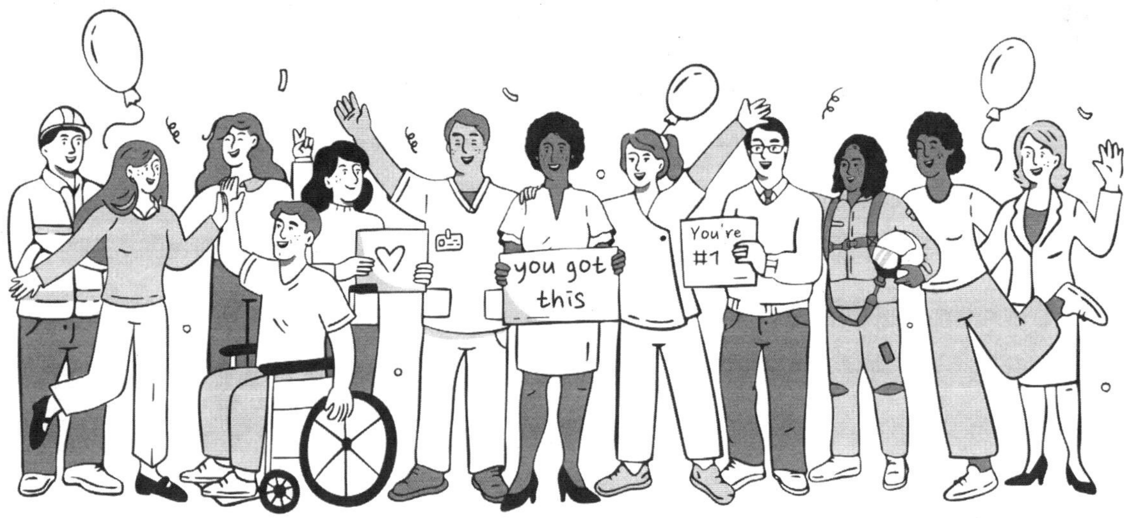

Share your story @mometrixtestpreparation